Transcultural Health and Social Care

For Elsevier:

Commissioning Editor: Susan Young
Development Editor: Catherine Jackson
Project Manager: Morven Dean
Designer: George Ajayi
Illustration Manager: Bruce Hogarth

Transcultural Health and Social Care

Development of Culturally Competent Practitioners

Edited by

Irena Papadopoulos PhD MA BA RN RM NDNCert DipN DipNEd RNT

Professor of Transcultural Health and Nursing, Head of Research Centre for Transcultural Studies in Health, School of Health and Social Sciences, Middlesex University, UK

Forewords by

Cecil Helman MBChB, FRCGP, Dip Soc Anthrop

Professor of Medical Anthropology, School of Social Sciences and Law, Brunel University and Senior Lecturer, Department of Primary Care and Population Sciences, Royal Free & University College Medical School, London, UK

Larry Purnell PhD, RN, FAAN

Professor Nursing, University of Delaware, Newark, DE, USA

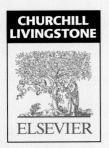

CHURCHILL
LIVINGSTONE

ELSEVIER

EDINBURGH   LONDON   NEW YORK   OXFORD   PHILADELPHIA   ST LOUIS   SYDNEY   TORONTO   2006

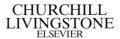

First published 2006

ISBN-13: 978 0 443 10131 1
ISBN-10: 0 443 10131 0

British Library Cataloguing in Publication Data
A catalogue record for this book is available from the British Library

Library of Congress Cataloging in Publication Data
A catalog record for this book is available from the Library of Congress

Notice
Knowledge and best practice in this field are constantly changing. As new research and experience broaden our knowledge, changes in practice, treatment and drug therapy may become necessary or appropriate. Readers are advised to check the most current information provided (i) on procedures featured or (ii) by the manufacturer of each product to be administered, to verify the recommended dose or formula, the method and duration of administration, and contraindications. It is the responsibility of the practitioner, relying on their own experience and knowledge of the patient, to make diagnoses, to determine dosages and the best treatment for each individual patient, and to take all appropriate safety precautions. To the fullest extent of the law, neither the publisher nor the editor assumes any liability for any injury and/or damage.

The Publisher

your source for books,
journals and multimedia
in the health sciences
www.elsevierhealth.com

The publisher's policy is to use paper manufactured from sustainable forests

Printed in China

I would like to dedicate this book to my late mother Panayiota, a great survivor and a strong mind, who despite becoming a refugee in her own country (Cyprus) in 1974, remained cheerful and supportive until her death. She taught me the importance of education, of having dreams, of working hard and of fighting for one's rights. I would also like to dedicate this book to my husband Costas and my sons Panikos and Chris who are my most faithful 'fans' and who provide me with constant unconditional love. Finally this book is dedicated to all who are oppressed, disadvantaged or excluded to whom I wish a fairer today and a brighter tomorrow.

Contents

Contributors

Silvia Garcia Barrios DipN, Degree in Nursing, Masters in Nursing Teaching, Teaching Cert
Director Exchange Coordinator, University College of Health Sciences, Málaga

Myfanwy M. Davies PhD MA MSc
AWARD Research Fellow, Department of General Practice, Cardiff University: Medical School, Cardiff, UK

Vered Delbar PhD MA BA ONS RN
Head of Nursing Department, Leon and Matilda Recanti School for Community Health Professions, Faculty of Health Sciences, Ben-Gurion University of the Negev, Israel

Zbys Fedorowicz MSC DPH BDS LDS RCS(Eng)
Director, UK Cochrane Centre, Bahrain Branch

Ann Gallagher PhD MA BA(Hons) PGCEA RMN RGN
Senior Research Fellow, Faculty of Health and Social Care Sciences, Kingston University and St George's University of London, UK

Alem Gebrehiwot MA BSc
Executive Director, Ethiopian Community Centre in the UK (ECCUK), London, UK

Monika Habermann DrPhil RN
Professor of Nursing; Head of the Centre of Nursing Research and Counselling, Hochschule Bremen, Germany

Athena Kalokerinou-Anagnostopoulou PhD BSc RN
Assistant Professor in Community Nursing, Department of Public Health, Faculty of Nursing, University of Athens, Athens, Greece

Marja Kaunomen PhD RN
Senior Assistant Professor, Department of Nursing Science, University of Tampere, Finland

Meeri Koivula PhD RN
Senior Lecturer, Department of Nursing Science, University of Tampere, Finland

Margaret Lay RMN RGN BA(Hons) Cert Counselling Skills
Research Fellow, Research Centre for Transcultural Studies in Health, School of Health and Social Science, Middlesex University, UK

Shelley Lees BSc RN MRes
Research Fellow, London School of Hygiene and Tropical Medicine, London, UK

M. Judith Lynam PhD RN
Associate Professor and Co-Director, Culture, Gender and Health Research Unit, School of Nursing, University of British Columbia, Vancouver, Canada

Akram Omeri PhD RN CTN MCN FRCNA
Adjunct Associate Professor, School of Nursing, Family and Community Nursing, University of Western Sydney, NSW, Australia

Chris Papadopoulos BSc (Hons)
Research Student/Teacher, School of Health and Social Sciences, Middlesex University, UK

Irena Papadopoulos PhD MA BA RN RM NDNCert DipN DipNEd RNT
Professor of Transcultural Health and Nursing, Head of Research Centre for Transcultural Studies in Health, School of Health and Social Sciences, Middlesex University, UK

Gina Taylor MSc BA PGDip CertFE DipN RN RCNT
Senior Lecturer, School of Health and Social Sciences, Middlesex University, UK

Mary Tilki PhD MSc BA RN RNT
Principal Lecturer, School of Health and Social Sciences, Middlesex University, UK

Thomas D. Walczyk BS DDS FAGD
United States Navy Dental Corps

Forewords

I have great pleasure in introducing *Transcultural Health and Social Care*, and in recommending it to all those who care for clients and communities from cultural backgrounds different to their own. The book is a landmark text, not only in the development of transcultural nursing, but also in the wider world of cross-cultural health care. A text such as this is much needed in the age of diversity – social, cultural, ethnic and religious – in which we now all live. For many health professionals this is a new, and sometimes confusing landscape. They find themselves working in a world in which, according the United Nations, some 175 million people (including about 15 million refugees) now live outside their countries of birth (a figure that was only 75 million in 1965), and where the patient population they encounter reflects the results these huge population movements. In the UK, for example, 4.3 million people (7.53 per cent of the total population) were born outside the country, and London schoolchildren now speak a total of 307 languages, with only two-thirds of them having English as a home language. In the United States, too, diversity is increasingly evident as nearly one in every five schoolchildren speak a language other than English at home, almost one in three Americans identifies themselves as belonging to a racial or ethnic minority, and in four states – California, Texas, Hawaii and New

Mexico – members of ethnic and racial minorities now account for more than half the total population.

This is the new environment in which nurses and doctors have to deliver health care in a compassionate, efficient, and culturally competent way. That is why *Transcultural Health and Social Care* is so valuable, and so timely. It combines a compassionate and humanitarian approach with intellectual rigour, and with relevant research data on transcultural nursing gathered from many different countries. It covers a wide range of crucial topics – from cultural attitudes to cancer, to the effects of inequality on health status, from the maternity needs of Arab women, to the ethics of culturally competent care. It deals with the nursing care of many different communities, and in many different countries, ranging from refugees, asylum-seekers and immigrants to the members of ethnic and religious minority groups. One great strength of the book is this global approach. It is not a parochial textbook, for it offers a wider view of the globalized world in which nurses now live and work, and the challenges and opportunities that they now encounter. Appropriately, too, the book's contributors are drawn not only from different countries, but also from a variety of professional backgrounds, and with a variety of perspectives on contemporary issues in transcultural nursing.

Another strength of the book is that its editor is Professor Irena Papadopoulos, a pioneer in the field of transcultural nursing, and one of the leading international experts in the subject. She brings to the book a well-deserved international reputation.

I predict that *Transcultural Health and Social Care* will become an international classic, a key text in transcultural nursing, not only in the UK but in many other countries as well.

Cecil Helman, 2005

Two very important worldwide movements are currently underway in the healthcare arena: culturally competent care and the elimination of racial and ethnic disparities. These movements have necessitated that the individual, the organization, and the healthcare system must address ethnocentrism, racism, and discrimination. Racism and discrimination, like ethnocentrism, are exceedingly complex and sometimes insidious; many people are not even aware that they are being ethnocentric or racist. This book, *Transcultural Health and Social Care,* addresses these very major concerns.

One of the most rewarding, exciting, and complex challenges for nurses and other healthcare providers worldwide in the 21st century is providing culturally competent care to patients, families, and communities and working with culturally diverse colleagues from multiple disciplines. As world migration and travel increases along with the movement of human capital, globalization increases the need for healthcare providers' cultural awareness, cultural sensitivity, and cultural competence.

For healthcare providers to take the journey toward cultural competence, they need to remember that culture is not border bound and that patients and staff bring their culture with them. Because healthcare providers cannot possibly know all the characteristics of the numerous worldwide ethnocultural groups, they need a framework, model, or theory for guidance in learning about culture and assessing and intervening in culturally consistent, competent manner. One such model, developed by Papadopoulos, Tilki, and Taylor, is used as a guide for the development of several chapters in this text. This model, developed in 1994, has proved its usefulness in education, in ethical decision making, and in research.

Societies around the world are increasingly hopeful that knowledge and opportunities can advance health promotion and wellness; illness, disease, and injury prevention; and health maintenance and restoration. One way to help bridge the gaps between healthcare providers and patients, between the rich and the poor, and between those who have power and those who do not have power, is through culturally competent care that includes the mind, body and spirit. *Transcultural Health and Social Care* addresses all of these issues on some level and thoroughly addresses the need for eliminating the health and healthcare inequities of race, migration, refugees, and asylum seekers, areas where research is just beginning.

Through cultural competence and policies for ensuring ethnic racial parity in healthcare, this unique book, *Transcultural Health and Social Care,* is an important addition to the literature and a rich source for practitioners, educators, administrators, and researchers, regardless of their practice settings and discipline.

Larry Purnell, 2005

Acknowledgements

I would like to thank, with all my heart, all the contributors to this book for their hard work and understanding. I also thank my development editor, Catherine Jackson, for her continuous support and encouragement. My final big 'thank you' goes to Professors Cecil Helman and Larry Purnell for honouring me and the book with their forewords.

Chapter 1

Introduction

Irena Papadopoulos

Most of the authors in this book (including myself) have been developing and implementing their transcultural work for a number of years. We are of differing cultural backgrounds, and live and work in a number of countries with people from diverse societies and different experiences. I have been extremely fortunate to have worked with many of them on a number of transcultural projects such as an Intensive European Programme in transcultural nursing, a Masters programme in European Nursing as well as in various research projects which I directed in the last five years. But the book is not just aimed at nurses in Britain and Europe; health and social care professionals across the world will benefit from the content of this volume, whose authors come from Europe, Canada, Australia and the Middle East.

The authors believe that transcultural or cultural competence (I will use both terms synonymously in this book) constitutes a health and social care imperative in the twenty-first century. Governments across the developed countries and increasingly in the developing world are expecting health and social care practitioners to deliver services and care that are culturally competent. There is also an expectation from the public that care should be sensitive to their cultural beliefs and values, appropriate to their needs, and free from discrimination. In the era of evidenced-based practice, cultural competence must also be deeply embedded in research and best practice.

The arguments for culturally competent health and social care are robustly presented and articulated in the chapters that follow. They illustrate the complexities, the challenges, and the legal and ethical issues related to cultural competence. Most importantly, they highlight the crucial interplay between culture and structure. And this is the heart of this book. For this is not another book about culture and health. The message of this book is that whilst our cultural backgrounds determine in many ways our behaviours and therefore our health, the structures of the society we live in – and increasingly the global structures of our shrinking world – impact on our lives and health with hugely significant effects.

The book aims to raise awareness about cultural competence, help you develop knowledge necessary for being a culturally competent practitioner, promote cultural sensitivity crucial for establishing transcultural communication and trusting relationships, and build on your existing skills so that you can deliver culturally competent care within an anti-discriminatory framework whilst valuing diversity.

The book is divided into four parts. The first deals with transcultural health care and the development of culture-generic competencies. Chapter 2 introduces you to the Papadopoulos, Tilki and Taylor model of developing cultural competence. In this chapter, I have, for the first time, expanded the model's principles, constructs and concepts. Within this model transcultural nursing and health care is defined as the study and research of cultural diversities and similarities in health and illness as well as their underpinning societal and organizational structures, in order to understand current practice and to contribute to its future development in a culturally responsive way. The model requires a commitment to the promotion of anti-oppressive, anti-discriminatory practices and emphasizes the importance of valuing diversity and empowering clients to participate in healthcare decisions. Cultural competence is the capacity to provide effective health care, taking into consideration people's cultural beliefs, behaviours and needs. Cultural competence is both a process and an output, and results from the synthesis of knowledge and skills which we acquire during our personal and professional lives and to which we are constantly adding.

The rest of the chapters in Part 1 develop in detail the underpinning guiding principles of the Papadopoulos, Tilki and Taylor model. In Chapter 3, Mary Tilki tackles the complex issues of human rights, whilst in Chapter 4 Gina Taylor focuses on inequalities suffered by migrants and refugees. But we must not forget that transcultural or culturally competent care is ethical care. In Chapter 5 Ann Gallagher discusses the ethical challenges faced by health and social care professionals in their everyday practice, highlighting the values and principles that can be used to enable us to make transculturally ethical decisions or cope with the ambiguity that exists in health and social care work in democratic, culturally diverse societies. Finally, in Chapter 6, I deal with the production, dissemination and utilization of culturally competent knowledge by advocating a new paradigm in health and social care research. Culturally competent research is needed in order to anchor culturally competent care and education in research evidence.

Part 2 addresses the need for developing culture-specific competencies. All the chapters in this part derive from research studies I have conducted with colleagues in the last five years. Thus the culture-specific knowledge you will find in this book differs from that in other textbooks where the information about cultural customs, healthcare traditions and other health-related behaviours in various cultural groups is invariably not research based. Chapter 7 presents culture-specific knowledge derived from three research studies which sought to investigate the cancer beliefs, knowledge and experiences among the Greek and Greek Cypriot community, the Chinese community, and those of male cancer sufferers and their wives from six different ethnic groups. Chapter 8 presents the findings of an investigation into the health and social care needs of Ethiopian refugees living in Britain, whilst Chapter 9 addresses the notions of motherhood and maternity needs of Arab Muslim women. Chapter 10 provides selected findings from two studies which sought to identify the knowledge, attitudes and drug habits of young Greek and Greek Cypriots. Finally, Chapter 11 deals with the important topic of health promotion. This investigation was carried out amongst minority ethnic groups, refugees and Gypsy Travellers living in Wales. Whilst all the studies in Part 2 deal with specific populations and issues and emphasize the importance of context, you will discover that there are themes that run through all of them which I believe you too will identify with in your particular context. For example, the lack of relevant and accessible health and welfare information, the importance of effective cross-cultural communication, the effects of marginalization and exclusion, the positive aspects of culturally competent care and so on.

Part 3 of the book is a collection of chapters which provide the European perspective on cultural competence. As the European Union continues to enlarge, more and more health and social care professionals are moving across national boundaries. Knowing about the culture, the healthcare systems and health and social challenges of the different European countries is now an urgent necessity for practitioners, educators and researchers. In Chapter 12 Marja Kaunonen and Meeri Koivula provide an account of some of Finland's cultural healthcare issues. They begin with an interesting outline of the ethnohistory of Finland which includes a fascinating glimpse into some culture-specific practices. Monika Habermann, in Chapter 13, deals with the cultural plurality in health and social care settings in Germany. Facts and figures about health and social care for migrants are given to underpin her critical review of the German healthcare system. Habermann acknowledges that in Germany, as in most other European countries, 'culture' is not yet a well-integrated part of nursing actions in the practice field and that transcultural nursing theories are not guiding the daily work of nurses. She highlights the need to educate nurses involved in direct care as well as supporting them in an interculturally open organization committed to diversity. In Chapter 14 Athena Kalokerinou-Anagnostopoulou illustrates the evolving nature of culture through a description of the Greek culture's history, geography and religion. In contemporary Greece this evolution is very evident within the family structure and values. Customs around marriage, choice of partner, family size, residence, familial obligations and norms around inheritance are continuously changing and inevitably are affecting the health and welfare of its people. Some of the challenges faced by the health services in multicultural Greece are presented and discussed. The final chapter in this part of the book comes from Spain. Silvia Garcia Barrios begins Chapter 15 with a brief ethnohistory of Spain. She describes the health needs of the new immigrants to Spain and of the Gypsy population, a long-standing minority ethnic group in Spain. The chapter explores the impact of Spanish immigration law and health policy on the health of these groups.

The final part of the book provides some global perspectives on cultural competence. In Chapter 16 Zbys Fedorowicz and Tom Walczyk explore the knowledge, attitudes and practices of healthcare providers and users in the Middle East within the framework of a trisomial concept of sociocultural and religious factors. This brings together social and cultural perspectives that are dominant in secular societies with religious factors that predominate in non-secular societies such as those of the Arab world. Chapter 17 looks at transcultural health care in Israel. Vered Delbar offers a useful account of the ethnohistory of Israel, its patterns of migration and its current programmes to respond to the needs of a multicultural state. Individual case studies are used to bring to life the differences in health needs, the differences in service access and utilization as well as the impact of culture and structure on individuals' health-seeking behaviours and compliance with healthcare interventions. In Chapter 18 Akram Omeri reminds us that one emerging characteristic of the globalized world is the obvious and growing disparity in health and social care. Writing from an Australian perspective she informs us that the current Australian policy of multiculturalism intends to enhance and foster social integration and fairness, yet respect difference. However, she argues, this intention has not yet extended to the health system where monoculturalism remains dominant and disparities and inequalities in service provision remain. She believes that the nature of Australian society's cultural diversity creates an urgent need for healthcare professionals to examine their knowledge and attitudes relating to cultural diversity and its importance in education and practice.

The culture and health discourses and practices in the Canadian context are provided by Judith Lynam in Chapter 19. A brief overview is provided of the ways history has shaped Canada's story of migration and in turn how policy decisions have set the context for the ways the discourse on culture and health has been taken up. Drawing from her personal research and practice she traces the ways the discourses on culture and health have developed and introduces the nature of health issues faced by immigrants and refugees and the ways these have been responded to. Lynam offers a fascinating account of Canada as both a colony and a colonizer which helps to illustrate the ways this history has contributed to both Canada's successes and challenges in addressing diversity. She argues that these two aspects of Canada's history have an ongoing influence on Canada's systems of governance, the definitions of individuals' rights and freedoms and the ways issues of culture and diversity are conceptualized or framed. Colonization is probably one of the earliest global phenomena. Therefore this theme applies to a number of countries and it is very relevant to transcultural nursing and health care, as Lynam so cogently illustrates. Finally, the book concludes with some reflections of mine on its themes and messages.

PART 1

Transcultural health care and the development of culture-generic competencies

PART CONTENTS

Chapter **2**

The Papadopoulos, Tilki and Taylor model of developing cultural competence

Irena Papadopoulos

LEARNING OBJECTIVES

After reading this chapter you should:
- be aware of the model's theoretical concepts
- understand the difference between culture-generic and culture-specific competencies
- consider the various levels of cultural competence
- appreciate the application of the model in health and social care education and practice.

INTRODUCTION

Movement across countries and continents has never been easier. At the same time, ethnic conflicts, wars, oppressive political regimes and natural phenomena continue to inflict poverty and illness on millions of people around the globe. Such disasters are largely responsible for an epidemic of mass migration that has affected almost every region of the world, including Europe. At the beginning of 2004, the number of people needing protection and assistance from the United Nations

High Commission for Refugees was just over 17 million (UNHCR 2005). Meanwhile, the creation of the European Union (EU) is enabling nationals of the 25 member states to move without difficulty within the EU.

In the last 25 years there has been a growing realization that our understanding of health and illness has to be considered not only in terms of biological factors, but also in terms of social and cultural determinants too. If we acknowledge that most of us live in culturally diverse societies, and if we agree that our cultural backgrounds play an important role in the construction of our health beliefs and practices, then nurses must be educated in ways that will enable them to provide care that is both efficient and culturally appropriate.

In response to the multicultural world, nursing in many countries is embracing the transcultural framework for preparing new practitioners and for continuing education. This means that the acquisition of transcultural skills and knowledge should lead to the provision of culturally competent nursing care.

DEFINING TRANSCULTURAL NURSING AND CULTURAL COMPETENCE

In America, Madeline Leininger defined transcultural nursing as:

A formal area of study and practice focused on comparative holistic culture, care, health, and illness patterns of people, with respect to differences and similarities in their cultural values, beliefs, and practices with the goal to provide culturally congruent, sensitive, and competent nursing care to people of diverse cultures. (Leininger 1995: 4)

In Britain, my colleagues and I have been working in the area of transcultural studies in health and nursing since the late 1980s. We defined this area as the study and research of *cultural* diversities and similarities in health and illness as well as their underpinning societal and organizational *structures*, in order to understand current practice and to contribute to its future development in a culturally responsive way. Further, we believe that transcultural nursing requires a commitment to the promotion of anti-oppressive, anti-discriminatory practices. Transcultural health and nursing emphasizes the importance of empowering clients to participate in healthcare decisions; therefore it is imperative that healthcare professionals recognize how society constructs and perpetuates power and disadvantage. In our view no other nursing philosophy and framework places so much emphasis in such an explicit way on the promotion of equality and the value of individuals as this one does (Papadopoulos & Alleyne 1995, Papadopoulos et al 1998, Papadopoulos & Lees 2002). These values and principles have now been made an explicit requirement of nursing education in Britain (NMC 2002, QAA 2001).

Section 2 of Professional Conduct for Nurses, Midwives and Health Visitors states:

2.1 You must recognise and respect the role of patients and clients as partners in their care and the contribution they can make to it.

This involves identifying their preferences regarding care and respecting these within the limits of professional practice, existing legislation, resources and the goals of the therapeutic relationship.

2.2 You are personally accountable for ensuring that you promote and protect the interests and dignity of patients and clients, irrespective of gender, age, race, ability, sexuality, economic status, lifestyle, culture and religious or political beliefs. (NMC 2002, section 2)

Another body charged with the benchmarking of the various higher education disciplines, the Quality Assurance Agency (QAA), produced benchmarks for Health Studies, Nursing and Midwifery. They all share a number of statements which health-related curricula should promote. For example, nurses should:

Practise in an anti-discriminatory, anti-oppressive manner; they should maintain relationships with patients/clients/carers that are culturally sensitive and respect their rights and special needs; use a range of assessment techniques appropriate to the situation and make provisional identification of relevant determinants of health and physical, psychological, social and cultural needs/problems; contribute to the promotion of social inclusion . . . (QAA 2001: 2–3)

Further support for the principles underpinning transcultural health care came from recent British legislation. The Race Relations (Amendment) Act 2000 requires that public authorities set out arrangements for training staff in the knowledge and skills they will need to carry out the general and specific duties required by the Act:

- General duties: elimination of unlawful discrimination, promotion of equality of opportunity, promotion of good relations between different racial groups.
- Specific duties: ethnic monitoring of advertising, recruitment, training, appraisals, promotions, complaints, dismissals, other reasons for leaving etc.

Other countries have similar nursing codes and evolving legislation as described in the chapters of Parts 3 and 4 of this book. However, let us also remember that the International Council of Nursing (ICN) also embraces the principles of transcultural nursing as advocated in its code of ethics for nurses. Specifically the ICN states that inherent in nursing is respect for human rights, including the right to life, to dignity and to be treated with respect. Nursing care is unrestricted by considerations of age, colour, creed, culture, disability or illness, gender, nationality, politics, race or social status (http://www.icn.ch/icncode.pdf).

THE GENESIS OF THE PAPADOPOULOS, TILKI, AND TAYLOR (PTT) MODEL FOR TRANSCULTURAL NURSING AND HEALTH

In 1998, in order to promote the inclusion of culture into the nursing curricula and help our students develop cultural competence, I and two colleagues – Mary Tilki and Gina Taylor – published for the first time our model of cultural competence which we had developed in 1994 following a research study into transcultural nursing education (Papadopoulos et al 1995). We defined *cultural competence* as the capacity to provide effective health care taking into consideration people's cultural beliefs, behaviours and needs. We argued that cultural competence is both a process and an output, and results from the synthesis of knowledge and skills which we acquire during our personal and professional lives and to which we are constantly adding. To give this knowledge and skills some structure and to facilitate its learning, we proposed the constructs and stages shown in Figure 2.1.

The underpinning values of the model, which were recently further refined and articulated (I Papadopoulos, S Lees, unpublished work, 2003), are based on human rights (see Chs 3 and 4), sociopolitical systems, intercultural relations, human ethics (see Ch. 5) and human caring. Specifically these are:

The individual. All individuals have inherent worth within themselves as well as sharing the fundamental human values of love, freedom, justice, growth, life, health and security.

Culture. All human beings are cultural beings. Culture is the shared way of life of a group of people that includes beliefs, values, ideas, language, communication, norms and visibly expressed forms such as customs, art, music, clothing and etiquette. Culture influences individuals' lifestyles, personal identity and their relationship with others both within and outside their culture. Cultures are dynamic and ever changing as individuals are influenced by and influence their culture, by different degrees.

Figure 2.1 The Papadopoulos, Tilki and Taylor model for developing cultural competence.

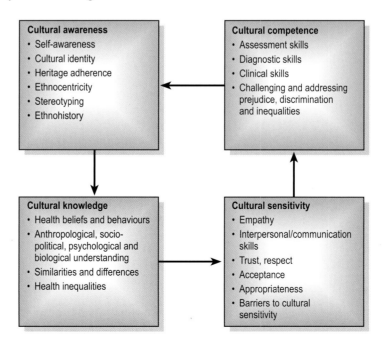

Structure. Societies, institutions and family are structures of power which can be enabling or disabling to an individual.

Health and illness. Health refers to a state of well-being that is culturally defined, valued and practised and which reflects the ability of individuals (or groups) to perform their daily role activities in culturally expressed, beneficial and patterned lifeways (Leininger 1991). Illness refers to an unwanted condition that is culturally defined and culturally responded to.

Caring. Caring is an activity that responds to the uniqueness of individuals in a culturally sensitive and compassionate way through the use of therapeutic communication.

Nursing. Nursing is a learned activity aiming at providing care to individuals in a culturally competent way.

Cultural competence. Cultural competence is a process one goes through in order to continuously develop and refine one's capacity to provide effective health care, taking into consideration people's cultural beliefs, behaviours and needs.

STAGES AND CONSTRUCTS OF THE MODEL

CULTURAL AWARENESS

The first stage in the model is *cultural awareness*, which begins with an examination of our personal value base and beliefs. The nature of construction of cultural identity as well as its influence on people's health beliefs and practices are viewed as necessary planks of our learning platform.

Simply put, our values and beliefs are the principles we use to guide our lives and to make decisions or judgements. They are the lenses through which we view the world. We develop our values from an early age and therefore our family, the culture of our family and our close social environment influence our values. If we compare what we value with a friend or fellow student who comes from a different cultural background to ours, we will soon discover that we have much in common. For example, we may discover that we both value love, life, justice, family life, health and so on. We will, however, discover that our interpretations of love, life, justice, family life and health differ to some degree. This difference will be due to a number of factors such as our different gender, different age, different cultural backgrounds and our different experiences in life. This will make us realize that even though all human beings have much in common, our small or subtle differences are important as they are the ones that define our uniqueness, our individuality.

Our individuality is closely linked to the notion of personal identity, which too is influenced by many factors. For example, important components of my identity, at the time of writing this chapter, are that I am a woman, a wife, a mother, a Greek Cypriot, a nurse, an academic, an immigrant, and a social activist within my ethnic community. At different times in my life, important components of my identity would have been: a refugee, a student, a Christian, and so on. If a friend was asked to describe me to someone who did not know me, she might say that I was a middle-aged, medium build, Greek woman who had been a nurse and now works in a university. People who do not know me at all may define me in completely different ways.

Some years ago I took my teenage son to the hospital. When I tried to ask what was happening to him, the nurses made it quite obvious that I would not understand the nature of the tests my son was having. They spoke to me slowly in brief sentences with a slightly raised voice which indicated to me that they thought my English was not very good. My examples illustrate that our identities are multifaceted and are never static. They also highlight that my ethnic and cultural background is one of the factors that defines 'me' whether I am doing the defining or others are doing it for me. The examples also demonstrate that health professionals' cultural assumptions are strongly influenced by the cultural norms of the society they live in.

Another important sub-construct related to cultural awareness is stereotyping. So, how did the health professionals stereotype me, in the example I used above? At the time of the incident, it was common for many Greek Cypriot women living in London to work as dressmakers in clothing factories often owned by Greek Cypriots, or to work from home. These women did not need to speak English to be economically active. Their world revolved around the confines of their family and their work, neither of which required them to speak English. Health professionals would often encounter Greek women whose ability to speak English was either absent or limited. The language barrier meant that misunderstandings would occur which were often attributed to the women's lack of education or even lack of intelligence. After all, would not an intelligent person living in another country recognize the importance of learning the new language? Since nobody in the hospital knew who I was, the stereotypical cultural assumptions about women who 'looked like me' came to the fore. When, in my worried state, I insisted on knowing what was happening to my son, I was ignored, the nurses' non-verbal behaviour seemed to me to be indicative of another stereotype, that of 'a temperamental Mediterranean mother'.

Returning to the notion of cultural self-awareness, it is important to understand that even if we are not consciously aware of our own values, beliefs and cultural identity, these do exist at a subconscious level and influence our behaviour towards others. Most of us have at one time or another judged people in negative ways, simply because their behaviour, lifestyle and so on, did not meet our own standards. When we assume that our values and those of our ethnic or cultural group are superior to those of people from different ethnic or cultural backgrounds, we are being ethnocentric. In my younger days, I was frequently ethnocentric. It was only when I stopped and thought why I often said such things as 'Greek people would never do that!' that I realized the years of primary and secondary education in Cyprus, as well as the pride of my parents in being Greek, filled me with romantic notions of the glorious Greek history, and the wondrous achievements of Greek philosophers and scientists who – according to my parents and teachers – gave civilization to the world. I was one of them, and so I felt superior to those who were not Greek. When all these notions became part of my conscious rather than unconscious self, I became less ethnocentric, without losing my pride in my Greek origins.

Therefore, before we attempt to understand the importance of the ethnic origins of other people, we must try and understand our own. Another important sub-construct related to cultural awareness or to cultural knowledge (the location of some of the sub-constructs in the model is arbitrary as there is a natural overlap between them and they are meant to be flexibly used to help not hinder our understanding), is that of ethnohistory.

Leininger (1995: 106) defined ethnohistory as 'all those past facts, events, instances, experiences of individuals, groups, cultures, and institutions that are primarily people-centred (ethno) and which describe, explain, and interpret human lifeways within particular cultural contexts and over short or long periods of time'. In practical terms this means that we must gain some understanding of the historical, geographical and sociocultural background of the people we care for. You will read examples of ethnohistory in some of the chapters that follow. I hope you find such information useful in helping you to understand the health issues of these countries. I agree with Leininger, who first highlighted the importance of ethnohistory, that it should form another of the building blocks of nurses' knowledge. For example, a nurse who calls a Turkish interpreter to help a Kurdish refugee who has language problems is in my view culturally incompetent, as she does not understand the ethnic conflict between Turkish and Kurdish people. Even if the Turkish interpreter is totally professional, in the eyes of the Kurdish refugee he represents the cause of her suffering and refugeedom. This incompetence will result in waste of resources and delays for the patient with sometimes dangerous consequences.

CULTURAL KNOWLEDGE

What is cultural knowledge and who produces it? If we take the definition I used earlier that 'Culture is the shared way of life of a group of people that includes beliefs, values, ideas, language, communication, norms and visibly expressed forms such as customs, art, music, clothing and etiquette. Culture influences individuals' lifestyles, personal identity and their relationship with others both within and outside their culture', and even more importantly, our definition of transcultural health and nursing 'as the study and research of *cultural* diversities and similarities in health and illness as well as their underpinning societal and organizational *structures*, in order to understand current practice and to contribute to its future development in a culturally responsive way', then we will see that cultural knowledge can be derived from almost all disciplines such as anthropology, sociology, psychology, biology, nursing, medicine, and the arts, and can be gained in a number of ways.

O'Hagan (2001) wrote that anthropology has been more preoccupied with culture than any other discipline and has provided by far the most illuminating theory on the subject. He cited the work of Edward Tylor (1832–1917) whose evolutionary theory argued that all cultures developed along similar ways because all human minds are similar and are governed by the same laws of cognition. Tylor's theory was criticized by Franz Boas (1858–1942), who believed in the historical uniqueness (particularism) of each culture and added cultural relativism to the body of anthropological theory. Margaret Mead (1901–1978) explored the cultural bases of personality; she believed that culture was much more significant than either race or biology in personality development. In general, the study of anthropology is important to a culturally competent health professional as this discipline helps us to know the cultural similarities and differences amongst cultural groups and understand why these exist and how they impact on our beliefs and practices.

Medical anthropologists such as Arthur Kleinman, Cecil Helman, Robert Hahn and Paul Farmer have furthered the anthropologists' theories by concentrating their efforts in understanding the impact of culture on our health and illness whilst at the same time raising our awareness of the undeniable interconnection of culture and structure. For example, Paul Farmer's latest book, *Pathologies of Power; Health, Human Rights and the New War on the Poor* (2003), provides a passionate critique of structural violence, the unequal distribution of power, which disregards human rights and results in social injustices and enormous health inequalities and suffering all around the world.

Power, its construction, its uses and abuses is a topic that has been investigated and written about by sociologists and is particularly relevant to the health inequalities which exist in different ethnic groups in European countries. Power lies at the heart of politics and governments who are responsible for the distribution of resources and influential in the way our societal institutions –including those providing health and social care – are structured. In the twenty-first century much preoccupation exists with the power and influence of global industries. Joseph Stiglitz, the Nobel Laureate for economics in 2001, exposes the powerful organizations that control our lives, such as the International Monetary Fund (IMF), the World Trade Organization (WTO) and the World Bank, in his best-selling book, *Globalization and its Discontents* (2002). Whilst, he argues, globalization can be a force for good, and that it has helped many millions of people attain higher standards of living, it is not working for many of the world's poor. It is not working for much of the environment and it is not working for the stability of the global economy. Social, political and economic forces at national and local level influence everyone, but people on the margins such as the poor, the disabled, the refugees and many migrants are affected the most. However, we must remember that global forces influence not only the underdeveloped countries, but all the countries in the world one way or another.

Poverty has long been considered as the main reason for ill health. The German philosopher Frederick Engels wrote of the poor of Manchester in 1844:

All conceivable evils are heaped upon the poor. They are given damp dwellings, cellar dens that are not waterproof from below or garrets that leak from above. They are supplied bad, tattered, or rotten clothing, adulterated and indigestible food. They are exposed to the most exciting changes of mental condition, the most violent vibrations between hope and fear . . . They are deprived of all enjoyments except sexual indulgence and drunkenness and are worked every day to the point of complete exhaustion of their mental and physical energies? (Engels 1887)

In 2001, nearly 160 years later, a group of public health scientists at the London Health Observatory published a report entitled *Mapping Health Inequalities Across London*. In summary, the report made the following points: The health gap between the rich and the poor in terms of life expectancy and infant mortality is widening – not closing – in the capital, a trend that is reflected across the country as a whole. A baby boy born in one of the poorest boroughs of London, Newham, is likely to die nearly six years earlier than a baby boy born in Westminster, one of the richest boroughs. A baby born in another of the poorest boroughs, Hackney, has more than double the risk of dying in the first year of life than a baby born in Bexley. Infant mortality among sole registered births (births to single mothers) is significantly higher than infant mortality in the manual social class group. In London as a whole, the infant mortality rate for sole registered births for 1993–1998 was 9.5 deaths per 1000 live births compared to 5.7 for births inside marriage or registered by both parents. Other groups with high infant mortality include births to mothers aged under 20 and births to mothers who were themselves born outside England and Wales. The report highlights that the average life expectancy for both males and females at borough level within London is closely related to deprivation. It concludes by stating that if trends continue at present levels, the gap is set to widen by 2010, not shrink.

The study of health inequalities forms an essential part of the Papadopoulos, Tilki and Taylor model of cultural competence. As explained earlier, the model apportions equal importance to both culture and structure. Health inequalities are more prevalent in minority cultural and ethnic groups, and the evidence points strongly to structural inequalities. Health inequality occurs when different groups defined by their social and demographic characteristics, such as income, education or ethnicity, have differences in access to health services or differences in health status. These differences are considered to be inequitable if they occur because the people concerned have limited choices in or access to resources for health or factors that affect health where these result in differences in health outcome. These differences are considered unfair or unjust, and have been the focus of health policy in many democratic governments around the world, as well as that of the World Health Organization (WHO). However, the slow progress of change begs a number of questions such as: how are these inequalities defined, who decides the priorities for dealing with them, how is policy translated into action at local level, and are individual practitioners able to understand their implications and equipped to make a difference? In terms of our model of cultural competence, these are questions related to the production of cultural knowledge, something that will be discussed more fully in Chapter 6, 'Promoting culturally competent research'.

The knowledge examples used above were derived by 'expert' anthropologists, sociologists, philosophers, and health scientists. Foucault (1980) stated that the truth-claim and the procedures for gaining access to that truth have historically privileged the pronouncements of trained experts over the discourses of "ordinary" people. Understanding human nature and the problems of living becomes the purview of scientists, rendering people dependent on experts to explain and oversee their life experiences (Berman 1981). Hence, the specialists dominate any debate concerning issues of public interest because ordinary people are unable to enter the scientized debate, as they lack the technical terminology and specialized language of argumentation (Habermas 1979).

It is important to balance – if not overturn – this domination of knowledge by enabling people to have a say in how they would like to see their world put together and run (Gaventa 1988). One way of doing this is through participatory research, an approach adopted by myself and colleagues in the last 10 years, albeit in a modified form as the examples in Chapters 7–11 illustrate. This approach is further discussed in Chapter 6. Whatever the source of the knowledge we access to enable us to care for our clients/patients in culturally competent ways, we must always ask ourselves: whose values were used to construct it? Notwithstanding the problematic nature of knowledge and its production within the various disciplinary traditions, another way of gaining knowledge is through meaningful contact with people from different cultural and ethnic groups. Lay cultural knowledge can enhance our understanding around health beliefs, behaviours and problems.

CULTURAL SENSITIVITY

Cultural sensitivity entails the crucial development of appropriate interpersonal relationships with our clients. An important element in achieving cultural sensitivity is how professionals view people in their care. Unless clients are considered as true partners, culturally sensitive care is not being achieved and we (nurses and other healthcare professionals) risk using our power in an oppressive way. Equal partnerships involve trust, acceptance and respect as well as facilitation and negotiation.

Culley (2001: 123) writes:

> Competent nursing practice must include being able to negotiate care in an encounter where at least some of the beliefs, values, attitudes and experiences of nurse and patient differ . . . But it must be recognised that because ethnic groups are not unified cultural wholes, because culture is complex and changing, because ethnic identity is to some degree situational and dynamic and because we live in a racist society, the task of providing good care is itself complex and fraught with difficulty. The nurse faces a tension between the need to recognise and respond to cultural difference and the necessity of doing this without recourse to stereotyping.

In the previous section we discussed the notion of power, identified some powerful agents and structures and contrasted this with the powerlessness of the poor and excluded. We also discussed the power of the 'expert' who both produces and uses knowledge in ways that exclude lay people. It is widely recognized that in a patient–healthcare professional encounter, the powerful one is the latter due to his/her expert knowledge; despite current efforts to make medical discourse more accessible to lay people, specialized medical knowledge remains the domain of the healthcare professional. Further, hierarchies are very common in all societies; not only are healthcare professionals often of higher social class than their patients but their position in the healthcare system affords them higher status than their patients. Evidence for this is provided regularly by the mass media in cases where, for example, doctors and nurses have abused their position with detrimental effects for the patient. It is because of this realization that the various professions have explicit codes of conduct, requiring their members to view their patients as partners in their care, something that must involve sharing of power and facilitating empowerment by providing understandable information and support.

The development of patient–healthcare professional partnership is based on the development of interpersonal relationships based on trust and effective communication. Husband & Hoffman (2003) proposed that all interpersonal communication contains the possibility of ambiguity and misunderstanding. The possibilities of misunderstanding and poor communication become much greater when we communicate across a cultural boundary.

Gerrish et al (1996) suggested that nursing professionals need to acquire and develop transcultural communicative competence which requires cultural competence in order to put their patients/clients at ease, and create an environment in which meanings, ideas, information and issues which are essential to professional care are efficiently exchanged. To achieve this, trust is required on both parts. Mayeroff (1972) explained that trusting the other is to let go, something which includes an element of risk and a leap into the unknown, both of which take courage.

Drawing on the work of Kim (1992), Gerrish et al (1996) identified two elements of transcultural communicative competence: (a) cultural communicative competence and (b) intercultural communication.

Cultural communicative competence, requires the nurse to learn to understand the cultural values, behavioural patterns and rules for interaction in specific cultures. This means developing specific knowledge and insights into a specific culture; and being prepared to draw upon that knowledge to guide one's understanding of the patient or colleague.

Intercultural communication is the generic ability to recognize the challenges of communication across cultural boundaries. It invites us to stay in touch with our own sense of authenticity, to recognize our anxiety about ambiguity in the situation, to recognize the potential and real challenges to our own values and expectations, and to remain committed to making the interaction effective.

Culley (2001: 124) concedes to the need for specific knowledge and insights into specific cultures but states:

This may present the nurse with a dilemma. Practitioners must avoid stereotypes, but must have sufficient prior knowledge to know what might be relevant to the caring encounter . . . Lack of such knowledge can lead not only to personal distress and offence but may have serious conse-quences for treatment . . . Rejecting what we have called essentialist views of culture does not mean rejecting the idea that aspects of culture can influence health and healthcare. However, nurses need to use communica-tion skills to ascertain rather than assume what preferences and practices are significant to patients.

At a more practical level, Purnell & Paulanka (1998) suggest that com-munication skills include verbal language skills (dominant language, dialects), paralanguage variations (voice volume, tone, intonations), non-verbal communications (eye contact, facial expressions, use of touch, body language, special distancing practices, acceptable greetings), tem-porality (past, present or future orientation of worldview), clock versus social time, and the degree of formality in the use of names. All these components may vary from culture to culture, and ignorance of them may result in barriers to communication. In numerous studies conducted by myself and colleagues, we found that communication barriers not only existed but were often one of the main causes of culturally incom-petent care. For example, doctors were reported to be insensitive in dis-closing patients' diagnoses (Papadopoulos & Lees 2004), information was not made available to people in accessible and appropriate formats (Papadopoulos et al 2004a), interpreters were not used but inappropriate use of family members was made (Papadopoulos & Worrall 1996), racist attitudes of health professionals prevented people from communicating their needs (Papadopoulos & Gebrehiwot 2002).

CULTURAL COMPETENCE

The achievement of the fourth stage (cultural competence) requires the synthesis and application of previously gained awareness, knowledge and sensitivity. Further focus is given to practical skills such as assess-ment of need, clinical diagnosis and other caring skills. A most important component of this stage of development is the ability to recognize and challenge racism and other forms of discrimination and oppressive practice.

Campinha-Bacote (1998) provides a comprehensive list of numerous models and tools developed to collect cultural data for patients' assess-ment of needs. Leininger (1995) writes about a culturological assessment using the major domains of her 'Sunrise' model, which are:

- worldview
- ethnohistory
- kinship and social factors
- cultural values, beliefs and lifeways
- religious, spiritual and philosophical factors
- technological factors
- economic factors
- political and legal factors

- educational factors
- language and communication
- professional and generic (folk or lay) care beliefs and practices
- general and specific nursing care.

In order to ensure a comprehensive assessment and to guide the nurse towards cultural competence in using the Sunrise model, Leininger suggested the following guiding principles:

- Show a genuine and sincere interest in the patient/client as you listen and learn from them.
- Pay attention to gender or class differences, communication needs and interpersonal space.
- Make sure you are completely familiar with the Sunrise model, its underpinning assumptions and its use in practice before commencing the transcultural nursing assessment.
- During the assessment remain fully conscious of your own cultural orientation, biases and prejudices.
- Remain aware that some patients/clients may belong to special groups, e.g. the homeless, the gay/lesbian community, drug users, the mentally ill. These groups need to be respected, and their rights understood and heard when being assessed in order to ensure culturally appropriate care.
- Be aware of your cultural competence or areas in need of development before using the assessment tool.
- Make sure you inform the patient/client and all significant others about the assessment, the date and time you intend to carry it out, in order to gain consent and to ensure full and complete understanding of the purpose of the transcultural assessment.
- Make sure you make an holistic assessment, i.e. use all appropriate parts of the Sunrise model.
- Remain an active listener throughout the assessment.
- Following the assessment, reflect on the information gathered in relation to your transcultural nursing knowledge.

Purnell's model of cultural competence (Purnell & Paulanka 1998) provides another framework for conducting a cultural assessment. Purnell's model has 12 domains which are common to all cultures:

- overview, inhabited localities, and topography
- communication
- family roles and organization
- workforce issues
- biocultural ecology
- high-risk behaviours
- nutrition
- pregnancy and childbearing practices
- death rituals
- spirituality
- healthcare practices
- healthcare practitioners.

Berlin & Fowkes (1982) proposed the LEARN model for conducting a cultural assessment. LEARN stands for 'listen' to the client's perception of his/her problem and then 'explain' your perception of the problem; then 'acknowledge' the similarities and differences between the two perceptions, and make 'recommendations' which must involve the client. Finally, 'negotiate' the treatment plan, considering that it is beneficial to incorporate selected aspects of the client's culture in providing culturally competent care.

Campinha-Bacote (1998) points out that conducting a cultural assessment is more than selecting a tool and asking the client the questions listed on the tool. This must be done in a culturally sensitive manner, bearing in mind the urgency of the patient's medical condition, your prior knowledge about the patient's culture so that for example, you avoid offence, or include the family in the process and so on. The same author suggests that an effective approach to cultural assessment would be to integrate relevant cultural content into the existing nursing documents. Therefore, culture is not seen as something extra but rather appropriately as a coherent part of the nursing process.

Sue Dyson (2003) provides an excellent example of how Roper et al's model of nursing and Giger and Davidhizar's model of transcultural nursing (Giger & Davidhizar 1995) can be integrated to provide a comprehensive assessment of the patient.

Papadopoulos et al (1998) give examples of how culturally appropriate nursing assessment, nursing diagnosis and clinical skills can be applied. As previously stated, the skills of a culturally competent healthcare professional are the practical expressions of his/her cultural awareness, cultural knowledge and cultural sensitivity. The amalgam of these three components will guide a health provider in knowing how to ask general and then more specific questions, how to overcome any communication barriers that may exist, how to effectively interact with the client's/patient's significant others, how to elicit information about health and illness beliefs, lifestyles and self-care practices, how to find out how important religion and religious practices are to the patient, whether he or she has any views about specific medical and nursing interventions such as blood transfusions, pain relief, resuscitation and so on, to more basic observational skills such as those involving the skin – the norms of which are based on white skin, for example pallor, cyanosis, jaundice, rashes, bruising – to food likes, dislikes and fasting practices. Some of the chapters that follow provide further information which will help you sharpen up your transcultural skills. But we must not forget that transcultural or culturally competent care is ethical care. In Chapter 5 Ann Gallagher discusses the ethical challenges faced by health and social care professionals in their everyday practice, highlighting the values and principles that can be used to enable us to make transculturally ethical decisions or cope with the characteristic ambiguity that exists in health and social care work in democratic culturally diverse societies.

In an ideal world, democratic multicultural societies are non-oppressive and afford all citizens equal rights. However, in the real world this perfection does not exist, despite efforts from governments to achieve this (Papadopoulos 2002). As discussed earlier, health inequalities are rife throughout the world. In Chapter 3, Mary Tilki tackles the complex issues of human rights, whilst in Chapter 4 Gina Taylor focuses on inequalities suffered by migrants and refugees, so I will not elaborate on this topic here. Ethnocentric and racist health and social care is a theme that can be found in many of the chapters in this book. The evidence provided illustrates how degrading and dangerous racist policies and practices can be and often are. It is therefore important that healthcare providers make every effort to eliminate practices that result in inequitable, ethnocentric or racist services; in other words it is time for them all to become culturally competent. And if, as was stated in the beginning of this chapter, we are all cultural beings, then culturally competent services and practitioners will benefit all of us.

CULTURE–GENERIC AND CULTURE–SPECIFIC COMPETENCIES

It is important to point out that throughout our professional lives, we develop and use a set of culturally generic competencies that are applicable across cultural groups (Gerrish & Papadopoulos 1999). These culture-generic competencies, such as the appreciation of how cultural identity mediates health, or a deeper understanding of the underpinning societal and organizational structures which promote or hinder culturally competent care, help us to acquire culture-specific competencies which are particular to specific cultural groups. It is obviously impossible for any nurse or other healthcare worker to know all about the numerous cultural groups that live in any one country or location. However, by using one's culture-generic competencies one can gather the relevant culture-specific information needed to care for the patient/client. Figure 2.2 depicts the dynamic relationship between culture-generic and culture-specific competencies.

Figure 2.2 The Papadopoulos and Lees culture-generic and culture-specific model of cultural competence.

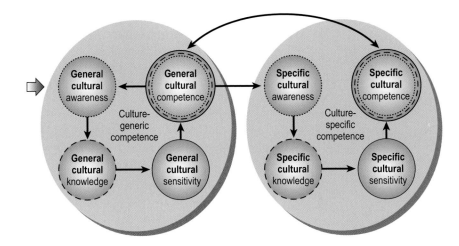

LEVELS OF CULTURAL COMPETENCE

In a recent study (Papadopoulos et al 2004b) which aimed at promoting cultural competence amongst mental health professionals (nurses, psychologists, psychiatrists, social workers and unqualified staff), we developed and delivered a programme of sessions based on our model. The programme consisted of two negotiated sessions for each of the four stages of the model: cultural awareness, cultural knowledge, cultural sensitivity and cultural competence. Prior to the delivery of the sessions we designed and validated a self-administered tool which measures an individual's level of cultural competence. This too was structured on the four stages of our model. Since we stress that cultural competence is continuously developing, this implies that healthcare workers function at different levels of cultural competence. Our assessment tool also takes into consideration the importance of cultural awareness as the first stage in this process as well as the importance of culture-generic competencies which must exist to facilitate the development of culture-specific competencies. We identified four different levels of culturally competent practice:

- level 1: culturally incompetent practice
- level 2: culturally aware practice
- level 3: culturally safe practice
- level 4: culturally competent practice.

We used these to measure the study participants' cultural competence levels prior to and after the intervention. We discovered that none were culturally incompetent prior to the intervention. The majority were operating at a cultural awareness level whilst a few provided culturally safe care. Only one person scored him/herself as culturally competent prior to the intervention. Most of the participants either remained at the same level or improved their levels of cultural competence following the intervention.

Although the number of participants in this study was small and the intervention probably too short, it nevertheless points out the benefits of appropriate educational input based on a sound framework. This study also illustrated that cultural competence is not an end point. It is a continuous process of learning; the more culture-generic competence we have the easier it is to attain culture-specific competence which is constantly evolving according to new cultural and healthcare contexts.

CONCLUSION

Culturally competent care is becoming a twenty-first century imperative for those responsible for providing healthcare services in multicultural societies. Being treated in a culturally competent manner is a reasonable expectation of all of us in the new millennium. It is no longer tenable to treat everyone in the same way, or to base the care we provide to individuals on norms drawn out of the majority culture. Culturally competent care is both a legal and a moral requirement for nurses (NMC 2002). Valuing diversity in health care enhances the delivery and effectiveness of health care for all people, whether they are members of a minority or a majority cultural group. It is evident that cultural and structural factors influence the quality of health and nursing care. If nursing fails to consider these factors, then it is failing to provide individualized care to all its clients.

Despite the progress we have made in the last 10 years, much work remains to be done. We need to develop better client assessment tools to include a 'cultural assessment'. We need to develop more efficient knowledge tools which do not stereotype but provide quick information in urgent situations. We need to achieve more efficient ways for cultural communication. We also need to develop more effective ways of assessing cultural competence, particularly in practice. And we need better, more detailed educational benchmarking for cultural competence. The Papadopoulos, Tilki and Taylor model provides a structure which, if applied, could improve nursing and other healthcare education and ultimately improve the quality of care for all of us, irrespective of the type of health services we may require.

REFLECTIVE QUESTIONS

1. Reflect on the focus of the Papadopoulos, Tilki and Taylor model for developing cultural competence and consider how this differs from other models of transcultural nursing.
2. Critically reflect on your culture-generic competencies and think of an occasion that you used them in order to develop your culture-specific competencies.

REFERENCES

Berlin E, Fowkes W 1982 A teaching framework for cross-cultural health care. Western Journal of Medicine 139(6):934–938

Berman M 1981 The re-enchantment of the world. Cornell University Press, New York

Campinha-Bacote J 1998 The process of cultural competence in the delivery of healthcare services. A culturally competent model of care. 3rd edn. Transcultural CARE Associates, Cincinnati

Culley L 2001 Nursing, culture and competence. In: Culley L, Dyson S (eds) Ethnicity and nursing practice. Palgrave, Houndmills, p 109–127

Dyson S 2003 Transcultural health care practice: Core practice module, chapter three: Transcultural nursing care of adults. Online. Available: http://www.rcn.org.uk/resources/transcultural/adulthealth/index.php 25 Jan 2005

Engels F 1887 Condition of the working class in England. American edn. Progress Publishers, New York

Farmer P 2003 Pathologies of power; health, human rights and the new war on the poor. University of California Press, Berkeley

Foucault M 1980 Power/knowledge: Selected interviews and other writings. Pantheon, New York

Gaventa J 1988 Participatory research in North America. Convergence 24(2–3):19–28

Gerrish K, Papadopoulos I 1999 Transcultural competence: the challenge for nurse education. British Journal of Nursing 8(21):1453–1457

Gerrish K, Husband C, Mackenzie J 1996 Nursing for a multi-ethnic society. Open University Press, Buckingham

Giger J N, Davidhizar R E 1995 Transcultural nursing. Assessment and intervention. 2nd edn. Mosby: St Louis

Habermas J 1979 Legitimation crisis in the modern society. Communication and the evolution of society. Beacon Press, Boston

Husband C, Hoffman E 2003 Transcultural health care practice: Transcultural communication and health care practice. Online. Available: http://www.rcn.org.uk/resources/transcultural/communication/index.php 25 Jan 2005

Kim Y Y 1992 Intercultural communication competence: a systems-theoretic view. In: Gudykunst W B, Kim Y Y (eds) Readings on communication with strangers. McGraw-Hill, New York

Leininger M M 1991 Culture care diversity and universality. A theory of nursing. NLN, New York

Leininger M M 1995 Transcultural nursing. Concepts, theories, research and practices. 2nd edn. McGraw-Hill, New York

Mayeroff M 1972 On caring. Harper Perennial, New York

Nursing and Midwifery Council (NMC) 2002 Professional conduct for nurses, midwives and health visitors. NMC, London

O'Hagan K 2001 Cultural competence in the caring professions. Jessica Kingsley, London

Papadopoulos I 2002 Meeting health care needs in culturally diverse societies. In: Daly J et al (eds) Contexts of nursing: an introduction. Blackwell Science, Oxford, p 196–208

Papadopoulos I, Alleyne J 1995 The need for nursing and midwifery programmes of education to address the health care needs of minority ethnic groups. Nurse Education Today 15:140–144

Papadopoulos I, Gebrehiwot A 2002 The EMBRACE UK Project: Ethiopian Migrants, their Beliefs, Refugeedom, Adaptation, Calamities, and Experiences in the United Kingdom. Research Centre for Transcultural Studies in Health, Middlesex University, London

Papadopoulos I, Lees S 2002 Developing culturally competent researchers. Journal of Advanced Nursing 37(3):258–264

Papadopoulos I, Lees S 2004 Cancer and communication: Similarities and differences of male cancer sufferers from six different ethnic groups. European Journal of Cancer Care 13(2):154–162

Papadopoulos I, Worrall L 1996 All health care is good until you have a problem. An examination of the primary health care needs of the Greek and Greek Cypriot women. GGCWE, London

Papadopoulos I, Alleyne J, Tilki M 1995 Teaching transcultural care. A report to the General Nursing Council. Research Centre for Transcultural Studies in Health. Middlesex University, London

Papadopoulos I, Lay M, Lees S 2005a Health ASERT Programme Wales: Enhancing the health promotion evidence base on Minority Ethnic Groups, Asylum Seekers/Refugees and Gypsy Travellers. Report 7. Full Length Primary Research Report. Cardiff: Welsh Assembly Government, Cardiff

Papadopoulos I, Tilki M, Lees S 2004b Promoting cultural competence in healthcare through a research-based intervention in the UK. Journal of Diversity in Health and Social Care 1(2):107–115

Papadopoulos I, Tilki M, Taylor G 1998 Transcultural care. A guide for health care professionals. Quay Books, Dinton

Purnell L D, Paulanka B J 1998 Transcultural health care. A culturally competent approach. F A Davies, Philadelphia

Quality Assurance Agency for Higher Education (QAA) 2001 Benchmark statement: Health care programmes – Nursing. QAA, Gloucester

Race Relations (Amendment) Act 2000 The Stationery Office, London

Stiglitz J 2002 Globalization and its discontents. Penguin, London

UNHCR 2005 Basic facts. Online. Available: http://www.unhcr.ch/cgi-bin/texis/vtx/basics 29 Mar 2005

Chapter **3**

Human rights and health inequalities: UK and EU policies and initiatives relating to the promotion of culturally competent care

Mary Tilki

LEARNING OBJECTIVES

After reading this chapter you should be able to:
- appreciate the relevance of human rights issues and culturally competent care for nurses in contemporary Europe
- increase your awareness of the development of human rights, how they are classified, promoted and protected, and their relationship to transcultural nursing
- consider the social determinants of health in Europe today and explore the potential of combined human rights and public health approaches in addressing health inequalities

- explore the legislation, policies and initiatives which aim to promote human rights and tackle discrimination, drawing on the example of the United Kingdom
- reflect on how examples of good practice in the UK might be adapted to meet local needs and address the needs of different cultural groups in other European countries.

INTRODUCTION

There is an inextricable link between human rights and health. The preamble to the World Health Organization constitution goes so far as to suggest that 'the enjoyment of the highest attainable standard of health is one of the fundamental rights of every human being without distinction of race, religion, political belief, economic or social condition' (WHO 1986: 2). There has been a vast expansion in the body of evidence about both health and human rights in the last two or three decades but although human rights issues have a clear impact on health, the relationship between the two has not always been fully exploited (Mann et al 1999).

With the expansion of the European Union, increasing levels of global migration and the persistence of famine and war in the developing world, it is important that nurses and health workers in Europe see human rights as an issue for them. Although the low turnout in the European elections in 2004 suggests that many citizens feel Europe is a remote concept of little relevance to their daily lives, the European Union has the capacity to be a catalyst for change which can deliver improvements in health. The need for change is not just a feature of an enlarged Europe but reflects the ageing population, changing epidemiological trends, a shift from institutional to community care, a concern with prevention rather than cure and a refocusing of responsibility from the state to the individual.

In early 2004, the existing 15 member states of the European Union (Austria, Belgium, Denmark, France, Finland, Germany, Greece, Ireland, Italy, Luxembourg, Netherlands, Portugal, Spain, Sweden, UK) were host to around 19 million immigrants of whom 6 million were from other EU countries. It was predicted that following the accession of 10 new states (Cyprus, Czech Republic, Estonia, Hungary, Latvia, Lithuania, Malta, Poland, Slovakia, Slovenia) in May of that year, a further 1.25 million would arrive in the old member countries (Coughlan 2004). Contrary to popular media reports, however, it appears that the predicted 'influx' of economic migrants from the new member states did not materialize. However, it is clear that increased population mobility will present Europe with a challenge over the next 25 years (Kastrissianakis 2004). The economic need for increased migration in the more industrial and economically developed countries in the coming years stems from the ageing of the population. The subsequent shrinking of the workforce is exacerbated by low birth rates and the failure of industrialized countries to invest adequately in professional and technical education. Some of the workforce shortfall can be made up temporarily by migration from the acceding states, where population age is somewhat lower, and unemployment is high or work is poorly remunerated. However, declining fertility rates in the 1990s mean that newly acceded countries too have an ageing population, so migration from outside the EU will continue to be necessary in years to come (Kastrissianakis 2004). While migration bridges gaps in the labour market, increasing arrival or settlement of people from different cultures has implications for welfare, housing, education and particularly health.

According to David Byrne, the former European Commissioner for Health and Consumer Protection, health is essential for economic prosperity. He argues that current health systems in Europe focus on illness despite an urgent need to do much more health promotion and prevention if existing health gaps across Europe are to be addressed (Byrne 2004). The health status of citizens of the 15 member states has improved, although class, gender and age-related inequalities still exist (European Commission 2003). The main causes of death in Europe are now heart disease, respiratory and digestive disorders, cancers and accidents and all are largely preventable. Health status has also improved in the newly acceded states, but the improvements are fewer and there are large differences between these states and the established member countries. In the newly acceded states there is a higher incidence of the same health problems as well as excesses of communicable diseases and violence (European Commission 2003).

Health inequalities are determined to a large extent by socio-economic and environmental factors and with freedom of movement across Europe it is foreseeable that some migrants will be from groups at most risk of poor health. However, contrary to media images, those moving across Europe and to Europe from other countries are more likely to be educated, skilled, motivated and healthy (Fahey 2004). Health can deteriorate in the process of migration, but the normal range of health problems experienced by any group may have different implications for individuals or health providers in a new society. Migrant receiving countries in Europe may be expecting an increase in culture-specific disorders such as thalassaemia and sickle cell disorder. However, they may be less prepared for the excess morbidity and premature mortality associated with heart disease, diabetes, stroke, limiting long-term illness, mental illness and suicide among people from different ethnic groups.

MIGRATION AND HEALTH

Evidence from the UK shows categorically that refugees, asylum seekers and minority ethnic groups (those who identify themselves or are identified by the wider community as separate from the majority) experience considerable health inequalities (Nazroo 1997, Acheson 1998). Culture shock may be a problem initially, but alienation, discrimination and hostility take their toll on health over time (Krieger 1990, 2000). Despite having professional or occupational qualifications and skills, labour shortages and discriminatory practices mean that newcomers are often forced into unskilled work. As members of lower socio-economic groups, their risk of social and health inequalities increases but this alone does not account for health disadvantage (Nazroo 1999). Lifestyle factors play a major role in the construction of ill health, and tobacco and alcohol consumption in particular contribute to significant mortality in the recently acceded countries (European Commission 2003). Cultural differences in smoking, diet, exercise and alcohol consumption influence health status and although causal links are much debated, research demonstrates a complex association between socio-economic status and ill health (Acheson 1998). For example, smoking and drinking alcohol are social activities people engage in to deal with loneliness and to cope with psychosocial distress (Tilki 2003).

There is clear evidence that racism impacts adversely on health (Krieger 1990, 2000) and that there is racism in health care (Tilki 2003, Sashidharan, 2001, 2003). A lack of knowledge due to ignorance, ethnocentricity, stereotyping or racial prejudice in receiving societies has the potential to deprive people of their human rights and preclude them from appropriate help and support. When migrants, refugees or minority ethnic groups do not access existing services it is easier to assume that they have chosen not to use them rather than examine the appropriateness of what is offered. It is clear, however, that language problems, an absence of cultural sensitivity and even outright hostility prevent people seeking effective health care when they have problems (Tilki 2003).

If the human rights of European citizens living in their own countries, those who move between member states and those who originate in third countries are to be met, there is a need for greater cultural awareness, knowledge, sensitivity and competence. Transcultural health care affords an approach which not only has the capacity to address human rights but provides the opportunity for more effective and acceptable care and measures to promote health.

THE BIRTH OF HUMAN RIGHTS

The history of human rights stretches back to the Enlightenment, and underpinned the French Declaration of the Rights of Man and the American Bill of Rights in the eighteenth century (McHale & Gallagher 2004). This era of human rights was concerned with liberty or civil and political rights.

The second era began when the European Convention on Human Rights (ECHR) was passed by the Council of Europe in 1950 following the Nazi atrocities of the Second World War. It gave people in European states civil rights which the Council of Europe believed every person in Europe should have. Signatory states were obliged to secure for everyone within their jurisdiction the civil and political rights and freedoms set out in the convention with the aim of eliminating future atrocities.

Although the protection of individual freedoms was evident in the convention, the acknowledgement that states and individuals had participated in the atrocities led to the inclusion of other values (McHale & Gallagher 2004). Values such as dignity, equality and community were central and required governments to take action to ensure social and economic rights in addition to the civil and political. Issues of discrimination and especially racial discrimination were central to the 1948 Universal Declaration of Human Rights (UDHR) in the wake of the Nazi Holocaust (Klug 2000).

A more recent third wave of human rights, referred to as solidarity or global solidarity rights, propose a reallocation of resources from rich countries to poorer ones to allow for the protection of human rights (Wilkinson & Caulfield 2000). They variously include the right to peace and a clean environment, and a growing emphasis on participation and mutuality (Klug 2000). As such, change is sought through trade agreements, education and persuasion rather than through litigation, and rights are presented not just as claims against governments but as obligations between individuals. McHale & Gallagher (2004) argue that the development of human rights has moved from an emphasis on individual liberty and freedom to an emphasis on equality and non-discrimination towards an era emphasizing mutuality and participation. This view of human rights includes human obligations and duties and is encompassed in contemporary treaties and conventions, many of which make reference to the right to health.

PROMOTION AND PROTECTION OF HUMAN RIGHTS

The promotion of human rights was identified as the principal purpose of the United Nations in 1945. In 1948 the Universal Declaration of Human Rights (UDHR) was adopted as a universal, common standard for all peoples and nations. The UDHR, the United Nations Charter, the International Covenant on Civil and Political Rights, its optional protocols and the International Covenant on Economic, Social and Cultural Rights form what is commonly known as the International Bill of Human Rights (Mann et al 1999). In addition, a large number of declarations and conventions have been adopted, focusing on issues such as racial discrimination or on specific groups such as women, children or those with mental illness or disability. Although the UDHR is not a legally binding document, many nations have endowed it with legitimacy and it forms the basis of a number of national constitutions, with governments frequently citing it when accusing other states of human rights violations.

The Council of Europe, founded in 1949, is Europe's oldest political organization and groups together 49 countries including 21 from central and eastern Europe. It is distinct from the European Union (EU) but no country has ever joined the EU without first belonging to the Council of Europe. The Council was set up to defend human rights, parliamentary democracy and the rule of law, to develop and standardize social and legal practices and to promote a European identity based on shared values across different cultures. Since 1989 it has, however, been more concerned with acting as human rights watcher for Europe's post-communist democracies (http://www.coe.int/T/e/CoM.about_coe/). It has assisted member states with the implementation and consolidation of political, legal, constitutional and economic reform and provided expertise on human rights, local democracy, education, culture and the environment. The Council of Europe oversees a number of different treaties, conventions and commissions which relate to human rights, democracy and the security of citizens, many of which impact indirectly on health. (Among the most significant treaties are the European Convention on Human Rights, the European Social Charter, the European Convention for the Prevention of Torture and Inhuman or Degrading Treatment or Punishment, the Framework Convention for the Protection of National Minorities, the European Commission against Racism and Intolerance.)

Enforcement of the European Convention on Human Rights (ECHR) and the investigation of abuses is the responsibility of the European Court of Human Rights in Strasbourg, where violations by individuals and governments can be tried. The Court comprises judges from every state signed up to the convention, who sit as individuals and not as representatives of their own country. With the exception of Ireland and Norway, signatory states have incorporated the ECHR into their own laws, thus enabling the domestic judiciary to consider alleged breaches of the convention, only seeking to involve Strasbourg when domestic remedies fail. Other organizations monitoring and publicizing human rights abuses include Amnesty International and Human Rights Watch, while the United Nations through its Commissioner for Human Rights investigates claims made by individuals and states.

CATEGORIES OF HUMAN RIGHTS AND CITIZENSHIP

The history of human rights demonstrates how the interpretation of rights evolved over time to relate to contemporary society rather than the mores of a previous era. Human rights are wide-ranging and while the aim is to ensure all persons have equality of rights, not all rights have the same status.

A useful example of how rights are classified is the UK Human Rights Act 1998, which describes three broad categories of absolute, limited and qualified rights. Absolute rights, such as the right to life, the prohibition of torture and degrading treatment, forced labour or slavery and the right to marry, cannot be restricted in any way. The second category, limited rights, takes account of issues such as liberty and security, the right to fair trial and abolition of the death penalty. These rights allow for exceptions such as the lawful detention of persons who are mentally ill or carrying infectious diseases or during circumstances of national emergency. The third category concerns a group of 'qualified' rights and includes the right to respect for private and family life, freedoms of conscience, religion and assembly. They also include rights to education and the peaceful enjoyment of property. Qualified rights may be restricted where there is conflict between individual needs and those of wider society or in the interests of national security, crime prevention or public safety. While the European Court of Human Rights provides a framework to protect human rights and some countries have incorporated them into domestic legislation, member states interpret rights differently and protect them in differing legislative ways.

Each category of human rights applies to health, but for justifiable reasons there has been more attention to absolute and limited rights. Absolute rights relating to torture and degrading treatment, reproduction and euthanasia are commonly debated in Europe. Limited rights such as those around the detention of people with mental illness are widely criticized (Morrall & Hazleton 2004). However, there is a need for greater attention to qualified rights, particularly in relation to people from different cultural groups whose beliefs, values and customs may differ from the majority community. Despite reference to the right to health in many European and UK policy documents, it is clear that no state can guarantee good health or protect against all causes of ill health. Consequently the right to health might best be understood as a qualified right dependent on the availability of services to facilitate health, inevitably implying cost constraint and prioritization of resources. However, as other chapters demonstrate, the right to work, housing, welfare and in many cases the right to health care is also dependent on citizenship status.

Citizenship is a contested term but perhaps the most influential definition is that of T.H. Marshall (1950), who envisaged citizenship involving civil, political and social elements. Citizenship is often likened to identity and although people living in Europe might describe themselves as Europeans, there is no clear picture of what the identity of a European citizen is. Given the geographical, cultural, ethnic and linguistic variety of Europe, any attempt to define European citizenship needs to include the notion of diversity. It is clear that a universal notion of citizenship is neither appropriate nor achievable. EU citizenship gives citizens of the EU member states civil, political and social rights, but since citizenship has evolved differently in the countries in Europe, the status afforded to people from outside Europe varies. While in theory all those from member states and some from outside Europe have formal citizenship status, personal, cultural and institutional racism may effectively limit their access to substantive citizenship rights.

HUMAN RIGHTS, TRANSCULTURAL NURSING AND PUBLIC HEALTH

The language of human rights frequently conjures up images of repressive regimes and political prisoners. The attention to persecution and torture reflects concerns about Nazi atrocities as well as recent and current events in many parts of the world. However, human rights also refer to basic everyday rights such as the dignity with which people are treated, fairness, freedom and equality. They are the essence of transcultural care and are particularly relevant to nursing and health care in contemporary Europe. It is the right of every human being to be treated with dignity and respect, and to have access to effective health care, and it is an essential component of the Papadopoulos, Tilki and Taylor model (1998) described in Chapter 2.

It is worth noting that this model considers cultural awareness in the practitioner as the cornerstone of cultural competence. The model's stance that awareness of ethnocentricity and ethnic reductionism is essential fits comfortably with a human rights approach aiming to respect and protect dignity, equality, culture and religious beliefs. The second element of the model relates to cultural knowledge and this is consistent with public health approaches that require understanding of the social context within which health and illness are shaped. Public health has a wide remit and relies on the cooperation between health and other policy areas such as income, housing, welfare and employment. While cultural knowledge is important to practitioners giving hands-on care, it is arguably crucial to those with a public health remit. Equally, cultural sensitivity and competence are critical aspects of clinical care, but they should also underpin strategies for the assessment of need and the development of services.

The failure to provide culturally appropriate services is not always deliberate but is underpinned by ethnocentricity which assumes that people from other cultures find mainstream provision acceptable and effective. For example, the way in which ethnicity is conceptualized in terms of skin colour in the UK neglects the fact that white minority ethnic groups can face the same difficulties as those who are visibly dark in colour. Attempting to provide culturally specific services either separately or within the mainstream can also be problematic since a homogeneous notion of any cultural group denies the diversity that exists within it. It neglects the extent to which people adhere to their culture or the different aspects of their heritage that they value. In particular, it can deny the way in which those born in the new society or those of mixed heritage identify with the culture of their parents. Just providing a dedicated service for a particular group will not in itself be sufficient since it can potentially ignore the barriers which prevent people accessing it or getting effective help. A lack of information about services is a real obstacle to uptake by people from minority ethnic or refugee groups. Policy-makers and professionals need to question why mainstream services are not widely used, when voluntary (non-governmental) organizations can barely cope with demands placed on them. It is mistakenly assumed that people choose not to use services, relying instead on self-help or support from family or lay healers. Services which deny, dismiss or pathologize culture or expect people to conform and adapt to local norms will not be used or at best used only in extreme circumstances. This cultural insensitivity is reflected in low, late or inappropriate use of services, which potentially leads to ill health. Therefore the failure to provide services which value, respect and dignify cultural difference breaches several limited and qualified human rights.

The cultural awareness and cultural knowledge domains of the Papadopoulos, Tilki and Taylor model (1998) provide a particularly useful framework for public health assessment in any culturally diverse environment. The link between the socio-economic factors and in particular poverty and health has been known for many years, but recent academic work across Europe and the United States of America has moved beyond description to explanation (Mackenbach & Bakker 2002). These explanations are particularly pertinent to human rights debates since they provide new understandings of the way in which wider social factors impact on health. Theoretical concepts such as relative deprivation (Wilkinson 1996, 1999), social cohesion (Stansfeld 1999, Wilkinson 1996, 1999, Kawachi et al 1997, 1999) psychosocial stress (Elstad 1998, Siegrist et al 1997) and the psychosocial environment of work (Bosma et al 1997, Brunner & Marmot 1999, Karasek & Theorell 1990, Marmot et al 1999) afford different understandings of health inequalities. Although there is little attention to migrants or minority ethnic people, this evidence is highly relevant since they are largely clustered in lower socio-economic groups.

However, tackling health inequalities in the population as a whole will not necessarily mean improvements for migrants or settled minorities because despite common socio-economic problems additional factors are involved. In particular, it is necessary to consider the impact of racism and discrimination and the relationship between identity, belonging and health (Karlsen & Nazroo 2000, 2002, Halpern & Nazroo 2000). There is evidence that positive ethnic identity (Cahill & Kelleher 1999) and ethnic support networks play an important part in the maintenance of health and recovery from illness (Halpern & Nazroo 2000, Karlsen & Nazroo, 2000, 2002) and that these are less sustainable in a racist, discriminatory society. In particular, dispersal strategies take scant account of the right to a sense of safety or belonging and frequently place vulnerable people in areas where there is little understanding, experience or will to help them.

Health services only play a part in improving health and addressing health inequality and the evidence is unequivocal about the need for public health to tackle a range of interrelated social factors which exclude certain groups of people and deny them equitable rights. Reducing health inequalities in Europe requires intervention through policies such as income, housing, environment, food, employment and working conditions, as well as health promotion and provision of services (Mackenbach & Bakker 2002). While health professionals in Europe invariably abhor the detention and abuse of people in other parts of the world, they may be less concerned about the way in which those seeking refuge and asylum are held in detention centres on arrival in different countries in Europe. Professional beliefs, attitudes or behaviours underpinned by negative messages about 'economic migrants' and 'bogus asylum seekers' collude with the withdrawal of meagre support when asylum claims are rejected. This exposes vulnerable people to further indignity and health risk and therefore conflicts with the fundamental principles of human rights. Given the importance of belonging and participating in community, tackling social exclusion and enhancing social cohesion are priorities for member states.

SOCIAL EXCLUSION, COHESION AND HEALTH

The problem of social exclusion is a central concern for the European Union and fits neatly within debates of human rights and health. It differs from previous notions of poverty and marginalization (Levitas 1998) but broadly refers to different ways in which people are excluded from participation as full citizens. It involves economic, political or spatial exclusion as well as access to information, housing, health care and education (Byrne 2004). It particularly reflects the absence of formal citizenship status or the gap between formal and substantive citizenship caused by discrimination and compounded by language or cultural differences.

Social cohesion refers to the way in which social inequalities, including income, power and status, have a fundamental influence on social relations and social interactions (Elstad 1998). Individuals cannot be understood without grasping the communities they are part of and inequalities or exclusion produce feelings of anger, resentment, and other negative emotions. The existence of mutual trust and respect between different sections of the community is a reflection of a socially cohesive society and contributes to health (Stansfeld 1999). Egalitarian societies have better social relations and greater evidence of trust, mutual respect and belonging, while a lack of social cohesion increases hostility and crime, giving rise to anxiety, fear and lack of trust (Kawachi et al 1997).

Reducing social exclusion and enhancing social cohesion are essential in an enlarged Europe, with increasing internal and external migration, a backdrop of extremism, racial and religious intolerance. It can therefore be argued that through enhanced social cohesion, not only can human rights be protected, but health improved, and hopefully prosperity increased and peace maintained.

PROMOTING SOCIAL INCLUSION AND HEALTH

The Council of Europe actively promotes social cohesion by guaranteeing social protection, improving employability, protecting the most vulnerable, and promoting equal opportunities. It aims to combat exclusion and discrimination and consolidate European policy on migration (http://www.coe.int.). The European Council comprises heads of member states and is the key decision-making, coordinating and guiding body of the European Union. The Lisbon European Council (2000) agreed a strategy to strengthen employment and economic reform and tackle social cohesion as part of a knowledge-based economy. One of its main aims was to invest in people, to combat poverty and social exclusion and required member states to set targets and objectives through National Action Plans. This is furthered by the European Committee for Social Exclusion and through instruments such as the European Social Charter, and the European Code of Social Security. Perhaps the most significant provision in the field of health was the Maastricht Treaty (1993), which encouraged cooperation between member states in disease prevention. This was later revised to focus on improving health and preventing disease through health information, education and incorporating health protection into other EU policies. In May 2000, the European Commission produced a new health strategy with key elements of community action in the field of public health (http://europa.eu.int/infonet/library/j/2000285/en). Health has been subsequently integrated into the Lisbon agenda and there is much more emphasis on poverty and exclusion among ethnic minorities and migrants (Byrne 2004). The responsibility for healthcare funding and provision lies with the member states and the quality and sustainability of health care has been acknowledged as one of the key issues for closer cooperation (European Commission 2003). There is also a need for greater synergy between health and other policies which influence the socio-economic and environmental determinants of health.

Although the European Commission, the Council of Europe and the Commissioner for Health all value collaboration between member states, the principle of subsidiarity means that each member state is responsible for the implementation of its own action plan. Despite all member states recognizing the vulnerability of refuges, migrants and ethnic minorities to poverty and social exclusion, there is still little evidence of attention to promoting access for these groups to income, housing, education or health care (Kastrissianakis 2004). The lack of data about people of migrant origin in the different countries in Europe impacts on policy. It is possible that as in the UK, one of the few states in Europe to monitor ethnicity data, they are badly recorded, the categories limited and information is not used to inform policy (Aspinall 1995). Several member states provide facilities and support services for different migrant groups, but they are generally assimilationist, focusing on induction, language and job finding (Kastrissianakis 2004). The majority emphasize the need for the migrant to adapt, but few consider the discriminatory attitudes, behaviours and practices which humiliate 'outsiders' and prevent them adapting. They invariably neglect the contribution of migrants to the economic prosperity and cultural richness of their country and fail to capture the skills, motivation and resourcefulness they bring (Fahey 2004).

THE UK HUMAN RIGHTS AND ANTI-DISCRIMINATION LEGISLATION

I will use the example of the United Kingdom (UK) to demonstrate how domestic legislation can take account of human rights and reinforce existing laws aimed at eliminating discrimination. The UK Human Rights Act 1998 gives effect to the rights and freedoms guaranteed under the European Convention on Human Rights. (McHale & Gallagher (2004) provide a useful account of how the Human Rights Act 1998 applies to nursing.) Sixteen rights are incorporated within the articles of the Act, mirroring those of the ECHR, and it has been operational since October

2000. It was hoped that the Act would generate a culture of respect for human rights, with public authorities taking the lead. The introduction of the Human Rights Act made no change to individual rights in the UK, but made it easier to challenge a public authority for alleged breaches without the need to take the case to European Court of Human Rights in Strasbourg. It arguably has more impact on the way in which public authorities are forced to balance rights and responsibilities when making policy decisions around the nature and provision of services.

Since the late 1960s the UK has had legislation aimed at preventing or tackling discrimination on grounds of race, gender or other social characteristics (Race Relations Act 1976, Sex Discrimination Act 1975, Disabled Persons Act 1986). However, the National Health Service and other public bodies remained outside the legislative framework of the Race Relations Act 1976 until the Race Relations Amendment Act 2000. Sadly the last decade has seen a number of large-scale inquiries into the treatment of people from minority ethnic groups by the police, social services and health authorities in Britain (Macpherson 1999, Blofeld 2003, Laming 2003). While these demonstrate evidence of prejudice, discrimination, ignorance and negligence at all levels of service provision, they also provide lessons for the UK and other European countries. Although not without their critics, these reports attempt to inform policy and practice in a strategic way and in the case of the Macpherson Inquiry have already influenced legislation.

The Race Relations Amendment Act 2000 was introduced in the wake of the Macpherson Inquiry, a government inquiry into the way in which the Metropolitan Police dealt with the death of the black youth Stephen Lawrence in London in the late 1990s. The Inquiry, headed by Sir William Macpherson of Cluny, demonstrated a catalogue of negligence and poor policing which led to the failure to follow up leads and gather sufficient evidence to convict the killers of the young man. The inquiry found that the Metropolitan Police failed to take seriously the racialized nature of the assault against Stephen. While there was evidence of overt racism in the police force, attitudes, organizational systems and policing practices were more a reflection of the stereotypes, ignorance and unchallenged prejudices held at all levels. Although the Macpherson Inquiry related to the Metropolitan Police, the report suggested that this was not unique to that organization and could be found in all major institutions in the UK. The report made clear recommendations not only for the Metropolitan Police Service but for local government agencies and other parts of the criminal justice system and was one of main drivers in the amendment to existing legislation on race relations.

The Race Relations Amendment Act 2000 required for the first time that over 25 000 public authorities such as the National Health Service, local authorities, social services departments, and professional regulatory bodies protect individuals and groups against racial discrimination. In addition, it placed a new, enforceable general duty on public authorities to promote racial equality and as such provide fair and accessible services, and to improve equal opportunities in employment and prevent unlawful discrimination. In practice, this means that public authorities

> **Box 3.1   Definition of institutional racism**
>
> Institutional racism consists of the collective failure of an organisation to provide an appropriate and professional service to people because of their colour, culture or ethnic origin. It can be seen or detected in processes, attitudes and behaviour which amount to discrimination through unwitting prejudice, ignorance, thoughtlessness and racist stereotyping which disadvantage minority ethnic clients. (Macpherson 1999)

must take account of racial equality in the everyday work of policy-making, service delivery, employment practice and other functions. In order to achieve this, each authority is required to put in place a coherent strategy for action called a Race Equality Scheme, to be later evaluated through a Race Impact Assessment. The Macpherson Inquiry recommendations and definitions are widely incorporated into the Race Equality Schemes of public authorities, with many in particular emphasizing the need to address institutional racism (Box 3.1).

Although the Macpherson (1999) and the more recent Laming (2003) and Blofeld (2003) inquiries have opened up the debate and raised awareness of issues faced by clients and practitioners in a multicultural society, it is arguable to what extent their recommendations tackle the organizational and professional cultures at the root of the problem. This reflects the resistance to acknowledge the racism and discrimination which exists in health services and the tendency to deny that the problem exists. The picture is not unique to the UK (Wrench 1996) and recent international research into racism in the workplace revealed similar problems in 15 European Union member states (Wrench et al 1999).

CULTURAL DIVERSITY, RACIAL EQUALITY AND THE UK HEALTH POLICY

The UK Department of Health (DH) has attempted to take the issue of cultural diversity and racial equality seriously and in the last decade commissioned research, introduced policy and implemented a range of initiatives to this end. A full search of the DH website (http://www.dh.gov.uk) will demonstrate the range of initiatives and activities in the field. While some of these were driven by the Macpherson Inquiry, concerns over negative publicity and fear of litigation provide opportunities to tackle health and access inequalities which persist in the UK. A number of the DH initiatives are concerned with workforce issues and are a key part of the agenda to reform and modernize the National Health Service (NHS) (e.g. 'The Vital Connection'; 'Equality and Diversity in the NHS Workforce'; 'Leadership – Breaking Through'; 'Positively Diverse'). The DH and its related organizations are also committed to the cultural competence of the care delivered to clients (e.g. 'Improving Health among Ethnic Minority Populations'; 'No Exclusion Clause Project: Opening Doors to Better Palliative Care for People from Culturally Diverse Communities'; 'Improving the Quality of Life of Ethnic Minority Children with Learning Disabilities'; 'Culturally Competent Primary Care Services: Project Dil, Leicester'). A trawl through the website highlights the myriad study days, workshops, courses and independent learning resources available to staff in the NHS. This chapter highlights a small number of initiatives concerned with cultural diversity and gives examples of collaborative partnerships which aim to improve the delivery of culturally appropriate care.

Mental health among people from minority ethnic groups is a major concern in the UK. There is widespread evidence of discrimination in mental health services and the quality of care leaves much to be desired (Sashidharan 2003). However, although the picture is still bleak, the DH has commissioned a number of initiatives aimed at improving services for minority ethnic mental health service users and carers. *Inside Outside: Improving Mental Health Services for Black and Ethnic Minority Communities in England* (Sashidharan 2003) is an attempt to address deficiencies and to inform the modernization of mental health provision. The report is the first national approach aimed at reducing inequalities in mental health and it makes a number of recommendations which may also be relevant to other EU healthcare systems. The need for change is two-fold: the 'inside' element requiring the current mental health system to reappraise its policies and practices, while the 'outside' element requires investment in enhancing the capacity of the community to deal with mental distress and ill health. In order to achieve these, three basic objectives have to be met. Firstly ethnic inequalities in experience and outcomes have to be reduced and eliminated. Actions to achieve this include ensuring accountability and ownership, developing cultural capability, setting national standards to improve access, care experience and outcomes, and enhancing the cultural relevance of research and development. Secondly a mental health workforce capable of delivering effective mental health services to a multicultural population has to be developed. This is to be achieved through training in cultural competence and ensuring a multicultural workforce. Lastly the capacity of black and minority communities and the voluntary sectors has to be built or enhanced. This is to be accomplished though the appointment of community development workers to enhance the capacity of community groups to deal with mental distress and tackle the deficiencies in existing services.

Although some of the actions are already under way, the real success of this groundbreaking report will be the extent to which its recommendations are adopted. *Delivering Race Equality: A Framework for Action, Mental Health Services Consultation Document* (2003) was widely disseminated for consultation between September 2003 and February 2004. It was hoped that the strategy would ensure the implementation of the recommendations of the *Inside Outside* report. However, community organizations, the voluntary sector and professionals expressed dissatisfaction with the plans proposed in the consultation document, believing the focus on community engagement did not address the persistent failure to provide a satisfactory service for people from minority ethnic groups. (The National Institute for Mental Health England website, www.nimhe.org.uk, includes *Delivering Race Equality: A Framework for*

Action, Mental Health Services Consultation Document (2003) and the *Inside Outside* report. A search of the site using the keyword 'social inclusion' will raise a list of projects which aim to address the exclusion of people with mental health problems from full participation in everyday life.) The final strategic document (DH 2005) was released in January 2005 as an action plan for reform of mental health services and incorporated the findings of the Blofeld Inquiry (2003) into the death of David (Rocky) Bennett (a young black man who died in a medium secure unit from a prolonged period of prone restraint following an aggressive episode which might have been prevented by culturally competent care). Despite many improvements it remains to be seen whether the action plan will bring true reform to mental health services in the UK.

The failure of the mental health system to provide an adequate, appropriate and acceptable service to people from minority ethnic groups has led to the emergence of community organizations providing advice, support and advocacy to particular cultural groups. Some have been able to provide culturally and linguistically specific counselling, psychological or complementary therapies from voluntary funds or more recently in partnerships with statutory providers. Although frequently unwilling to use mainstream services, people from minority ethnic groups appear very willing to use these services and some organizations have difficulty coping with the demand. One example is the Chinese Mental Health Association in Birmingham (Box 3.2).

There is widespread evidence that people from minority ethnic groups in Britain experience high levels of heart disease and stroke. There are many causal factors but smoking is a particular problem in some communities and appears to be resistant to conventional health promotion initiatives (Erens et al 2001). An example of culturally appropriate approaches to health promotion is described in Box 3.3 and the principles underpinning this could be adapted and adopted more widely to deal with different health issues among diverse cultural groups.

Other strategies to tackle health inequalities in Britain since 1999 include the National Lottery funding for Healthy Living Centres. (Further details can be found at http://www.ohn.gov.uk.partnerships/hlc.htm and www.hda-online.org.uk.) They involve a range of partnerships between voluntary, public and private sectors working with each other,

---

Box 3.2   The Chinese Mental Health Association

The Chinese Mental Health Association is a registered charity in the UK dedicated to serving the Chinese community in the UK. The Association is actively involved in providing direct services, increasing mental health awareness, and representing Chinese mental health issues in public forums. It lobbies for better mental health services to improve the quality of life for Chinese people and their carers. It helps users access services provided by statutory and voluntary organizations as well as offering services run by Chinese workers specifically trained in mental health care.

Further information can be obtained from the Chinese Mental Health Association website at http://www.cmha.org.uk.

> **Box 3.3   Smoking cessation and Asian communities**
>
> The DH endeavoured to tackle smoking cessation in the Asian community in 2000 by providing the NHS Asian Tobacco Helpline, which offered services in different community languages such as Gujarati, Urdu, Hindi, Punjabi and Bengali. Advertising the Helpline coincided with the start of the Muslim Holy Month of Ramadan and the Hindu celebration of Diwali. It aimed to tackle the problems of higher smoking rates and lower awareness of the serious health risks associated with tobacco use amongst some Asian communities in England.
>
> In the 2001 Brick Lane Mela, a major festival in the heart of the Bengali community in East London, the NHS Asian Tobacco Helpline was endorsed by local and international Bengali film stars and performers, to raise awareness of the dedicated help that is available to those wanting to give up tobacco usage. Staff handed out self-help literature and 'Tip' cards in mother tongue languages to help tobacco users kick the habit.
>
> Details of these campaigns can be found on the DH website at www.doh.gov.uk.

> **Box 3.4   Healthy living for the Irish community in Camden**
>
> The Healthy Living Centre at the London Irish Centre offers individual and group sessions on smoking cessation, substance misuse, healthy eating, exercise, and mental health awareness. Because of the older age profile of the Irish in London, the maintenance of health in the presence of limiting long-term illness, the management of medication and prevention of falls have high priority. The Centre also provides a range of published information which takes account of the customs, habits and preferences of Irish people and is conscious of sensitivities around religion, alcohol or general stereotypes of Irish people in Britain.
>
> Further information about the background to the service and the facilities provided can be found on http://www.irishcentre.org.

and with general practitioners and local people. There is no blueprint for projects and schemes are designed to be flexible so that they can be specifically tailored to meet the needs of different communities. Priority is given to areas of deprivation, to communities that are normally excluded or who have significant health problems.

The Irish in Britain are one such community who, as a result of the conceptualizations of ethnicity in terms of skin colour, are frequently not recognized as a minority ethnic group because they are predominantly white (Box 3.4). The age profile is older and health status is similar or worse than that of visible minorities, with high levels of heart disease, stroke, respiratory disorders, mental illness and the highest mortality from cancers in the UK (Tilki 2003).

SUMMARY

The chapter's perspectives were: The Papadopoulos, Tilki and Taylor (1998) model of cultural competence and the European Union. The model emphasizes the importance of understanding and respecting each other and the necessity to strive towards the elimination of health inequalities. This chapter therefore attempted to make the essential link between human rights and health equality. It is hoped that it raised your awareness, enriched your cultural knowledge and helped you to understand the importance of human rights in your everyday endeavours to provide culturally competent care.

The former EU Health Commissioner David Byrne stated that the strength of the European Union depends on its ability to build an active, open and just society, to mobilize the energies and talents of its people and to improve their quality of life and health. Investing in health brings substantial benefits for the economy (Byrne 2004). There has been extensive work around both public health and human rights in the latter half of the twentieth century and the interface between them offers complementary ways of improving health and health care. While greater mobility across the EU might pose some risks, greater political and economic power and cross-cutting structures facilitate new opportunities for protecting human rights and improving health. There are many pan-European policies and collaborative initiatives across member states and there are joint projects with non-European partners. While there is still much to be achieved, lessons can be learned from countries like the UK who have lengthier histories of mobility and migration. However, there is also much to be gained from understanding about health and health care in other cultures and social systems. Nurses and other health professionals can and must contribute to a wider recognition of the benefits and costs associated with failure to respect human rights and dignity. Respect for human rights and dignity can enhance health and those who are healthy are better equipped to participate fully and benefit from the opportunities afforded by the European Union.

REFLECTIVE QUESTIONS

1. Reflect on the different categories of human rights and identify the ways in which the rights of individuals might be infringed in your own practice or the healthcare organization within which you work.
2. Reflect on the threats to social cohesion which exist within an enlarged Europe and explore the implications of these for nurses.
3. Look at the definition of institutional racism suggested by Macpherson (1999) and reflect on the extent to which it exists in your healthcare organization or in your professional practice.
4. To what extent are the recommendations of the *Inside Outside* report (Sashidharan 2003) relevant to other countries in Europe?

REFERENCES

Acheson D (Chair) 1998 Independent inquiry into inequalities in health. The Stationery Office, London

Aspinall P 1995 Department of Health's requirement for mandatory collection of data on ethnic groups of in-patients. British Medical Journal 311:1006–1009

Blofeld J (Chair) 2003 Independent inquiry into the death of David Bennett. Department of Health, London

Bosma H, Marmot M G, Hemingway H et al 1997 Low job control and risk of coronary heart disease in Whitehall II (prospective cohort) study. British Medical Journal 314:558–565

Brunner E, Marmot M 1999 Social organisation, stress and health. In: Marmot M, Wilkinson R (eds) Social determinants of health. Oxford University Press, Oxford

Byrne D 2004 Enabling good health for all: a reflection process for a new health strategy. Online. Available: http://europa.eu.int/comm/health/ph_overview/strategy/health_strategy_en.htm 26 Oct 2004

Cahill G, Kelleher D 1999 The health of the Irish: Stress and the negotiation of a contested identity. Paper to British Sociological Association Medical Sociology Conference, 24–26 September 1999, University of York

Chinese Mental Health Association 2005 Online. Available: http://www.cmha.org.uk 27 Mar 2005

Coughlan M 2004 Opening speech: The role of employment and social policy. Irish presidency conference on reconciling mobility and social inclusion. Bundoran, 1 and 2 April 2004

Council of Europe Portal. Online. Available: http://www.coe.int 27 Mar 2005

Council of Europe. Human rights: protection, promotion and prevention. Online. Available: http://www.coe.int/T/E/Com/About_coe/Human_rights.asp 27 Mar 2005

Department of Health Portal. Online. Available: http://www.doh.gov.uk. 27 Mar 2005

DH 2005 Delivering race equality in mental health care: An action plan for reform inside and outside services and the government's response to the independent inquiry into the death of David Bennett. Department of Health Publications, London

Elstad J 1998 The psychosocial perspective on social inequalities in health. In: Bartley M, Blane D, Davey Smith G (eds) The sociology of health inequalities. Blackwell, London

Erens B, Primatesta P, Prior G 2001 The health survey for England 1999. The Stationery Office, London

European Commission 2003 In brief: The social situation in the European Union 2003. Directorate General for employment and social affairs/Eurostat. European Commission, Belgium

Fahey F 2004 The role of employment and social policy. Irish presidency conference on reconciling mobility and social inclusion. Bundoran, 1 and 2 April 2004

Halpern D, Nazroo J 2000 The ethnic density effect: results from a community survey of England and Wales. International Journal of Psychiatry 46(1):34–46

Human Rights Act 1998 HMSO, London

Karasek R, Theorell T 1990 Healthy work: Stress, productivity and the reconstruction of working life. Basic Books, New York

Karlsen S, Nazroo J 2000 Identity and structure: Rethinking ethnic inequalities in health. In: Graham H (ed) Understanding health inequalities. Open University, Buckingham

Karlsen S, Nazroo J 2002 Agency and structure: The impact of ethnic identity and racism on the health of ethnic minority people. Sociology of Health and Illness 24(1):1–20

Kastrissianakis A 2004 The role of employment and social policy. Irish presidency conference on reconciling mobility and social inclusion. Bundoran, 1 and 2 April, 2004

Kawachi I, Kennedy B, Gupta V et al 1997 Social capital, income inequality and mortality. American Journal of Public Health 87:1491–1498

Kawachi I, Kennedy B, Wilkinson R 1999 Income inequality and health: A reader. New Press, New York

Klug F 2000 Values for a godless age – the story of the United Kingdom's new bill of rights. Penguin Books, London

Krieger N 1990 Racial and gender discrimination: risk factors for high blood pressure? Social Science Medicine 30(12):273–1281

Krieger N 2000 Discrimination and health. In: Berkman L, Kawachi I (eds) Social epidemiology. Oxford University Press, Oxford

Laming H (Chair) 2003 The Victoria Climbie Inquiry. Department of Health, London

Levitas R 1998 The inclusive society? Social exclusion and New Labour. Macmillan, Basingstoke

London Irish Centre (Healthy Living Centre). Online. Available: http://www.irishcentre.org 27 Mar 2005

McHale J, Gallagher A 2004 Nursing and human rights. Butterworth Heinemann, London

Mackenback J, Bakker M (eds) 2002 Reducing inequalities in health: a European perspective. Routledge, London

Macpherson W (Chair) 1999 The Stephen Lawrence inquiry. Report of an inquiry by Sir William Macpherson of Cluny. The Stationery Office, London

Mann J, Gruskin S, Grodin M (eds) 1999 Health and human rights: a reader. Routledge, London

Marmot M, Siegrist J. Theorell T, Feeney A 1999 Health and the psychosocial environment at work. In: Marmot M, Wilkinson R (eds) Social determinants of health. Oxford University Press, Oxford, p 105–131

Marshall T H 1950 Citizenship and social class. Pluto, London

Morrall P, Hazleton M 2004 Global policies and human rights. Whurr, London

Nazroo J 1997 The health of Britain's ethnic minorities. Policy Studies Institute, London

Nazroo J 1999 Ethnic inequalities in health. In: Gordon D et al (eds) Inequalities in health. The evidence presented to the independent inquiry into inequalities in health chaired by Sir Donald Acheson. The Policy Press, Bristol

Ottawa Charter for Health Promotion 1986 World Health Organization, Geneva

Papadopoulos I, Tilki M, Taylor G 1998 Transcultural care: a guide for health care professionals. Quay Books, Dinton

Sashidharan S 2001 Institutional racism in British psychiatry. Psychiatric Bulletin 25:244–247

Sashidharan S 2003 Inside outside: improving mental health services for black and minority ethnic communities in England. National Institute for Mental Health/Department of Health, Leeds

Siegrist J, Peter R, Cremer P, Seidel D 1997 Chronic work stress is associated with atherogenic lipids and elevated fibrinogen in middle aged men. Journal of Internal Medicine 242:149–156

Stansfeld S 1999 Social support and social cohesion. In: Marmot M, Wilkinson R (eds) The social determinants of health. Oxford University Press, Oxford

Tilki M 2003 A study of the health of Irish born people in London: The relevance of social and economic factors, health beliefs and behaviour. Unpublished PhD thesis. Middlesex University, London

Wilkinson R 1996 Unhealthy societies: the afflictions of inequality. Routledge, London

Wilkinson R 1999 Putting the picture together: prosperity, redistribution, health and welfare. In: Marmot M, Wilkinson R (eds) Social determinants of health. Oxford University Press, Oxford

Wilkinson R, Caulfield H 2000 The Human Rights Act: a practical guide for nurses. Whurr, London

WHO 1986 World Health Organization Constitution. WHO, Geneva. Online. Available: http://www.who.int/library/historical/access/who/index.en.shtml 25 Feb 2005

Wrench J 1996 Preventing racism at the workplace: a report of 16 European countries. Office for Official Publications of the European Communities, Luxembourg

Wrench J, Rea A, Ouali N (eds) 1999 Migrants, ethnic minorities and the labour market: integration and exclusion in Europe. Macmillan, London

Chapter 4

Migrants and refugees

Gina Taylor

LEARNING OBJECTIVES

Having read this chapter, you should be able to:
- discuss reasons why people migrate
- differentiate between the terms refugee and asylum seeker
- describe immigration and asylum policy in the UK
- reflect on the 'refugee experience'
- recall factors that can influence the health of refugees and asylum seekers
- utilize the knowledge gained when caring for refugees and asylum seekers

WHY PEOPLE MIGRATE

There is a long history of migration both within European countries and from countries outside of Europe. However, over the years, patterns of migration have changed. Various theories account for migrations, but one commonly cited theory relates to 'push' and 'pull' factors. Demographic changes, low standards of living, lack of opportunities or political oppression 'push' people to leave their countries of origin. 'Pull' factors are the converse of these; demand for labour, good economic opportunities and political freedoms will attract people to receiving countries (Castles & Miller 2003).

Between 1945 and the 1970s large numbers of migrant workers were drawn from less developed countries to fill labour shortages in the fast expanding industrial areas of western Europe, North America and Australia (Castles & Miller 2003, Hansen 2003). Such labour migration took the form of guest worker policies in Germany and migration from former colonies in Britain and France (Hansen 2003). Following the oil crisis and slowdown in economic growth in 1973–1974, labour migration ceased to be encouraged by western European governments as the price of oil rose dramatically, having an effect on western European economies and contributing to recession. However, family reunion and permanent settlement continued.

While each migratory movement has its own characteristics, Castles & Miller (2003) argue that some general patterns can be detected. Labour recruitment, particularly of young men, has often formed the initial impetus to migrate, followed by family formation which results in long-term settlement.

There does not appear to be a defining point at which migrants become members of minority ethnic groups, but the above model would appear to account for the patterns of migration and settlement seen during the period of 1945 to the mid-1970s. Following family reunion and permanent settlement, second and third generations have grown up as members of minority ethnic groups in Western countries.

ACCULTURATION

When people migrate from one country to another they have to adjust to being in contact with different cultures; this process has been called acculturation. Doná & Berry (1999: 172) have defined it as 'a multidimensional phenomenon that includes one's orientation towards one's ethnic group, towards the larger society and possibly towards other ethnic cultures'.

Berry (1980, cited in Doná & Berry 1999) describes different strategies for acculturation, as migrants consider the extent to which they wish to retain their cultural identity and the extent to which they wish to interact with the dominant society. Depending on their wishes, settlement in a host country can result in assimilation, when migrants relinquish their cultural identity and merge into the host society. An assimilationist approach is adopted in France, where migrants can be regarded as French, provided they espouse French cultural values and behave like French people. Alternatively, settlement in a host country can result in integration, where individuals retain their cultural identities but also become part of the wider society. Integration is the approach adopted in the United Kingdom. If migrants choose to retain their cultural identity and not become part of the wider society then separation occurs; whereas if migrants choose not to retain their own cultural identity but also not to become part of the wider society, then marginalization occurs, resulting in loss of contact both with their own communities and the host society (Doná & Berry 1999). For Castles & Miller (2003) these strategies are influenced by the stance taken towards migrants by the host community; the approach of the government and the people of the host country will determine whether permanent settlement is characterized by the formation of ethnic communities which are seen as part of a multicultural society and where cultural diversity is accepted and valued, or by the formation of ethnic minorities that are socially excluded.

REFUGEES AND ASYLUM SEEKERS

The 1980s saw a new wave of migrants to Europe in the form of refugees. Castles & Miller (2003) argue that push–pull theories have limitations, concentrating on economic and market factors to the relative neglect of social factors. In terms or refugees and asylum seekers, factors such as persecution, human rights abuses and breakdown of infrastructures need to be considered as push factors. The situation of refugees and asylum seekers is very different from that of voluntary migrants, their migration usually being forced upon them. Refugees and asylum seekers are not new to Europe, or other Western countries, but since the 1980s migration flows have accelerated and have become more diverse (Castles 2000).

The term 'refugee' has a precise legal definition. The United Nations Convention relating to the status of refugees in 1951, and its 1967 Protocol, stated that a refugee is a person who:

> Owing to a well-founded fear of being persecuted for reasons of race, religion, nationality, membership of a particular social group or political opinion, is outside the country of his nationality and is unable, or owing to such fear, is unwilling to avail himself of the protection of that country; or who, not having a nationality and being outside the country of his former habitual residence as a result of such events, is unable or, owing to such fear, is unwilling to return to it. (UNHCR 1961, cited in Kushner & Knox 1999: 10)

However, it is necessary to distinguish clearly between the terms refugee and asylum seeker, as their respective statuses and associated rights are different. Therefore, a refugee is someone whose status is officially recognized by the country of asylum under the terms of the 1951 Geneva Convention, and who has been granted refugee status in the host country. Refugee status therefore confers some degree of security. On the other hand, an asylum seeker is someone who has applied for refugee status and is awaiting a decision on the application. This status is very uncertain.

HUMAN RIGHTS, EU AND UK LEGISLATION AND POLICY

The definition of a refugee cited above was originally confined to people who had become refugees as a result of the events that took place before 1 January 1951, that is the Second World War and its aftermath. As a result of the continued movement of refugees a protocol was introduced in 1967 which made the Convention universal. These two legal instruments enshrine the rights of asylum seekers and refugees, preventing them being returned to countries where they fear persecution (Rutter 1994). However, states differ in their interpretation and implementation of these instruments, declaring some states 'safe' and returning asylum seekers to these states. Also, within Europe, some countries apply a narrow definition of who can qualify as a refugee, excluding people who have suffered at the hands of 'non-state agents' like rebels or religious extremists; for example, those fleeing Afghanistan's Taliban, Bosnian Muslims and Somalis were excluded from claiming refugee status (Kumin 1998). Despite well-documented atrocities involved in ethnic cleansing policies in former Yugoslavia, a majority of the displaced Bosnians were not regarded as Convention refugees.

The European Convention on Human Rights also affords protection to refugees and asylum seekers and has been used by some immigration lawyers in Europe, as it contains commitments preventing the return of people to countries where they would be subject to 'cruel and degrading treatment' (Rutter 1994).

Most of the world's refugees and displaced persons are found in Africa and Asia. Displaced persons are those who have been forced to flee but have not crossed a border (Adelman 1999). Many displaced people seek refuge in neighbouring countries and some 'refugee-producing' countries, e.g. Ethiopia, Congo, are also recipients of refugees and asylum seekers from other countries (Westin 1999). By the end of 2003, the United Nations High Commission for Refugees (UNHCR 2004) estimated the global number of refugees as 9.7 million people. This number has been falling over the last two years as a result of durable solutions to the refugee problem, for example repatriation. Although most refugees remain in developing countries, Europe hosted 25% of all refugees in 2003 (UNHCR 2004).

While western European countries had been familiar with people seeking asylum from other European countries, in the 1970s asylum seekers from developing nations started to appear in Europe. In 1972 Ugandan Asians arrived in Britain, in 1973 asylum seekers from Chile arrived in Europe and in the late 1970s Vietnamese boat people and other Indochinese refugees formed the first large-scale group of non-European people to seek asylum in Europe (Kumin 1998, Westin 1999). By the mid-1980s the numbers of asylum seekers were increasing and more applications came from Africa, Asia and the Middle East (Kumin 1998). By the end of the 1980s all European governments had become more restrictive with their asylum procedures (Kumin 1998, Westin 1999). This was achieved by employing deterrent policies, such as reducing social benefits and detaining asylum seekers. Kumin (1998: 6) describes how the emphasis had shifted from one of protecting refugees to one of exclusion and control, and claims that 'Today, Europe's doors to asylum seekers are, at best, ajar'. Thus, an increase in the numbers of people seeking asylum in the late 1980s coincided with an increase in EU policies aimed at restricting the entry of non-EU nationals (Sales 2002). This also coincided with increasing social exclusion of asylum seekers, as a result of a general trend towards reduced rights.

The UNHCR (2004) cited the following as the main countries of origin of refugees in 2003: Afghanistan, Sudan, Burundi, Democratic Republic of Congo, Palestine, Somalia, Iraq, Vietnam, Liberia and Angola.

While individual countries employ their own policies on immigration and asylum, there has been a tendency towards harmonization of such policies across member states of the European Union (EU). In 1997 the Treaty of Amsterdam (Article 63) established community competence in the area of migration and asylum and principles for a common policy were laid down by the European Council (Castles & Miller 2003). The Dublin Convention on asylum, which came into force in 1997, decrees that asylum seekers can be returned to the country which first allowed them to enter the EU (Watt 2001). The member states of the EU have been committed to creating a common European asylum system since the Tampere Summit in 1999. In January 2003, EU ministers adopted the directive on reception conditions for asylum seekers, marking the start of a common EU asylum system. This directive sets out minimum standards for access to employment, education, health care and rights to family reunion and the free movement of asylum seekers (Kerrigan 2003). However, this directive also aims to reduce numbers of asylum seekers by strengthening controls on the EU's borders, via a regulation known as 'Dublin II'. The country that first allowed asylum seekers into the EU is still responsible for considering claims for asylum and the regulation continues to allow states to send asylum applicants back to other EU states where they may have fewer chances of being recognized as being in need of protection (Kerrigan 2003).

An important feature of membership of the EU is European citizenship. Article 8 of the Maastricht Treaty of European Union states that every person holding the nationality of a member state of the EU shall be a citizen of the EU. European citizens are entitled to vote in local government and European Parliament elections in the state in which they reside. European citizens have freedom of movement and residence in the territory of the member states and the right to diplomatic protection in a third country. They also have the right to petition the European Parliament as well as the possibility to appeal to an Ombudsman, who has the powers to investigate maladministration in EU institutions. Further, discrimination is proscribed against citizens of member states on grounds of nationality. Rights and duties of citizenship of the EU are limited to the nationals of member states. Many European countries have substantial populations of people who are nationals of non-member states who will not be citizens in the European context and will thus be excluded from the above rights.

SEEKING ASYLUM IN THE UNITED KINGDOM

As 'programme refugees', e.g. Vietnamese in the 1980s, gave way to 'spontaneous refugees' in the 1990s, it has become increasingly difficult to successfully claim asylum as an individual in the UK (Duke et al 1999).

UK policy relating to immigration and asylum is frequently changing. While UK immigration policy recognizes international law in relation to refugees and aims to meet obligations towards refugees, it also aims to reduce the misuse of asylum procedures (Coleman 1996). The Immigration and Asylum Acts of 1993 and 1996 restricted social rights of asylum seekers (Sales 2002). Asylum seekers are expected to claim asylum at the port of entry into the UK. Depending on the availability of an interpreter, applicants are interviewed about their history of persecution, following which they have to collect evidence to substantiate their claim (in English). The application is then sent to the Home Office's Immigration and Nationality Directorate for a decision. Asylum seekers have fewer rights than those who have been granted refugee status. Under the Immigration and Asylum Act 1999, asylum seekers requiring support may be dispersed to different parts of the UK. This is in order to relieve pressure on local authorities in London and the Southeast as these are areas in which asylum seekers have traditionally attempted to settle as they are more likely to find members of their own communities in these areas. The result is that asylum seekers may find themselves in areas where there is no support from a relevant community group. Support from the state is dependent on asylum seekers staying in the areas to which they have been dispersed. The government also provides financial support at around 70% of income support levels, so placing asylum seekers at a distinct disadvantage relative to the rest of society and contributing to their social exclusion. Further, asylum seekers are not able to work on arrival in the UK, but can apply for eligibility to work after 6 months' residence. Again, this places asylum seekers at a disadvantage as employment has been found to be crucial in resettlement (Bloch 1999).

Legislation relating to refugees and asylum seekers in the UK continues to be both deterrent and restrictive in nature. The Nationality, Immigration and Asylum Act 2002 concentrated on the control and removal of refused asylum seekers, but also proposed pilot accommodation centres to house asylum seekers who await decisions on their applications. These centres may include health and education facilities on site: children will be educated on site rather than in schools. The legislation also promotes the importance of citizenship via the introduction of English language tests, citizenship ceremonies and a new citizenship oath for those wishing to acquire British citizenship. Further legislation, the Asylum and Immigration Act 2004, has rendered it a criminal offence to enter the UK without documents demonstrating identity and nationality without a good reason. This makes it more difficult for asylum seekers to reach the UK and does not heed the situation of asylum seekers who are forced to flee their home countries without such documents.

The UK is party to international treaties and conventions that seek to guarantee certain rights. Rights to health have long been established in international rights documents (Montgomery 1992). For example, the right to protection of health (Article 11) is enshrined in the European Social Charter of the Council of Europe (drawn up to deal with the social and economic aspect of the United Nations Declaration of Human Rights), to which the UK is a party (Lewis & Seneviratne 1992).

Refugees and asylum seekers are entitled to free treatment from the National Health Service, in the same way as UK citizens; however, in reality, it has not always been possible for these groups to gain access to health care.

THE CONTRIBUTION OF NON-GOVERNMENTAL ORGANIZATIONS (NGOS)

The UK has not developed an enduring strategy for the reception and settlement of refugees and asylum seekers. Instead, responses to the arrival of different groups of refugees and asylum seekers have been ad hoc. The UK government has always relied heavily on the contribution of non-governmental organizations in this area. Such organizations provide advice on rights and how to gain assistance. These organizations are not necessarily made up of refugees and asylum seekers, but may be attached to local churches or welfare groups (Zetter & Pearl 2000). Some NGOs may be more formal and enjoy registered charitable status, operating at national or local level. The leading national organization in the UK is the Refugee Council, which receives some funding from the Home Office, and provides reception support, advocacy, training and information services (Zetter & Pearl 2000).

There is a long history of refugee community-based organizations in the UK (Zetter & Pearl 2000). These are organizations established by groups of refugees themselves. Refugee community-based organizations can assist members in using mainstream services, they can provide employment for members of the community and can also promote cultural awareness in healthcare professionals (Carey-Wood 1997). The main link with wider society for most newcomers is often the local community group (Carey-Wood et al 1995). These groups provide practical help, emotional support and cultural activities as well as serving as a forum for association. Those refugees who had been in the country longer often spent a large proportion of their time doing voluntary work on behalf of their community (Carey-Wood et al 1995).

MAIN HEALTH AND SOCIAL CARE ISSUES

Migrant populations have specific health needs for several reasons. Their patterns of disease may be different from those seen in the indigenous populations, but also migrants are often on the margins of society and thus at increased risk of the diseases associated with poverty (Abel-Smith et al 1995). Migrants often have reduced access to health services due to communication problems, lack of knowledge of available services and, for some, fear that health services may be linked with immigration officialdom (Abel-Smith et al 1995).

THE WORLD HEALTH ORGANIZATION AND HEALTH

The World Health Organization (1998) has retained its goal to achieve full health potential for all in the European Region 'Health 21' policy. Following on from the previous 'Health for All' policy (WHO 1992), the current policy views health as a fundamental human right and continues to stress the need for equity in health, and also for individual and community participation in health development. 'Health 21' (WHO 1998) draws attention to the effects of poverty on health and the wide health gap between the richer and poorer parts of the European Region. While there is a health gap between countries, there is also a similar gap within countries where richer people live longer and have fewer illnesses than poorer people (WHO 1998).

In both the UK and other European countries the goals of public health are placing greater emphasis on tackling inequalities in health (Graham 2004). Health inequalities, in relation to social class, exist in all western European countries, though the causes of death differ between countries (Fox 1989, Kunst et al 1998, Macintyre 1997, Power 1994). Difficulties also exist when attempting a systematic comparison of socio-economic differences in mortality across countries, as each country has its own classification system and these are not necessarily directly comparable (Kunst et al 1998, Leon 1998). However, Kunst et al (1998) were able to demonstrate higher mortality in manual classes than non-manual classes in 11 western European countries. What is more important is that other authors (Brunner & Marmot 1999, Levine 1995, Power 1994) have identified the absence of a clear distinction between 'privileged' and 'underprivileged' people in terms of health status and the presence of a step-wise gradient with increasing morbidity and mortality with declining socio-economic status. People from minority ethnic groups are likely to experience poverty and disadvantage, as identified by higher unemployment rates, a greater reliance on social housing, lower incomes and lower car ownership (HEA 1994, Nazroo 1998, Smaje 1995). Thus members of minority ethnic groups are likely to be located in lower socio-economic groups.

MIGRATION AND HEALTH

There is not a clear picture in relation to the effects of migration on health. Evidence suggests that following migration, migrants' mortality rates either stay the same, increase or decrease, in relation to mortality rates in their home countries (McKay et al 2003). Mortality rates among international immigrants can be influenced by their country of origin, their destination and by the process of migration itself (McKay et al 2003). A similar picture exists concerning mental health; migration does not necessarily cause mental illness, but migrants may find the experience of migration stressful and will benefit from social support from both the already established migrant community and the host community (McKay et al 2003).

Bollini & Siem (1995), of the International Organization for Migration, reviewed the available evidence on access to health care and the two health outcomes of perinatal mortality and accident/disability for migrant and minority ethnic groups in selected receiving industrialized countries. They cite a publication from the European Office of the World Health Organization which made an interim evaluation of the performance of various European countries towards the achievement of 'Health for All by the year 2000', which indicated that, in spite of an overall health improvement in Europe, no real progress was made towards equity during the 1980s. Higher rates of perinatal mortality and accidents/disability were observed in many migrant groups compared to the native populations. Bollini & Siem argue that poor health outcomes for migrants and minority ethnic groups are linked to the lower entitlements for these groups in the receiving societies, arguing that migrants and minority ethnic groups are exposed to poor working and living conditions and they also have reduced access to health care for a number of political, administrative and cultural reasons, for example due to barriers resulting from language problems, different concepts of health and disease or racism. The authors advocate the involvement of members of ethnic communities in designing health promotion campaigns and service delivery schemes.

Data relating to ethnicity and health in Britain have been sparse until recently. While patterns of health and illness relating to ethnicity are emerging, for example the high rates of coronary heart disease among the Asian population, Ahmad (1997) points to a 'glaringly obvious gap' in research and health, particularly among the 'forgotten minorities' such as numerically small groups of people like those from Somalia and Ethiopia.

Diseases of minority ethnic populations do not differ fundamentally from those faced by majority populations (Smaje 1995). Cardiovascular disease is the leading cause of death in both developed and developing countries, with marked variations between populations (McKay et al 2003). However, it is known that rates of ill health and mortality among minority ethnic groups differ from those of the white majority population and differences exist between the ethnic groups.

One early and important study in Britain (Balarajan & Soni Raleigh 1993) identified the biggest difference in health and illness in relation to coronary heart disease, mortality from coronary heart disease being higher among people born in the Indian subcontinent than among the white majority population and also than among other minority ethnic groups. However, later studies (Balarajan 1996, Bhopal et al 1999) were able to demonstrate that grouping disparate ethnic groups under one heading can be misleading. When people born in the Indian subcontinent were identified in separate groupings it was found that mortality from coronary heart disease was highest among Bangladeshis, followed by Pakistanis, and then Indians. There is a tendency for Indians to enjoy a better socio-economic profile than Pakistanis and Bangladeshis, leading Balarajan to suggest social class as a mediating factor among the determinants of coronary heart disease.

In relation to the other major causes of premature death, such as cancers, variations are seen in cancer mortality rates of different immigrant groups in different countries. Cancer mortality is governed by genetic and/or environmental factors (McKay et al 2003). Marmot & Wilkinson (1999) stress the importance of the environment in determining health and illness, referring to studies investigating the patterns of heart disease and stroke in men of Japanese ancestry which found that, for Japanese men living in California, the rate of heart disease increased with the degree of acculturation. Generally, deaths from cancer are lower among minority ethnic groups than indigenous populations, but the incidence may be changing as members of minority ethnic groups adopt some of the lifestyles of the indigenous populations (Balarajan & Soni Raleigh 1993, Smaje 1995), again, a feature of acculturation.

The issue of mental health and illness and ethnicity is a complex and controversial one. Studies in Britain have identified higher admission rates to psychiatric hospitals among members of minority ethnic groups than among the white majority population (Balarajan & Soni Raleigh 1993, Smaje 1995). The boundary between mental health and mental disorder is concerned with the question of normality, which is culturally relative (Fernando 2002). Helman (2000) notes that as well as having higher rates of mental illness than the indigenous populations, immigrants also have higher rates of mental illness than the populations of their countries of origin. Material deprivation, discrimination and language difficulties may all play a part in the attribution of the diagnosis of mental illness to members of minority ethnic groups, but Helman also highlights the influence that culture has on psychiatric diagnosis, which is particularly important when the psychiatrist is white and middle class. Berthoud & Nazroo (1997) further point out that the questions used to diagnose mental illness may be unreliable when used cross-culturally. A study in Britain (Thomas et al 1993) concerning compulsory psychiatric admissions found that the rate of schizophrenia was 9 times higher in second-generation (UK born) Afro-Caribbean people than in white people. However, this could largely be explained by their greater socio-economic disadvantage, with poor inner-city housing and higher rates of unemployment, rather than psychiatric misdiagnosis.

THE REFUGEE EXPERIENCE

Migrants to western European countries may thus experience problems similar to those of people in low social classes and members of minority ethnic groups. However, refugees and asylum seekers will have added problems relating to their 'refugee experience' and their health will thus be placed in 'triple jeopardy'. It is further important to remember that for refugees and asylum seekers migration will have been forced; there will have been little choice whether to leave their home countries or to stay. Likewise, there will often have been little choice concerning destination.

There are no systematic arrangements in place in the UK to deal with the health and social problems of refugees and asylum seekers. There is also a lack of information on the demographic characteristics of different refugee groups, their health problems and health and social welfare service use.

The health of refugees and asylum seekers can be affected by many factors relating to their experience before flight, during flight and after arrival in a host country. However, on arrival in a western European country refugees and asylum seekers are situated in societies that are characterized by health inequalities. Any existing health problems that refugees and asylum seekers face will be compounded by their experience in the host country.

'Refugee experience' is defined as 'the human consequences – personal, social, economic, cultural and political – of forced migration' (Ager 1999: 2). There are many aspects of the 'refugee experience' that can affect health. Ager (1999) describes discrete phases within forced migration: pre-flight, flight, reception, settlement and resettlement. The health of refugees and asylum seekers can be harmed at all of these phases. This framework is used here to consider the threats to the health of refugees and asylum seekers.

PRE-FLIGHT

Apart from the direct effects of conflict on the health of refugees and asylum seekers, economic hardship may result in disruption to livelihoods either as a result of political persecution or breakdown in the country's economy, or both (Ager 1999, Kalipeni & Oppong 1998). Social disruption can become so widespread that food supplies are interrupted and schools and health facilities may cease to function (Ager 1999, Coker 2001, Kalipeni & Oppong 1998, Rutter 1994). Political oppression can result in powerlessness and resultant detrimental effects on mental health.

FLIGHT

The whole process of flight can be traumatic as often family members are left behind. The experience of passage can also be dangerous (Muecke 1992). Women and children are particularly vulnerable and can become the victims of rape and sexual exploitation (Coker 2001, Kalipeni & Oppong 1998). Such risks are not confined to the period of flight but extend throughout the entire refugee experience.

RECEPTION

Reception occurs in the first country of asylum (Ager 1999). This is often a neighbouring country and the first 'safe haven' might be a refugee camp. Camps are often near the borders of the countries from which asylum seekers flee. The conditions in refugee camps are often poor; they often have inadequate sanitation and nutritional support, contaminated water supplies and severe overcrowding. These conditions are ideal for the transmission of infectious diseases (Clinton-Davis & Fassil 1992, Dick 1984, Gellert 1993, Kalipeni & Oppong 1998, Weekers & Siem 1997). Women are, again, particularly at risk of sexual violence (Callamard 1999, Coker 2001, Forbes Martin 1992). Reception might also occur in Western countries and the experience is characterized by registration procedures.

SETTLEMENT

Many refugees and asylum seekers do not remain in the country of first asylum (Ager 1999); they might move on to another country where the temporary period of settlement will occur. Kemp (1993), writing from experience in the USA, claims that the health of refugees and asylum seekers is generally compromised on arrival in a host country. Frequently encountered problems include untreated communicable diseases, chronic conditions exacerbated by lack of health care and nutritional problems resulting from the disruption of food supplies (Coker 2001, Kemp 1993). Typically refugees and asylum seekers migrate to countries where residents have little exposure to communicable diseases such as malaria and tuberculosis and medical professionals may not suspect such diseases (Weekers & Siem 1997). Migrating communities are also exposed to new diseases (Dick 1984). There is also the problem of psychosocial distress resulting from torture to the refugees and asylum seekers themselves, or to their relatives, or from the experience of flight (Coker 2001, Kemp 1993). Access to health care may present a problem due to lack of knowledge concerning how to access care and communication problems if access is achieved (Coker 2001, Woodhead 2000). In particular, in the UK, refugees and asylum seekers have experienced problems and dissatisfaction when attempting to gain access to health care, resulting from their lack of familiarity with the GP gate-keeping system.

Health and health care are not always initial priorities for refugees and asylum seekers because of preoccupation with asylum, housing, employment and finances (Clinton-Davis & Fassil 1992, Kemp 1993, Hargreaves et al 2001, Papadopoulos et al 2004, Woodhead 2000).

RESETTLEMENT

The attitudes of both the refugees and asylum seekers and the host country will influence the extent and manner of resettlement adopted by refugees and asylum seekers (Ager 1999). However, it is important to remember that refugees and asylum seekers may experience greater difficulty adjusting to their host country than voluntary migrants (Kemp 1993). Of particular importance are issues relating to cultural identity and relationships with other groups of people. Baker et al (1994) conducted a phenomenological study in Canada to explore the experience of resettlement for migrants who did not have access to a community of their own culture. Their informants, who included refugees, described feelings such as powerlessness, inability to understand people, feeling bewildered and unable to understand customs. The informants did express a strong commitment to adjust to their host society and were receptive to support from others. Informants reported somatic problems such as headaches, anxiety and tension. These problems frequently arise in research relating to the health of refugees and asylum seekers.

The first systematic national study performed in relation to refugees by the Home Office in the UK involved people who had been granted refugee status or exceptional leave to remain and investigated how they had fared over the last decade in terms of settling into the community (Carey-Wood et al 1995). This took the form of a large-scale survey. Many of the findings have been supported by smaller-scale qualitative studies concerning specific groups of refugees and asylum seekers. Key issues in resettlement included the following:

- Language, or rather the inability to communicate effectively in English, emerged as a major problem in many studies (Brent and Harrow 1995, Carey-Wood et al 1995, Gammell et al 1993, Haringey Council 1997, Papadopoulos & Gebrehiwot 2002, Taylor, unpublished work, 2005).
- For asylum seekers there was an overwhelming concern with immigration status (Directorate of Public Health, Croydon Health Authority 1999, Papadopoulos & Gebrehiwot 2002, Taylor, unpublished work, 2005). Those who have been granted refugee status express enormous relief.
- Poverty has been reported in some studies (Carey-Wood et al 1995, Jones 1999, Papadopoulos & Gebrehiwot 2002, Taylor, unpublished work, 2005). The effects of poverty on health have been documented.
- Employment is also a key issue in resettlement (Bloch 1999, Brent and Harrow 1995, Carey-Wood et al 1995, Haringey Council 1997, Gammell et al 1993, Taylor, unpublished work, 2005). Carey-Wood et al (1995) found that the unemployment rate among refugees was above that for minority ethnic groups in general. It is recognized that unemployed people have worse health than those in employment (Harkins & Stead 2002, Townsend et al 1992).
- Accommodation is a major issue in resettlement (Carey-Wood et al 1995); the majority of respondents were renting accommodation in the public sector and dissatisfaction was expressed with this accommodation. Such sentiments were echoed in other studies (Brent & Harrow 1995, Haringey Council 1997, Papadopoulos & Gebrehiwot 2002, Taylor, unpublished work, 2005).

Traditional family patterns may be disrupted as family members may be lost and some, particularly women and children, may be forced to take on new roles. Children often become interpreters (Forbes Martin 1992) and intergenerational conflict can occur.

Refugee children face threats to their development and survival (Ahearn et al 1999). They may suffer physical health problems in a similar way as adults, but separation from family is particularly traumatic. Schooling may be disrupted, both pre-flight and during flight. Some children act out their distress and there are reports of school children hiding under tables when aircraft fly overhead (Marchant 1994). Refugee children's drawings often convey stories of trauma and pain. However, Ahearn et al (1999) also stress that most refugee children adapt to their host countries and have productive and satisfying lives.

Refugees and asylum seekers also suffer an inordinate amount of loss (Coker 2001, Kemp 1993). Loss relates to the past as lifestyles change in order to survive in a new culture, leading Kemp (1993: 22) to ask 'What value is the village elder in urban Paris, London, or New York?' Loss also relates to the present as role, status and employment patterns change and children begin to adopt values of the host community.

THE HEALTH OF REFUGEES AND ASYLUM SEEKERS

Carey-Wood et al (1995) found that the physical and mental health of a refugee may be one of the most significant factors affecting settlement. It is important to remember that this study concerned refugees, and not asylum seekers, and there is an important difference in the two statuses. In Carey-Wood et al's study, 10% of respondents reported wide-ranging disabilities sufficient to affect their daily lives. There were also high levels of stress, anxiety and depression, attributed mainly to problems in their home countries and worry about lack of work.

PHYSICAL HEALTH

Refugees and asylum seekers are a fairly young population (Aldous et al 1999). Evidence suggests that most refugees and asylum seekers arrive in Britain in reasonably good health (Aldous et al 1999, Woodhead, 2000). However, the evidence is varied. In the study of settled refugees (Carey-Wood et al 1995), 16% of the sample were suffering from physical health problems sufficient to affect their way of life.

MENTAL HEALTH

There is no doubt that refugees and asylum seekers are susceptible to psychological problems following their varied and extraordinary experiences pre-flight, during flight and post-flight in their host countries (Ahearn 2000). In the study of settled refugees (Carey-Wood et al 1995), two-thirds of respondents said that they had experienced anxiety or depression; problems in their home countries were the main reason for depression. However, there is a debate concerning the diagnosis, and extent, of clinical mental illness in refugees and asylum seekers. From research conducted after the Second World War, it has been accepted that those who have been forcibly uprooted are at greater risk of mental ill health than those who voluntarily migrate (Harrell-Bond 2000). Shackman (1995) describes exile as a kind of bereavement; as such, various psychological reactions can be expected. Summerfield (1994) warns of the dangers of employing a Western discourse to address mental health issues of refugees and asylum seekers, as doing so can result in mental illness becoming a self-fulfilling prophecy and capable of incapacitating refugees.

> *What constitutes psychological knowledge is the product of a particular culture at a particular point in time and there is more than one true description of the world. (Summerfield 1999: 1455)*

Of particular concern is the concept, and possible diagnosis, of post-traumatic stress disorder (PTSD), which was recognized as a distinct psychiatric category in 1980 following the war in Vietnam (Summerfield 1999, Watters 2001).

Some refugees and asylum seekers will have been exposed to traumatic experiences beyond the imagination of the average western European, and it is important not to mistake natural distress for mental pathology (Burnett & Peel 2001, Summerfield 1994). Summerfield (1999) acknowledges the misery engendered by war and the potential long-term effects but claims that there is a lack of evidence to demonstrate increased rates of psychiatric morbidity among refugees and asylum seekers. Equally he claims that there is a lack of evidence that talk therapies are preventive, particularly as many non-Western cultures have little place for the revelation of intimate material outside a close family circle. Indeed, Summerfield (1999) claims that when most refugees are asked what would help their situation they are much more likely to point to social and economic factors than psychological help. On the other hand, Thompson (2001), writing in Britain, estimates that refugees experience up to five times more incidence of mental illness than the general population and yet they are not well served by statutory services. This is partly due a lack of familiarity with counselling but also due to a reluctance to report their mental distress. Many refugees and asylum seekers come from societies that stigmatize mental illness. A study in Cardiff (Ruddy 1992) concerning Somali refugees and asylum seekers found significant mental distress and disease but the sufferers were not seeking help as mental illness is believed to bring shame on the family. However, Thompson (2001) also asserts that it is important that professionals do not rush to label those with severe distress as having a clinically defined mental illness.

Muecke (1992) and Watters (2001) point to the danger of locating the problem within the individual and negating the psychological impact of specific policies directed towards refugees. For example, Silove et al (1997) report on interviews with 40 asylum seekers attending a community resource centre in Sydney, Australia; the authors argue that post-migration stresses faced by asylum seekers, such as waiting for a decision on their application for asylum and lack of work permits, may interact with and possibly exacerbate their existing problems. In a similar vein, Gorst-Unsworth & Goldenberg (1998) interviewed 84 Iraqi refugees in Britain and found that social factors in exile, particularly the level of social support, proved important in determining the severity of both PTSD and depressive reactions. They concluded that poor social support is a stronger predictor of depressive illness than trauma factors. Also, Lavik et al (1996) interviewed 231 refugees and asylum seekers in Oslo,

Norway, and commented on the destructive effects of being without employment or having educational possibilities in exile. It would appear, then, that some of the most important factors in producing psychological morbidity in refugees may be alleviated by planned, integrated rehabilitation programmes and attention to social support and family reunion (Gorst-Unsworth & Goldenberg 1998).

ACCESS TO HEALTH SERVICES

While refugees and asylum seekers are entitled to use the National Health Service in Britain, many have experienced difficulties accessing services (Jobbins 1997). Carey-Wood et al (1995) report high levels of registration with GPs; however, only 40% of respondents who said they had a medical or psychological problem actually sought help from their GP. In Britain registration of refugees and asylum seekers with GPs is reasonably high, but there are reports of problems achieving this registration (Aldous et al 1999).

PROVIDING CULTURALLY AND LINGUISTICALLY COMPETENT SERVICES TO MIGRANTS AND REFUGEES

CULTURAL AWARENESS

It is important to be aware that refugees and asylum seekers do not form a homogeneous group, but come from a wide variety of different cultures. It is important, therefore, not to stereotype refugees and asylum seekers. While refugees and asylum seekers might share some problems in common, e.g. oppression, persecution, the cultures of the different groups will vary. Cultural awareness is therefore necessary in order to be prepared for new arrivals of refugees and asylum seekers as patterns of asylum seeking are liable to change over short periods of time. When examining their own personal values, professionals might like to consider what it might feel like to be forced to flee their own country and to leave behind everything they hold dear, e.g. family, friends, home, work, indeed a whole way of life. Refugees and asylum seekers might even have been persecuted in their home countries because of their cultural identity; for example, Kurdish people in Turkey have been denied the right to sing Kurdish songs (Budak 1993).

CULTURAL KNOWLEDGE

As well as learning from refugees and asylum seekers about their varied cultures, it is important to acquire knowledge about the 'refugee experience'. Knowledge about the situations from which refugees and asylum seekers have fled will help with understanding of their needs. However, it is important to acknowledge the shared experience of refugees and asylum seekers, but also to be aware that they will still present with different illnesses. Refugees and asylum seekers have claimed that some professionals assume that they all have the same problems relating to their refugee experience (Taylor, unpublished work, 2005). Working with groups of refugees and asylum seekers will facilitate the advance of cultural knowledge; for example, in a participatory health needs assessment exercise, health professionals will gain cultural knowledge from the particular refugee community. In turn, the members of the community will gain skills in research and health needs assessment.

CULTURAL SENSITIVITY

Cultural sensitivity will be enhanced by the appropriate use of interpreters to assist in overcoming the language problems cited by so many informants in the various studies cited above. It is clear that communication problems can result in a very unsatisfactory encounter for both patients and health professionals. Bischoff et al (2003) set out to determine whether language barriers during screening interviews affected the reporting of asylum seekers' health problems and their referral to further health care. These authors found that the detection of traumatic events in the patients' histories increased drastically when there was good language concordance between nurses and asylum seekers. Good language concordance also significantly improved the appropriate referral to further health care. It was also felt that relatives might not be able to provide the necessary cultural mediation between the two cultures – that of healthcare providers and that of migrants. Cultural sensitivity naturally goes beyond the mere use of language to encompass non-verbal communication, taboo subject areas and etiquette.

CULTURAL COMPETENCE

In conclusion, cultural competence in relation to refugees and asylum seekers involves the synthesis of cultural awareness, knowledge and sensitivity. As such, cultural competence takes time to develop and health professionals will be challenged by new waves of people seeking asylum. Preparedness to listen to patients, awareness of possible aspects of the 'refugee experience' and an understanding of the fear that refugees and asylum seekers might have of people in authority will assist professionals in encounters with refugees and asylum seekers. Reflection on each new encounter should help professionals towards cultural competence.

REFLECTIVE QUESTIONS

1. Recall an occasion when you were a newcomer or a 'stranger'. This might have been an experience of entering a new environment, e.g. starting at college, a new job, or going on holiday to another country.
2. What thoughts and emotions did the feeling of being a 'stranger' evoke?
3. How were all those things you had previously taken for granted challenged by this new situation?
4. Do you think a migrant who has recently arrived in your country might experience similar thoughts and emotions?
5. How did your previous life experience equip you to cope with the new situation?
6. Consider the experiences of refugees and asylum seekers who might have been persecuted or oppressed, and how these particular experiences might influence their coping mechanisms in a new situation.
7. What are the implications of being a 'stranger' for health and the provision of health care?

REFERENCES

Abel-Smith B, Figueras J, Holland W et al 1995 Choices in health policy: an agenda for the European Union. Dartmouth, Aldershot

Adelman H 1999 Modernity, globalization, refugees and displacement. In: Ager A (ed) Refugees. Perspectives on the experience of forced migration. Pinter, London

Ager A 1999 Perspectives on the refugee experience. In: Ager A (ed) Refugees. Perspectives on the experience of forced migration. Pinter, London

Ahearn F L Jr 2000 Conclusions and implications for future research. In: Ahearn F L Jr (ed) Psychosocial wellness of refugees. Issues in qualitative and quantitative research. Studies in Forced migration 7. Berghahn Books, Oxford

Ahearn F, Loughry M, Ager M 1999 The experience of refugee children. In: Ager A (ed) Refugees. Perspectives on the experience of forced migration. Pinter, London

Ahmad W I U 1997 Foreword. In: Nazroo J Y The health of Britain's ethnic minorities. Policy Studies Institute, London

Aldous J, Bardsley M, Daniell R et al 1999 Refugee health in London. Key issues for public health. The Health of Londoners Project, London

Baker C, Arseneault A M, Gallant G 1994 Resettlement without the support of an ethnocultural community. Journal of Advanced Nursing 20:1064–1072

Balarajan R 1996 Ethnicity and variations in mortality from coronary heart disease. Health Trends 28(2):45–51

Balarajan R, Soni Raleigh V 1993 Ethnicity and health. A guide for the NHS. Department of Health, London

Berthoud R, Nazroo J 1997 The mental health of ethnic minorities. New Community 23(3):309–324

Bhopal R, Unwin N, White M et al 1999 Heterogeneity of coronary heart disease risk factors in Indian, Pakistani, Bangladeshi and European origin populations: cross sectional study. British Medical Journal 319:215–219

Bischoff A, Bovier P A, Isah R et al 2003 Language barriers between nurses and asylum seekers: their impact on symptom reporting and referral. Social Science and Medicine 57:503–512

Bloch A 1999 Refugees in the job market: a case of unused skills in the British economy. In: Bloch A, Levy C (eds) Refugees, citizenship and social policy in Europe. Macmillan, Basingstoke

Bollini P, Siem H 1995 No real progress towards equity: Health of migrants and ethnic minorities on the eve of the year 2000. Social Science and Medicine 41(6):819–828

Brent & Harrow Health Agency, Brent & Harrow Refugee Groups, Northwest London Training & Enterprise Council 1995 Brent & Harrow refugee survey. Brent & Harrow Health Agency, London

Brunner E, Marmot M 1999 Social organization, stress, and health. In: Marmot M, Wilkinson R G (eds) Social determinants of health. Oxford University Press, Oxford

Budak N (1993) Health needs of Kurdish refugees in Haringey. New River Health Authority, London

Burnett A, Peel M 2001 The health of survivors of torture and organised violence. British Medical Journal 322:606–609

Callamard A 1999 Refugee women: a gendered and political analysis of the refugee experience. In: Ager A (ed) Refugees. Perspectives on the experience of forced migration. Pinter, London

Carey-Wood J 1997 Meeting refugees' needs in Britain: the role of refugee-specific initiatives. HMSO, London

Carey-Wood J, Duke K, Karn V et al 1995 The settlement of refugees in Britain. Home Office Research Study No 141. HMSO, London

Castles S 2000 International migration at the beginning of the twenty-first century: global trends and issues. International Social Science Journal 52(165)269–281

Castles S, Miller M J 2003 The age of migration. International population movements in the modern world. 3rd edn. Palgrave, Basingstoke

Clinton-Davis Lord, Fassil Y 1992 Health and social problems of refugees. Social Science and Medicine 35(4):507–513

Coker N 2001 Asylum seekers' and refugees' health experience. In: Appleby J, Harrison A (eds) Health Care UK. Winter 2001. The King's Fund review of health policy. King's Fund, London

Coleman D A 1996 UK Immigration policy: 'Firm but Fair', and Failing? Policy Studies 17(3):195–214

Dick B 1984 Diseases of refugees – causes, effects and control. Transactions of the Royal Society of Tropical Medicine and Hygiene 78:734–741

Directorate of Public Health, Croydon Health Authority 1999 Refugee health in Croydon. Croydon Health Authority, Croydon

Doná G, Berry J W 1999 Refugee acculturation and re-acculturation. In: Ager A (ed) Refugees. Perspectives on the experience of forced migration. Pinter, London

Duke K, Sales R, Gregory J 1999 Refugee settlement in Europe. In: Bloch A, Levy C (eds) Refugees, citizenship and social policy in Europe. Macmillan, Basingstoke

Fernando S 2002 Mental health, race and culture. 2nd edn. Palgrave, Basingstoke

Forbes Martin S 1992 Refugee women. Zed Books, London

Fox J (ed) 1989 Health inequalities in European countries. Gower, Aldershot

Gammell H, Ndahiro A, Nicholas N et al 1993 Refugees (political asylum seekers): service provision and access to the NHS. College of Health & Newham Health Authority, London

Gellert G A 1993 International migration and control of communicable diseases. Social Science and Medicine 37(12):1489–1499

Gorst-Unsworth C, Goldenberg E 1998 Psychological sequelae of torture and organised violence suffered by refugees from Iraq. Trauma-related factors compared with social factors in exile. British Journal of Psychiatry 172:90–94

Graham H 2004 Tackling inequalities in health in England: remedying health disadvantages, narrowing health gaps or reducing health gradients. Journal of Social Policy 33(1):115–131

Hansen R 2003 Migration to Europe since 1945: its history and its lessons. In: Spencer S (ed) The politics of migration. Managing opportunity, conflict and change. Blackwell, Oxford

Hargreaves S, Holmes A, Friedland J S 2001 Europe's health-care lottery. Lancet 357:1434–1435

Haringey Council 1997 Refugees and asylum seekers in Haringey: Research project report. Haringey Council, London

Harkins D, Stead M 2002 Opportunities for improving health through regeneration. In: Adams L, Amos M, Munro J (eds) Promoting health. Politics and practice. Sage, London

Harrell-Bond B 2000 Foreword. In: Ahearn F L Jr (ed) Psychosocial wellness of refugees. Issues in qualitative and quantitative research. Studies in Forced Migration, Vol 7. Berghahn Books, Oxford

Health Education Authority 1994 Black and minority ethnic groups in England: health and lifestyles. Health Education Authority, London

Helman C 2000 Culture, health and illness. 4th edn. Butterworth Heinemann, Oxford

Jobbins D 1997 The impact of the Asylum and Immigration Act (1996) on the health of refugees and asylum-seekers in the UK. Share 16:5–6

Jones J A 1999 Refugees and asylum seekers in Enfield and Haringey. A health needs assessment/service provision review with recommendations for Health Authority action. Directorate of Public Health, Haringey

Kalipeni E, Oppong J 1998 The refugee crisis in Africa and implications for health and disease: A political ecology approach. Social Science and Medicine 46(12):1637–1653

Kemp C 1993 Health services for refugees in countries of second asylum. International Nursing Review 40(1):21–24

Kerrigan S 2003 Welcome to Europe: the truth about asylum responsibility sharing in the European Union. Inexile 25:4–5

Kumin J 1998 An uncertain direction . . . Refugees 2(113):4–9

Kunst A E, Groenhof F, Mackenbach J P et al 1998 Occupational class and cause specific mortality in middle aged men in 11 European countries: comparison of population-based studies. British Medical Journal 316:1636–1642

Kushner T, Knox K 1999 Refugees in an age of genocide. Frank Cass, London

Lavik N J, Hauff E, Skrondal A et al 1996 Mental disorder among refugees and the impact of persecution and exile: Some findings from an out-patient population. British Journal of Psychiatry 169:726–732

Leon D A 1998 Commentary: unequal inequalities across Europe. British Medical Journal 316:1642

Levine S 1995 The meanings of health, illness and quality of life. In: Guggenmoos-Holzmann I, Bloomfield K, Brenner H et al (eds) Quality of life and health. Concepts, methods and applications. Blackwell, London

Lewis N, Seneviratne M 1992 A social charter for Britain. In: Coote A (ed) The welfare of citizens. Developing new social rights. IPPR/Rivers Oram Press, London

Macintyre S 1997 The Black Report and beyond. What are the issues? Social Science and Medicine 44(6):723–745

McKay L, Macintyre S, Ellaway A 2003 Migration and health: A review of the international literature. Medical Research Council Social and Public Health Sciences Unit, Glasgow

Marchant C 1994 Risky future. Community Care 24:16–17

Marmot M, Wilkinson R G (eds) 1999 Social determinants of health. Oxford University Press, Oxford

Montgomery J 1992 Rights to health and health care. In: Coote A (ed) The welfare of citizens. Developing new social rights. IPPR/Rivers Oram Press, London

Muecke M A 1992 New paradigms for refugee health problems. Social Science and Medicine 35(4):515–523

Nazroo J Y 1998 Genetic, cultural or socio-economic vulnerability? Explaining ethnic inequalities in health. Sociology of Health and Illness 10(5):710–730

Papadopoulos I, Gebrehiwot A (eds) 2002 The EMBRACE Project. The Ethiopian migrants, their beliefs, refugeedom, adaptation, calamities, and experiences in the United Kingdom. Middlesex University, London

Papadopoulos I, Lees S, Lay M, Gebrehiwot A 2004 Ethiopian Refugees in the UK: their adaptation and settlement experiences and their relationship to health. Ethnicity and Health 9(1):55–73

Power C 1994 Health and social inequality in Europe. British Medical Journal 308:1153–1156

Ruddy B 1992 Any port in a storm. Health Service Journal 102(5330):29

Rutter J 1994 Refugee children in the classroom. Trentham, Stoke on Trent

Sales R 2002 Migration policy in Europe: contradictions and continuities. In: Sykes R, Bochel C, Ellison N (eds) Social Policy Review 14. Development and Debates: 2001–2002. Policy Press, Bristol

Shackman J 1995 On defeating exile. Open Mind 73:18–19

Silove D, Sinnerbrink I, Field A et al 1997 Anxiety, depression and PTSD in asylum-seekers: associations with pre-migration trauma and post-migration stressors. British Journal of Psychiatry 170:351–357

Smaje C 1995 Health, 'Race' and ethnicity. Making sense of the evidence. King's Fund, London

Summerfield D 1994 Post traumatic stress and mental health. Symposium on Refugee Health Issues, Selby Centre, Tottenham, 6 May 1994

Summerfield D 1999 A critique of seven assumptions behind psychological trauma programmes in war-affected areas. Social Science and Medicine 48:1449–1462

Thomas C S, Stone K, Osborn M et al 1993 Psychiatric morbidity and compulsory admission among UK-born Europeans, Afro-Caribbeans and Asians in Central Manchester. British Journal of Psychiatry 163:91–99

Thompson A 2001 Refugees and mental health. Diverse Minds Magazine 9:6–7

Townsend P, Davidson N, Whitehead M 1992 Inequalities in health. The Black Report and the Health Divide. Penguin, Harmondsworth

UNHCR 2004 Global Refugee Trends. Overview of Refugee Populations, New Arrivals, Durable Solution, Asylum-seekers and other persons of concern to UNHCR. UNHCR, Geneva. Online.. Available: http//www.unhcr.ch/statistics 11 Apr 2005

Watt N 2001 Asylum seekers to be 'sent back'. The Guardian 6 Feb 2001, p 1–2

Watters C 2001 Emerging paradigms in the mental health care of refugees. Social Science and Medicine 52:1709–1718

Weekers J, Siem H 1997 Overseas screening of migrants: justifiable? Public Health Reports 112:397–402

Westin C 1999 Regional analysis of refugee movements: origins and response. In: Ager A (ed) Refugees. Perspectives on the experience of forced migration. Pinter, London

Woodhead D 2000 The health and well-being of asylum seekers and refugees. King's Fund, London

World Health Organization 1992 Targets for health for all. The health policy for Europe. Summary of the updated edition. September 1991. WHO, Copenhagen

World Health Organization 1998 Health 21 – health for all in the 21st century. WHO, Copenhagen

Zetter R, Pearl M 2000 The minority within the minority: refugee community-based organisations in the UK and the impact of restrictionism on asylum-seekers. Journal of Ethnic and Migration Studies 26(4):675–697

Chapter 5

The ethics of culturally competent health and social care

Ann Gallagher

LEARNING OBJECTIVES

After reading this chapter you should be able to:
- outline different approaches to ethics
- discuss five ethical challenges that arise in relation to cultural competence in health and social care:
    relativism versus universalism
    the paradox of multiculturalism
    cultural aspects of information-giving
    the limits of respect for autonomy in relation to cultural preferences
    the potential for cultural complacency.

INTRODUCTION

Ethics is unavoidable. In relationships with other people, other species and with the environment we act or omit to act in certain ways, we have values or beliefs we may or may not express and we use language such as 'right', 'wrong', 'good', 'bad', 'just' and 'unjust'. We also talk about qualities such as honesty, trustworthiness, compassion and integrity. All of this is the territory of ethics. With some reflection it becomes clear that ethics is inextricably linked with our personal and professional lives. It is not, however, something everyone agrees upon and this is particularly so in relation to culture.

This chapter is concerned with the ethics of culturally competent care. A good deal has already been discussed regarding culture and cultural competence. Culture has been described as a way of life of a group, class or community (Papadopoulos et al 1998, O'Hagan 2001). Culture concerns the ideas, values, activities or practices and, fundamentally, the identities of individuals. Cultural competence is described as an amalgam of cultural awareness, knowledge and sensitivity (Papadopoulos et al 1998).

Demonstrating cultural competence in health and social care requires ethical actions and the demonstration of ethical or moral qualities. Given the diversity of ethical accounts and approaches that coexist in a multicultural society a range of theoretical and practical challenges arise. First, which or whose account of ethics should inform the practice of workers in health and social care? Given the range of views, can anything be agreed and considered 'universal' or is ethics merely 'relative' to individuals and groups? If workers are committed to diversity and to cultural competence, they may conclude that values are culturally relative so nothing can be agreed and nothing universal can be said about ethics at all. They may, in fact, conclude that talk of values or ethics in relation to other cultures is racist or colonialist. Second, how might a worker negotiate different views – in relation to information-giving, for example – within cultural groups? Here, respect for the autonomy of the individual may conflict with respect for family decision-making. Third, what is a worker to do when there is a request for an intervention in keeping with cultural practices but contrary to the worker's professional ethics? Workers may flounder when confronted with an issue where respect for a culture as a whole compromises the rights of individuals or subgroups within it. Hence, there is a 'paradox of multiculturalism'. The fourth challenge also relates to choice. How should a worker respond when an individual's cultural preferences compromise the rights of others, be they workers or other patients/service users? Finally, how can workers who have undertaken training in cultural competence avoid complacency and cultural stereotyping? The final challenge relates to a potential consequence of workers embracing cultural competence in an unreflective manner. They may become complacent or engage in cultural stereotyping, compromising a holistic approach to the individual.

Vignettes are introduced to illustrate each of these challenges. The chapter concludes with a discussion regarding the possibility of a 'transcultural ethics'.

WHICH ETHICS? WHOSE ETHICS?

Ethics can be subdivided as normative and non-normative ethics. *Normative ethics* includes general normative ethics derived from philosophical, religious and cultural norms and practical or applied ethics.

One key question is: 'which general moral norms for the guidance and evaluation of conduct should we accept and why?' (Beauchamp & Childress 2001: 2). One view is that practical or applied ethics refers to the implementation or application of theories to real 'problems, practices and policies in professions, institutions and public policy' (Beauchamp & Childress 2001: 2). Practical or applied ethics has then much to do with workers in health and social care concerned to respond appropriately in practice and to understand the theoretical underpinning for their actions.

Non-normative ethics includes metaethics and descriptive or empirical ethics and is concerned with the analytic and descriptive components of ethics. *Metaethics* involves the analysis of ethical language and discussion of the basis of ethical theory. Metaethical questions include: what are we doing when we engage in ethical judgements or argument? Is this akin to a scientific endeavour or the expression of emotion? On what basis can we claim that moral judgements are true or false? What do words such as 'good', 'right', 'virtue', 'obligation' and so on mean? Metaethics comprises theories *about* ethics, not theories *of* ethics (Singer 1993: xiv). The term suggests examining ethics, not engaging in it (the latter involves exploring what should be done or how people should be). Metaethics includes the debate about the possibility of ethics in a multicultural society: Can there be agreement about ethics? Can there be universal values? Or, is ethics relative to cultural groups? The last two questions will be discussed in the next section.

There is now a good deal of consensus that workers in health and social care require some understanding of ethics. Most professions now have codes of ethics or conduct providing guidance and prescriptions for practice, as have many organizations – statutory and voluntary. What theory or approach underpins these documents is not always made explicit. However, a range of perspectives can be identified. In the General Medical Council's *Good Medical Practice* (1995) there is evidence of duty-based and rights-based ethics. Doctors have a duty to 'respect patients' dignity and privacy' and must 'respect the rights of patients to be fully involved in decisions about their care'. In relation to 'maintaining trust' the following clauses have particular relevance to cultural issues:

> 12. *You must not allow your views about a patient's lifestyle, culture, beliefs, race, colour, sexuality, age, social status or perceived economic worth to prejudice the treatment you give or arrange.*

> 13. *If you feel that your beliefs might affect the treatment you provide, you must explain this to patients, and tell them of their right to see another doctor.*

There is also evidence of duty- and rights-based ethics in the Code of Practice for Social Care Workers (Social Care Council 2002). Clauses state, for example, that workers must 'protect the rights and promote the interests of service users and carers' (section 2), also respect and maintain 'the dignity and privacy of service users' (1.4) and communicate in 'an appropriate, open, accurate and straightforward way' (2.2). Culture is made explicit in the following clause, which specifies rights protection and the promotion of interests by:

1.6 Respecting diversity and different cultures and values.

The Nursing and Midwifery Council (NMC) Code (2004) also points to duties and rights, for example, 'All patients and clients have a right to receive information about their condition. You must be sensitive to their needs and respect the wishes of those who refuse or are unable to receive information about their condition'. Culture is referred to as follows:

2.2 You are personally accountable for ensuring that you promote and protect the interests and dignity of patients and clients, irrespective of gender, age, race, ability, sexuality, economic status, lifestyle, culture and religious or political beliefs.

Common themes are identifiable in these codes for health and social care workers, most significantly, the protection of rights, respect for dignity and autonomy (in terms of information-giving, for example) and respect and non-discrimination on the basis of culture. There is also common ground in terms of the moral qualities or character traits necessary for health and social care. The NMC Code (2002) states 'be trustworthy'. The GMC (1995) states 'be honest and trustworthy' and the code for social care workers states that workers need to be 'honest and trustworthy'.

Duty-based and rights-based ethics are very common in the health and social care literature and focus primarily on action, directing that workers should do whatever it is their duty to do and should respect the rights of service users or patients. There is also discussion of worker rights (in relation to working conditions, for example) and service user or patient duties (in relation to lifestyle and compliance with treatment, for example). Other common approaches providing ethical guidance are *principle-based ethics* and *consequence-based ethics*. These approaches have their origins primarily in Western philosophical approaches. Before considering alternative frameworks something will be said about each of these approaches.

In Chapter 3 of this text there was discussion of *rights-based* ethics. Rights have been defined as 'justified claims which individuals or groups can make upon other individuals or upon society; to have a right is to be in a position to determine, by one's choices, what others should do or need not do' (Beauchamp & Childress 2001: 357). The Human Rights Act 1998 in the United Kingdom has urged a renewed consideration of moral and legal rights.

'Human rights' have a long and distinguished history but their existence also reminds us of human potential for cruelty and as, Glover (1999: 3) puts it, 'man-made horrors'. He says:

To talk of the twentieth-century atrocities is in one way misleading. It is a myth that barbarism is unique to the twentieth century: the whole of human history includes wars, massacres, and every kind of torture and cruelty: there are grounds for thinking that over much of the world the changes of the last hundred years or so have been towards a psychological climate more humane than at any previous time. But it is still right that much of twentieth-century history has been a very unpleasant surprise. Technology has made a difference. The decisions of a few people can mean horror and death for hundreds of thousands, even millions of other people.

Some of the grossest violations of human rights were directed towards specific cultural groups. There is also evidence that workers in health and social care were implicated (see, for example, Steppe 1997 and Lifton 1986, 1988). Research and recent reports confirm that abuse and harm continue in health and social care settings (BBC 2003, Lawrence 2001). These are violations of human rights.

The British Medical Association in its publication *The Medical Profession and Human Rights: Handbook for a Changing Agenda* (2001) points to a range of roles for professionals in relation to human rights. It states, for example (2001: xxiii):

Health professionals are among the first in society to encounter evidence of human rights violations. Doctors have been assigned particular impor-tance in efforts to reduce gross human rights abuses, by acting as whistleblowers.

Speaking out about human rights violations is not an easy matter and there are high profile examples of health and social care workers who have blown the whistle, for example nurse Graham Pink and Bristol Royal Infirmary doctor Stephen Bolsin (Pink 1994, Bosely 1998).

Ethical conduct, on a rights-based view, consists then of respecting the rights of others. There may not be agreement as to what these rights are nor about what they mean – for example, in different contexts – and also challenges when rights conflict as, for example, in abortion. A 'human rights' perspective is, however, advantageous in relation to professional ethics as it requires a looking outwards, a less parochial and morally myopic view and a consideration of issues beyond national boundaries. The ethical concepts or values of dignity and autonomy are much in evidence in a rights perspective. Rights do not necessarily resolve ethical challenges. One such, discussed below, is female genital mutilation which appears to place cultural rights against human rights and result in a 'paradox of multiculturalism'.

The work of the eighteenth century German philosopher Immanuel Kant is referred to primarily in discussions of *duty-based* or *deontological ethics*. The good will and the role of practical reason are central to Kant's philosophy. Actions are, on this account, right or wrong in themselves and not dependent on consequences. The duties that are arrived at by reason are absolute. Kant's 'categorical imperative' has three formula-tions: First, 'act as if the maxim of your action was to become through your will a universal law of nature' (Paton 1948: 30). This means that individuals must always act in a way that they would will everyone else to act, in a way they would will this to be a general law for everyone.

Second, 'act in such a way that you always treat humanity, whether in your own person or in the person of any other, never simply as a means, but always at the same time as an end' (Paton 1948: 32). This is taken to mean that people should never be treated as a means to an end but rather as an end in themselves. Thirdly, 'so act as if you were through your maxims a law-making member of a kingdom of ends' (Paton 1948: 34) What Kant is said to envisage is rational agents who act as if they were making laws, on the basis of reason, for themselves and if they are able to do this they become law-making members of a kingdom of ends (Vardy & Grosch 1999, Paton 1948).

On this view, good conduct consists in doing what it is our duty to do. It consists in treating people as ends rather than means. There is clearly much appeal in an ethics that prioritizes respect, autonomy, dignity and treating people as ends in themselves. These are values that are much apparent in professional ethics. The prioritization of these ethical values is a strength of Kantian ethics.

The slogan 'the greatest happiness of the greatest number' is commonly taken to refer to the central principles of utilitarianism. *Consequence-based* ethics was popularized by Jeremy Bentham and John Stuart Mill in the nineteenth century. Unlike a duty-based perspective, utilitarianism is primarily concerned with consequences, with the outcome of action. Mill (1962 edition: 257) writes:

> *The creed which accepts as the foundation of morals, Utility, or the Greatest Happiness Principle, holds that actions are right in proportion as they tend to promote happiness, wrong as they tend to produce the reverse of happiness. By happiness is intended pleasure, and the absence of pain; by unhappiness, pain and the privation of pleasure.*

In health and social care, there is evidence of utilitarian thinking at a macro-level in relation to, for example, resource allocation and at a micro-level in relation to issues such as confidentiality (Harris 1985: 227). Utilitarian ethics may prioritize the 'happiness' of the majority over minorities. This has potentially negative consequences for ethnic and cultural minorities. Having said this, there is also a role for autonomy in Mill's version of utilitarianism. In On Liberty it is clear that individual freedom is also prized highly. Constraints on what is, effectively, autonomy are in relation to the freedoms and interests of others (Mill 1962: 208–209).

Unlike the three perspectives thus far considered, *principle-based* ethics qualifies as an approach rather than a theory. Principles are evident in the theories just discussed – the principle of utility, for example. The four principles of biomedical ethics or 'principlism' promoted by Beauchamp & Childress (2001) and Gillon (1986) are said to express the basic values binding on all persons in all places. Beauchamp & Childress (2001: 15) state:

> *Our four clusters or principles do not constitute a general moral theory. They provide only a framework for identifying and reflecting on moral problems.*

The principles are: respect for autonomy, beneficence, non-maleficence and justice.

They have been generally taken to be derived from theories such as deontology (duty-based ethics) or utilitarianism (consequence-based ethics) and are described as 'mid-level' principles. They are less specific than rules and more specific than theories.

Roughly, autonomy refers to respect for the autonomous actions of individuals/patients. Beauchamp & Childress (2001: 59) consider autonomous action in relation to the individual's ability to: act intentionally; with understanding; and without controlling influences. Beneficence and non-maleficence equate with doing good and minimizing or avoiding harm. Justice relates to fairness and is usually considered in relation to distribution in health care. There is a range of distributive justice principles within the principle of justice. Interpreting all these principles in relation to healthcare practice is not, of course, always an easy matter.

Good conduct, on a principle-based approach, consists of specifying and balancing principles. It consists of respecting the autonomy of patients or service users, of doing good, avoiding or minimizing harm and treating patients fairly or justly. This is no mean feat in relation to culture and the challenges which may arise from it. How, for example, is autonomy to be understood in cultures where family decision-making is most common? Are we well placed to say what counts as benefit or harm in cultures we know little about? What counts as fairness when dealing with refugees or asylum seekers? In relation to culturally competent care the fair or just distribution of resources can present real challenges, for example in the provision of interpreting services and in the training of workers.

Thus far, four perspectives on professional ethics have been outlined: duty-based ethics, which is evident in professional codes and which specifies right conduct as the fulfilment of duties; rights-based ethics, also evident in codes, which encourages professionals to consider ethics more broadly as 'human rights'; consequence-based ethics, which defines right conduct in terms of maximizing happiness or utility; and a principle-based approach, which promotes a version of right conduct that consists in respecting autonomy, beneficence, non-maleficence and justice. All of these approaches focus on the actions of the worker in health and social care.

It has already been said that a range of moral qualities or character traits such as honesty and trustworthiness are recommended in the codes of health and social care workers. These point to another approach to ethics, one that focuses on character rather than action or conduct. Virtue or *character-based ethics* focuses on the moral qualities or virtues of individuals. It is as concerned with who the individual is, their internal world, their motives, with how they live their lives overall as with their conduct or action (Devettere 2002). A wide range of qualities or virtues has been proposed in relation to workers in health and social care.

This section raised the questions Which ethics? Whose ethics? The five perspectives sketched so far have their origins in European and American writing, in other words, in Western philosophical traditions. Are these approaches appropriate for a discussion of cultural competence? Are they not ethnocentric? How do they compare with other traditional and non-Western approaches to ethics, for example based on religious frameworks such as Buddhist, Jewish and Islamic ethics and those identifiable within national boundaries such as Indian and Chinese ethics.

There are significant differences within non-Western philosophical and spiritual or religious systems that underpin ethics and also between Western and non-Western approaches to ethics. Indian ethics, for example, encompasses a variety of ethical systems. These include Brahmanical-Hindu ethics, the Jaina tradition and Gandhian ethics. These all differ in their philosophical underpinning and their practical recommendations (Bilimoria 1991). Buddhist ethics is also embedded in a complex system and contains doctrines of impermanence, suffering and egolessness, noble truths and a noble eightfold path (De Silva 1999). Both Indian and Buddhist ethics provide guidance for right conduct or action and point to virtues or character traits. Many of these values are identifiable in Western ethics and others seem unique to that approach. In the Jaina tradition, for example, there are vows relating to non-harming and truthfulness. Both traditions also make reference to virtues found in Western approaches such as courage and compassion whereas others – 'loving kindness', for example – are less familiar.

Differences are also apparent between classical Chinese ethics and Western ethics and between different systems of Chinese ethics. Hansen (1991: 69) points out:

> The differences between Chinese and Western ethics are broad and deep. Our inherited Greek psychology divides the ego into the rational and the emotional. It explains all human mental processing via belief and desire. Our concept of morality involves reference to the human faculty of reason. Chinese thinkers view human action in a different way. They appeal to no such faculty nor to beliefs and desires as reasons for action.
>
> The Chinese approach is initially more social. Humanity is social. A social dao ('way') guides us. Chinese ethical thinkers reflect on how to preserve, transmit or change this way – the public, guiding discourse. When modern Chinese writers sought a translation for 'ethics', they chose the compound dao de – ways and virtues. Dao is public, objective guidance. De ('virtue') consists of the character trains. Skills and dispositions induced by exposure to a dao.

Different schools of Chinese ethics have different ideas about 'which way was the way' (Hansen 1991: 69). There is evidence of duty-based and consequence-based ethics in the different varieties of Chinese ethics and also evidence of virtue-based ethics. Jewish ethics is similarly complex with disagreement amongst its proponents. Kellner (1991: 89) states that:

> One can find Jewish thinkers who maintain that Jewish ethics is essentially autonomous in the Kantian sense and others who glory in the fact that it is, was, and should be absolutely heteronomous. . . . Every possible posi-

tion on the question of the relation between ethics and Halakhah [Jewish law] is forcefully maintained by different thinkers as being the authoritative position of the Jewish tradition.

Cultural aspects of Islam are discussed in Chapter 16 of this text. The values of Islamic ethics are derived from two primary sources – the Qur'an and the Sunnah (Nanji 1991). As with other traditions, Islamic ethics deserves much more attention than can be allocated here. There are also different traditions within Islam, for example the Shi'a and Sufi perspectives. Whilst some values appear to be distinctively Islamic others resonate with Western perspectives, for example a focus on redressing economic and social injustice (Nanji 1991: 108). What should become clear is that there is as much diversity, in fact probably more, in non-Western approaches as there is in Western approaches and the possibility of consensus in relation to ethics is as challenging. Non-Western approaches to ethics are embedded in complex philosophical and religious systems. What cultural competence would seem to amount to in relation to non-Western approaches is to acquire some knowledge of the key ideas in the particular system that underpins the ethics of colleagues, service users or patients and families.

Given how much diversity there is in Western and non-Western approaches it might be said that nothing can be agreed, all ethics is culturally relative and nothing universal can be said about ethics. It is to this issue I turn next.

UNIVERSALISM VERSUS RELATIVISM

Consider the following vignette:

(a) Dave is a student social worker who describes himself as 'British' and 'atheist'. He is currently on placement in an area where service users are primarily Asian and either Hindu or Muslim. In a supervision session with his tutor he says that in his work he is wary of making recommendations or giving advice as most issues are culturally or religiously influenced. He says he feels he is interfering and his interventions may be considered racist. He says that when it comes to values or ethics everything is 'relative' to the particular culture and it is wrong of workers to try to impose their values on service users.

So how is Dave's position to be understood? How should his supervisor respond? Is his role as social worker merely to respond uncritically and willingly to the culturally determined wishes of service users? To ascertain and act on these ethical views whatever these might be?

Dave's plight gets to the crux of one of the most challenging issues relating to ethics and culture. Ruth Macklin (1999: v) puts it as follows:

A long-standing debate in ethics and public policy focuses on the fact that ethical beliefs and practices may vary from one place to another, giving rise to the question whether there are any overarching or universal ethical precepts.

Cultural relativism, the view that appraisals of behaviours should be judged only from within cultures, raises profound challenges for workers in health and social care. Baker (1997: 3) outlines the positions taken by those who agree and disagree with cultural relativism:

Its proponents argue that it buffers against parochialism, encourages openness to others, and results in flexibility when cultural differences are encountered. But critics have called cultural relativism a nihilistic doctrine that undermines any condemnation of the violation of human rights or of repression in cultures other than one's own.

Dave's reluctance to make recommendations or give advice to those from different cultures and his fear that such behaviour may be construed as racist has some foundation. Ruth Macklin (1999: viii) discusses a response to an article she had written about sex determination preference for sons in India where her comments were described as 'rather colonial and racist'. She says:

What I think is going on in identifying certain language as 'racist' and 'colonialist' is the unspoken premise that people from one culture are not qualified to discuss the beliefs, attitudes and behaviour of people from another culture. Americans may not discuss women in India, men may not discuss problems of women, white people may not write about black people. Those who adhere to this view share some sort of code that they use to identify violators who deign to write about the 'other'. Invariably, our language will betray us as 'racist' or 'colonialist' because we are, in fact, outsiders.

Macklin does not permit such views to silence her in her writing and she points to violations in human rights emerging from culture. She says:

It remains true that cultural beliefs and practices in some parts of the world depart from the tenets that have come to embody respect for human rights in a large part of the modern world.

If Dave continues to be wary of making recommendations, giving advice or making interventions as a social worker it seems likely that, professionally, he will be ineffective and may even contravene his professional code and legal obligations. However much he may wish to be respectful of the cultural values and practices of service users he also has professional and legal obligations. To this end Dave needs to understand the *raison d'être* of his chosen profession (social work), the prescriptions in his professional code and also the relevant law and policies. His code sets out his profession-specific duties in relation to service users, families and his colleagues. Legal and policy issues impacting on social work practice are complex and wide-ranging, for example, relating to child protection, vulnerable adults, professional duty of care, mental health and human rights. Human rights straddle both ethics and the law and provide a particularly helpful framework for discussion of culture and health and social care. Most particularly, human rights challenge an extreme cultural relativism. Macklin (1999: 243) again:

> *If human rights is a meaningful concept, and if there are any human rights, then normative ethical relativism must be false. Human rights are, by definition, rights that belong to all people. Wherever they may dwell and what ever may be the political system or the cultural traditions of their country or region of the world. The doctrine of normative ethical relativism holds that all moral norms and rules derive from specific cultures. It therefore must deny that there are any universal ethical standards that are (or ought to be) binding on cultural groups or nations despite their igno- rance or rejection of these standards. Because human rights embody one such set of universal ethical standards, to remain consistent the ethical relativist must deny that there are any human rights.*

This is not to say, however, that professionals should ignore cultural values. On the contrary, they need to be knowledgeable, sensitive and discerning – balancing cultural norms with professional duties and a commitment to human rights. The next section discusses a second chal- lenge in relation to ethics and culture.

THE PARADOX OF MULTICULTURALISM

Consider the following vignette:

> (b) Comfort is a newly qualified midwife working in the labour ward of a London hospital. She describes herself as South African. A woman she is allocated to is in labour and is accompanied by her husband. During the vaginal examination Comfort discovers that the woman has been 'circumcised'. The woman's husband tells Comfort that his wife would like to be 're-stitched as before' following the birth of their child. Comfort discusses the situation with her supervisor. She says that although she thinks the practice of female genital mutilation is abhor- rent she is unsure how to proceed.

Female genital mutilation (FGM) is one of the most troubling issues relating to culture and ethics. The BMA (2001: 361) defines FGM as:

> *. . . a collective term used for a range of practices involving the removal of parts of healthy female genitalia; from the removal of the head of the clitoris to the total amputation of the clitoris and labia minora and part of the labia majora, the remainder of which is stitched together leaving a matchstick- sized opening for the passage of urine and menstrual blood.*

It is usually performed on girls between infancy and puberty. It is estimated by the World Health Organization that some 2 million girls may have the operation every year (Sala & Manara 2001). The prevalence of FGM is estimated to be 98% in some countries (BMA 2001: 361). It takes place in South-east Asia, the Middle East and in many African countries. The cultural rationale for this practice is described (Sala & Manara 2001: 248) as follows:

> *These procedures are intended to have several aims, the most important being the preservation of female chastity, because, after the operation, women cannot have sexual intercourse. A girl, once infibulated, is 're-opened' surgically so that her husband may have sexual intercourse with her, reassured that he is the first and only man to do so. This is essential both for the man's sense of pride and the woman's respectability and virtue. Men from areas where the practice is used hold uncircumcised women in contempt as immoral and disgusting. It meets a cultural requirement because it has social, moral and religious implications.*

The health implications of FGM are wide-ranging and potentially fatal. In addition to severe pain, bleeding and infection, women experience problems with urination, menstruation and intercourse. It also impacts on their reproductive health and may result in infertility and difficulties in childbirth. There is an increased risk of stillbirth, bleeding and maternal death (BMA 2001: 362).

Comfort is clearly in a difficult position. It may be that she knows a good deal about FGM from her personal or cultural experience and may be culturally competent in terms of knowledge, awareness and sensitivity. However, she now works as a midwife in the United Kingdom. It is most likely that she will be aware that FGM is against British law. She may well be committed to human rights but also have views about the importance of cultural rights even though she considers this practice 'abhorrent'. So how is Comfort to think of this situation? What is she to do? What should health professionals generally do in such a situation?

Comfort's dilemma also raises issues of cultural relativism and universalism. The situation can also be framed in terms of 'a paradox of multicultural societies'; John Harris (1982) introduces this as follows:

> *Most obviously culture is an important source of a person's sense of her own identity, of who she is and where, and to what, she belongs. Cultures are classically centred on a religion or on some other set of deeply held beliefs, but culture ranges far wider than this. Acceptance of other cultures' equal rights to exist, or to co-exist, involves not simply their freedom to believe, but also to be.*

Disrespect for culture is not only insulting but also injurious including the 'injury of suffering injustice' (Harris 1982: 223). Harris points to the ethical imperative to respect cultures equally. There is, however, a problem or a 'paradox'. Harris outlines it as follows:

> *The problem arises in connection with any culture which does not equally respect its own members. It looks as though a society committed to equality and containing such cultures or sub-cultures within it, is caught in a genuine and uncomfortable dilemma. If the society wishes to show to each*

individual the same concern and respect that it accords to any, then it may be required to outlaw, frustrate or at the very least condemn, important features of a constituent and discriminatory culture. While if it respects all cultures equally a society may find itself endorsing culturally enshrined inequalities.

FGM is one such activity that illustrates the nature of this 'paradox of multiculturalism'. As has been discussed above, professional codes of workers in health and social care direct them to treat service users and patients fairly and with dignity. These are key values within a multicultural society. However, whilst there appears to be some cultural rationale for FGM it seriously impacts on the health of women, is carried out on children below the age of consent and is discriminatory in that it subjects girls and women to torturous practices compromising their general and sexual health.

Paradoxes and dilemmas are not easily or readily resolvable. This is certainly not something Comfort can or should respond to alone. It will be necessary to discuss the issue in the multiprofessional team and to consider local, national and international policies. Comfort's situation is also not unique. As the BMA (2001: 363) states:

In the UK too doctors may have to provide after-care and continuing care for such patients [those who have undergone FGM]. In addition, they may come into contact with requests for re-infibulation after a woman has given birth. Custom demands that a woman be re-infibulated – the labia stitched together again – after each childbirth. To comply with such requires breaches of standards of medical ethics and possibly the law. UK law, for example, which prohibits FGM, also prohibits the repair of the vulva in this way.

The BMA recommends that the first priority is to counsel the woman and her husband, if this is possible, to 'ensure that they understand the effects and risks of infibulation' (2001: 363). It is pointed out that a discussion with the couple is more likely to be effective.

Despite efforts by women's groups, the World Health Organization and health professional groups, FGM continues to be one of the most challenging and culturally entrenched practices which compromises the health and, arguably, the dignity and human rights of women. Sala & Manara (2001: 256) have this to say in concluding their discussion of the role of nurses in relation to FGM:

Our conclusion is that tolerance in practice and relativism at the epistemological level are not enough to cope with value and cultural conflicts. An example of such conflict is the question of infibulation. Tolerance is necessary for peaceful coexistence, but this is not sufficient.

Indeed, we must be able to recognise all cultural features without prejudice. Respect for culture is an expression of respect for people independent of their race, culture and sex. Everybody has the right to be treated as an equal; equality must include respect for individual differences. However, we must first respect human rights and dignity. Individual rights and dignity must be defended, even against a cultural group.

The next issue to be discussed regarding ethics and culture is less dramatic than FGM but it is no less challenging. It is the everyday issue of information-giving.

CULTURAL ASPECTS OF INFORMATION-GIVING

(c) Mr Achilleas is 75 years old, describes himself as Greek and speaks little English. He has been admitted to hospital for tests following weight loss and abdominal pain. During his admission he develops a rapport with his named nurse, Carmelina, who speaks Greek. He tells her: 'If the tests come back positive and I have cancer, I want to know. I know my family has told you not to tell me, but pay no attention to what they say.' Mr Achilleas' family, however, tell Carmelina: 'If our father's tests reveal that he has cancer, we must be told and under no circumstances is he to be told. We know him and this news will kill him. The family is best placed to handle this information.' (Adapted from Johnstone (1999: 152–153).)

The professional codes referred to in earlier sections pointed to the importance of information-giving, of respect for autonomy and of workers in health and social care demonstrating the ethical qualities of honesty and trustworthiness. Generally, information-giving in health and social care highlights a range of questions relevant to different ethical approaches: Will sharing negative information or bad news result in more harm than good? Will the good consequences outweigh the bad? Do health and social care workers have a duty to tell the truth, the whole truth and nothing but the truth? When cultural issues are thrown into the ethical equation things become even more complex. In some cultures individual autonomy is thought to be a lesser ethical consideration than family decision-making. Such appears to be the case in Mr Achilleas' situation.

Carmelina has a dilemma. If she respects Mr Achilleas' wishes she goes against the wishes of the family. If she respects the family's wishes she is going against Mr Achilleas' request. If Carmelina has knowledge of certain aspects of Greek culture she may hesitate to follow the directives in the Nursing and Midwifery Code (2004) emphasizing a patient's right to have information about his condition. A similar situation is discussed by Megan-Jane Johnstone where a doctor discloses the diagnosis with the patient. The close involvement of the family is likely to be valued by people from a traditional cultural background, particularly during periods of illness or suffering. Family involvement is considered an important part of the therapeutic process and this appears to be the case in the situation of Mr Achilleas.

Johnstone discusses empirical research suggesting that sharing a diagnosis of cancer with a patient who comes from a traditional background such as that, perhaps, of Mr Achilleas may result in premature death. She explains what is called 'the nocebo phenomenon' described as the 'negative effect on health of beliefs and expectations – and therefore the exact reverse of the "placebo" phenomenon' (Johnstone 1999: 148). It seems that during the 1950s and 1960s there were few hospitals in rural Greece and little effective treatment available, resulting in painful deaths from cancer. It is thought that, due to this experience, receiving a diagnosis of cancer can be devastating. Johnstone (1999: 149) points out:

> . . . even mentioning the word 'cancer' is sufficient to trigger in ill persons an overwhelming sense of hopelessness which ultimately finds its expression in their losing their will to live. Under these circumstances, to tell such patients, would probably be sufficient to trigger the nocebo phenomenon, resulting in the ill person's premature death.

So in the light of this what is Carmelina to do? Should she assume that Mr Achilleas is likely to succumb to the 'nocebo phenomenon' and conclude that his diagnosis should be withheld from him and shared with his family instead? Cultural competence does not mean drawing conclusions about one person's care on the basis of a statement of preferences and some knowledge or evidence is needed which relates to *this* person's situation.

There are then alternative strategies. One is to have a discussion – in collaboration with other members of the multiprofessional team – with Mr Achilleas and his family, early in his admission, to discuss information-giving generally. It may then be established what the rationale is for the preferences expressed. Carmelina would also then be in a position to share with patient and family what her professional duties require in terms of honesty and trustworthiness. In addition to the challenges relating to individual autonomy and family decision-making autonomous choice can present other challenges. This is the focus of the next section.

THE LIMITS OF RESPECT FOR AUTONOMY IN RELATION TO CULTURAL PREFERENCES

> (d) Mr McLaughlin is an older person who lives in a rural part of Scotland. Following a visit from Shirin, a social worker who describes herself as 'Mauritian', he phones the social services office. He complains that this 'young woman can't understand me. Can I have a Scottish social worker instead?'

However culturally competent workers in health and social care may be, it is not always the case that patients or service users will respond positively. In the discussion earlier regarding rights and duties it was pointed out that whilst there is much focus on patient or service user rights and worker duties, rights also apply to workers and arguably, duties to patients and service users. There is, at least, anecdotal evidence that workers encounter racism in their day-to-day work. Some hospitals in the UK have also formulated policies banning repeatedly violent or abusive patients from their premises. But is this what is at issue here? What should Shirin's manager do? Should she encourage Shirin to persist in attempting to form a therapeutic relationship with Mr McLaughlin? Or should she replace Shirin with a worker of the same cultural background as Mr McLaughlin?

It is unclear why Mr McLaughlin is expressing a preference for a 'Scottish social worker'. Is he expressing racism or has there been some misunderstanding with Shirin? Rather than making assumptions on little information, Shirin's manager needs to find out more. It may have been the case that Shirin was not sufficiently culturally competent, paying insufficient attention to her own cultural identity or that of Mr McLaughlin. It may be that he is indeed expressing prejudice towards a worker with a different cultural identity. More details are, of course, required to understand this situation. Perhaps if he had had an opportunity to discuss his discomfort with Shirin then there would have been no complaint. It may, of course, also be the case that Mr McLaughlin might become aggressive should his request be refused and Shirin's safety is compromised on a future visit.

A number of ethical issues arise in relation to this situation. There are again issues of autonomy (does Mr McLaughlin have a right to choose?), dignity (how is acknowledgement of the value of worth of both best demonstrated?) and a balancing of benefit and harm. Are Mr McLaughlin and Shirin likely to benefit or be harmed as a result of the continuation of the relationship? There are also justice issues in terms of resources. Is it just or fair or, given scarce human resources, to permit services users or patients to select a worker of their choice? Or does this necessarily result in condoning discriminatory practice.

There are no easy responses to these questions or to the dilemma emerging from the vignette. Workers are equally deserving of rights and need to have their well-being and interests safeguarded. Not all service users or patients will have had the same exposure to the positive aspects of a multicultural society. Living in a rural part of Scotland, service users like Mr McLaughlin, for example, may have had no previous contact with non-British health or social care workers. The issue of the cultural competence of service users is an interesting one. Requiring that patients or service users have training in this area seems unrealistic but it does seem sensible to do some preparatory work when it is anticipated that there may be cultural barriers to the development of worker/service user relationships.

Whilst having training in cultural competence is likely to enhance workers' knowledge, awareness and sensitivity to cultural aspects of their practice, it does not guarantee it. The next section discusses the challenge of cultural complacency.

AVOIDING CULTURAL COMPLACENCY

> (e) Joanne is an occupational therapist in mental health and has just completed training in cultural competence. She comes back to work full of enthusiasm and keenness to share what she has learnt. She tells colleagues that she would like to take referrals from patients from culturally diverse backgrounds because 'I've learnt all about them'. Joanne makes it clear that she is less interested in, what she calls, 'indigenous' patients.

This final example is included as a cautionary vignette. Workers and educators need to be alert to the potential dangers of complacency and perhaps arrogance which may be an undesirable and unintended consequence of undertaking a training or education programme relating to cultural competence. In Joanne's case there appears to be an over-confidence regarding what she believes she has learnt. It is clearly not possible to 'learn all about' all cultural groups. It is crucially important that individuals are treated as such – as individuals with complex histories and possibly a range of cultural identities. Joanne also errs in indicating an interest in non-'indigenous' patients, suggesting perhaps that 'indigenous' patients were less interesting or less in need of culturally competent health or social care. This is misguided. Everywhere there is culture and everywhere cultures interacting. Cultural competence is not required only for the exotic but also for the everyday.

These ideas are echoed by Seibert et al (2002: 143), who share their experience of challenges that may arise in teaching:

> *Labelling and generalising those who are different, based on global and ignorant stereotypes, are major contributors to the problem of being culturally uneducated. One could argue that labelling assists in grouping people for sampling or organising, but when considering a person as an individual, it is inaccurate and largely unfair. We were recently amused to hear a person who had enrolled in a workshop focused on American Indian culture say that she was 'going to learn about how Indians think'. The world would be very simple indeed if a person could attend a single workshop and miraculously learn how all members of a particular group think.*

The last word in this section, which would serve as a response to Joanne, goes to O'Hagan (2001: 243), who states:

> *Some writers and researchers restrict their learning efforts to one particular culture. They may know the culture thoroughly, belong to it, speak the language and be able to function as an interpreter. They are truly experts and will have no difficulty in working effectively within that culture. This does not necessarily mean that they will be culturally competent working within and providing a service for all cultures. If they are uninterested in*

other cultures which they encounter in their work they cannot be cultur-
ally competent. Cultural competence, as Leigh (1998) states, is about
demonstrating the capacity to form and sustain relationships with people
from contrasting cultures. It is about sincerity, effort and openness in
response to all cultures encountered in one's professional practice.

CONCLUSION – TOWARDS A TRANSCULTURAL ETHICS?

This chapter has provided an overview of five ethical perspectives commonly referred to in relation to the conduct or actions and character of
health and social care professions. It has been emphasized that the predominant Western approaches to ethics need to be considered in relation
to non-Western approaches. There appears to be some common ground
in the different approaches but also significant differences in the philosophical and religious systems in which ethics is embedded.

A range of challenges have been discussed in relation to ethics and
culture and it has been suggested that there is a place for duty-based and
rights-based perspectives in particular. A human rights framework is
necessary but this does not mean there is no scope for a consideration of
the specificity of cultures and individuals' situations. All of the approaches
to ethics outlined here and the values therein need to be interpreted in
relation to the cultural context. So can there be a transcultural ethics,
an ethics that transcends cultural differences and provides guidance for
all health and social care workers?

Megan-Jane Johnstone (1999: 159–160) proposes the following definition of a transcultural approach to ethics:

Transcultural ethics, like feminist ethics, recognises the inherent difficul-
ties associated with genuine moral problems in human life . . . It also rec-
ognises the inability of abstract and decontextualised moral thinking to
provide concrete answers to complex questions concerning a range of
human experiences. Key among these experiences are: human pain and
suffering, intense and sometimes conflicting human emotions, ambivalent
and ambiguous human relationships, and, not least, differing cultural
world views about the value and meaning of life – all of which often (too
often) have to be dealt with in the face of overwhelming uncertainty, the
unpredictability of probable outcomes (positive and negative), fallible
modes of communication, and the fallibilities of decision-makers [. . .]
Unlike other moral critiques, however, transcultural ethics offers an opti-
mistic outlook. Its suggestion that acceptance of – and achieving a harmony
of – moral diversity offers the key to sustaining the existence and purpose
of morality provides an important basis upon which we can all develop,
not just our moral thinking and sensibilities, but our ability to actually
be moral in a world characterised by diverse and competing valid world
views. This is not merely compromise, as some might believe, or even toler-
ance – the blinded eye of an indiscriminate mind [. . .] Nor is it confusion.
Rather, it is celebration. In particular, it is the celebration of the 'other' as

*different, but not inferior or fallacious or superstitious – as having some-
thing worthwhile to share, not as being something worthless to be marginalized, trivialized and ignored. If we accept this, we will all be in a
much better position to judge what is really unethical as opposed to being
merely disliked; what is truly wrong, as opposed to being merely unfamiliar and strange; and what is really confusion as opposed to simple misunderstanding of another's moral language with which we are not familiar.*

Johnstone's view of transcultural ethics has a number of strengths:

- There is recognition of the challenging nature of everyday ethical
  issues.
- There is an acknowledgement of the limitations of approaches to ethics
  that focus solely on abstract thinking, ignoring contexts.
- Attention is drawn to the complexity of human experience and
  relationships.
- It is accepted that there is much uncertainty and unpredictability in
  everyday life and that humans are fallible.
- The value of moral diversity is celebrated.

What Johnstone proposes does not seem to contradict the pluralist
perspective on ethics adopted in this chapter. A range of ethical
approaches coexist in relation to health and social care. These are primarily Western approaches. Common values are identifiable in these quite
diverse approaches, for example dignity, autonomy, justice, promoting
good and working towards diminishing harm. Cultural competence also
requires some familiarity with non-Western approaches and a commitment to identifying common ground and areas of divergence. Ethical
approaches, be they Western or non-Western, offer no panacea towards
the resolution of ethical challenges. What an understanding of theoretical
and professional approaches does do is contribute to reflective practice.
It is essential that practitioners are not complacent, can tolerate uncertainty and ambiguity and have the humility and honesty to engage in
self-scrutiny and demonstrate a commitment to working towards ethical
and cultural competence.

**REFLECTIVE
QUESTIONS**

1. Consider your own views of ethics – do you tend to focus on actions
   or moral qualities and character?
2. What ethical approaches are you aware of in your everyday work in
   health and social care?
3. What ethical challenges have you encountered in your personal and/
   or professional life?
4. Do you think ethics or values are relative to individual cultures or do
   you think they are universal?
5. How would you have responded to the situation or views of the
   workers in each of the five vignettes?
6. Reflect on your learning from this chapter – how might this contribute
   to culturally competent health and social care?

Acknowledgements I would like to thank the Editor, Professor Irena Papadopoulos, and Sarah Banles for their helpful and generous comments on this chapter.

REFERENCES

Baker C 1997 Cultural relativism and cultural diversity: Implications for nursing practice. Advances in Nursing Science 20(1):3–11

BBC 2003 Fears over elderly mental health care. Online. Available: http://news.bbc.co.uk/1/hi/england/manchester/1313334.stm 24 Sep 2003

Beauchamp T L, Childress J F 2001 Principles of biomedical ethics. 5th edn. Oxford University Press, Oxford

British Medical Association 2001 The medical profession and human rights: Handbook for a changing agenda. Zed Books in association with the BMA, London

Bilimoria P 1991 Indian ethics. In: Singer P (ed) A companion to ethics. Blackwell, Oxford

Bosely S 1998 Arrogance let babies die – now a chance to mend NHS. The Guardian 19 July 19, front page

De Silva P 199 Buddhist ethics. In: Singer P (ed) A companion to ethics. Blackwell, Oxford

Devettere R J 2002 Introduction to virtue ethics: insights of the ancient Greeks. Georgetown University Press, Washington

General Medical Council 1995 Good medical practice: guidance from the General Medical Council. London

Glover J 1999 Humanity – a moral history of the twentieth century. Jonathon Cape, London

Hansen C 1991 Classical Chinese ethics. In: Singer P (ed) A companion to ethics. Blackwell, Oxford

Harris J 1982 A paradox of multicultural societies. Journal of Philosophy of Education 16(2):223–229

Harris J 1985 The value of life: An introduction to medical ethics. Routledge, London

Human Rights Act 1998 HMSO, London

Johnstone M-J 1999 Bioethics: a nursing perspective. 3rd edn. Harcourt Saunders, Sydney

Kellner M 1991 Jewish ethics. In: Singer P (ed) A companion to ethics. Blackwell, Oxford

Lawrence J 2001 Routine abuse of elderly in NHS care. The Independent 28 March

Leigh J 1998 Communication for cultural competence. Allyn and Bacon, Sydney.

Lifton R J 1986 The Nazi doctors: A study of the psychology of evil. Macmillan, London

Lifton R J 1988 The Nazi doctors: Medical killing and the psychology of genocide. Basic Books, New York

Macklin R 1999 Against relativism: Cultural diversity and the search for ethical universals in medicine. Oxford University Press, New York

Mill J S 1962 Utilitarianism. Fontana Press

Nanji A 1991 Islamic ethics. In: Singer P (ed) A companion to ethics. Blackwell, Oxford

Nursing and Midwifery Council (2004) Code of professional conduct. NMC, London

O'Hagan K 2001 Cultural competence in the caring professions. Jessica Kingsley, London

Papadopoulos I, Tilki M, Taylor G 1998 Transcultural care. A guide for health care professionals. Quay Books, Dinton

Paton H J 1948 The moral law: Kant's groundwork of the metaphysic of morals. Hutchinson, London

Pink G 1994 The price of truth. British Medical Journal 309:1700–1705

Sala R, Manara D 2001 Nurses and requests for female genital mutilation: Cultural rights versus human rights. Nursing Ethics 8(3):247–258

Seibert P, S, Stridh-Igo P, Zimmerman C G 2002 A checklist to facilitate cultural awareness and sensitivity. Journal of Medical Ethics 28:143–146

Singer P (ed) 1993 A companion to ethics. Blackwell, Oxford

Social Care Council 2002 Code of practice for social care workers. Online. Available: http://www.gscc.org.uk/codes_practice.htm 28 Dec 2004

Steppe H 1997 Nursing under totalitarian regimes: the case of national socialism. In: Rafferty A M, Robinson J, Elkan R (eds) Nursing history and the politics of welfare. Routledge, London

Vardy P, Grosch P 1999 The puzzle of ethics. Fount/Harper Collins, London

Chapter **6**

Promoting culturally competent research

Irena Papadopoulos

LEARNING OBJECTIVES

Having read this chapter, you should be able to:
• understand the relevance of culturally competent research to the construction of knowledge in the twenty-first century
• define culturally competent research
• list the main constructs of the Papadopoulos model of culturally competent research
• discuss the underpinning principles and characteristics of culturally competent research.

INTRODUCTION

I have defined culturally competent research as research that both utilizes and develops knowledge and skills which promote the delivery of health care that is sensitive and appropriate to individuals' needs, whatever their cultural background (Papadopoulos 2005).

Despite the cultural diversity of most societies in today's world, Porter & Villarruel (1993) argue that a unicultural perspective in research prevails, which assumes that concepts, and explanations of relationships between concepts, are universally applicable across different cultures. Research continues to exclude 'culture', and its related concept of 'ethnicity', as essential variables even though in the last 25 years there has been a growing realization that our understanding of health and illness has to be considered not only in terms of biological factors, but also in terms of social and cultural determinants (Dahlgren & Whitehead 1991). One reason for this has been the continuing domination of the health research agenda by positivistic approaches with a focus on objective measurement, emphasis on facts, prediction, and production of value-free, universal truths. Further, most of the research in the UK (and other developed countries) continues to be focused on the majority culture and is primarily undertaken by researchers who belong to the majority culture. This inevitably has affected the way research priorities and research problems are conceptualized, defined and funded.

However, the research agenda is very slowly becoming more balanced, primarily due to the persisting health inequalities worldwide, which are forcing governments to invest in research that aims to understand the impact of socio-economic and cultural factors on health. In addition, the pluralistic nature of our society has heightened awareness of the need for research paradigms that can deal with the needs of culturally and ethnically diverse populations, in more effective and sensitive ways. The need for new paradigms is also becoming more evident and compelling in a global world. Health problems in one country quickly become problems of all countries. The recent outbreak of SARS in China amply demonstrated the importance of generating knowledge across national and cultural divides. Irrespective of the scale of the research projects – international, national or local – researchers need to understand the world views of their collaborators and target populations; otherwise the chances of generating invalid results are high.

It is important to clarify at this point that we are all cultural beings. Therefore a culturally competent research approach is not aimed only at researching the health needs and problems of minority ethnic groups. It is also important to realize that such an approach not only applies to qualitative research, but also equally to quantitative research designs.

A MODEL FOR THE DEVELOPMENT OF CULTURALLY COMPETENT RESEARCHERS

Papadopoulos et al (1998) first proposed a model for developing culturally competent health practitioners, which consisted of the four constructs: cultural awareness, cultural knowledge, cultural sensitivity and cultural competence (see Ch. 2 for an expanded explanation of the model). Papadopoulos & Lees (2002) have adapted these constructs to address culturally competent research as they believe that a framework, rather than a 'pot-pourri', approach to training is far more preferable and effective (Fig. 6.1).

CULTURAL AWARENESS

This begins with the researchers examining, reflecting on, and challenging their own personal value base and understanding how these values are socially and culturally constructed. This means that culturally com-

Figure 6.1   Concepts of culturally competent research. Adapted from Papadopoulos et al (1998).

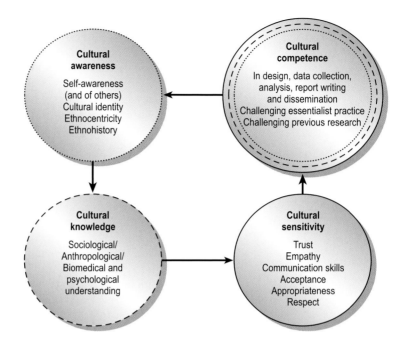

petent research is reflexive research. It requires researchers to be conscious of and to make explicit their positions in the research process, irrespective of their chosen research design. We are all products of, and members of, dynamic cultures. We all hold cultural values and cultural biases and can be ethnocentric. However, we are not always fully aware of our cultural values or may be deluding ourselves that our values are universal. And if we lack cultural self-awareness then we most probably are not aware of our biases and ethnocentricity. I suggest that cultural self-awareness is a prerequisite to understanding the cultural values of others. Since research is about the production of knowledge and since no knowledge is neutral and its objectivity can be challenged, it becomes imperative that researchers make every effort to become culturally aware and to make their cultural and value positions absolutely clear during all stages of the research process. Leininger (1995) points out that without cultural awareness researchers tend to impose their beliefs, values and patterns of behaviour upon cultures other than their own. She suggests that this leads to invalid research. To avoid invalid research we need to become culturally competent reflexive researchers who acknowledge the impact of our own history, identity, experiences, beliefs and culture on the processes and outcomes of inquiry.

When cultural self-awareness is achieved, researchers aspiring to be culturally competent should endeavour to become aware of the cultural values and norms of those they wish to study. One way to reach this is by making a serious effort to understand the ethnohistory of the population under study. This means that historical, geographical, political and sociocultural information must be studied during the preparation of the research proposal and at the start of the project. If we fail to do this we should seriously question ourselves as to whether we are using the best methods to collect data, whether we are sensitive and effective enough during the data collection stages, and whether our analysis and interpretation is valid.

Ethnohistorical information is not only important for the researcher, it is also useful for the reader of the research report or articles which may result from the research study. Ethnohistory provides background and context and helps the reader to make sense of the findings, discussion and conclusions.

CULTURAL KNOWLEDGE

You may find it strange when I say that cultural knowledge is not only about culture! This is because within the context of the Papadopoulos et al (1998) model 'cultural knowledge' is about the acquisition of all kinds of knowledge which will enable us to become culturally competent. Relevant knowledge can be drawn or produced by different disciplines such as anthropology, sociology, psychology, nursing, medicine, biology and so on. In Chapter 2, I explained that transcultural health and nursing is the study and research of *cultural* diversities and similarities in health and illness as well as their underpinning societal and organizational *structures*, in order to understand current practice and to contribute to its future development in a culturally responsive way. I went on to provide some examples of how the various disciplines contributed to the development of knowledge aimed at understanding people's health and illness. One of my chosen examples from sociology is knowledge about the construction, the use and abuse of power and its relevance to health professionals who wish to become culturally competent. However, as I mentioned earlier, much of the knowledge we use in nursing and the health field in general has been produced using research paradigms that are researcher/expert driven, and which value objectivity and generalizable knowledge. Community activists, particularly in the developing countries, have been questioning this approach to research for some time. In their view, the research activity and thus the construction of knowledge should be more relevant to ordinary people, who have been excluded in this process due to the scientific language used by researchers in all stages of research, from the articulation of the problem, to the construction of research tools, to the analysis and dissemination of findings which were (and continue to be) inaccessible to most ordinary people.

In the last 20 years (probably more) a new research paradigm which addresses the above concerns has emerged. This is called *participatory research* (PR). This approach is not proposing the use of different or new methods for collecting data such as surveys, interviews, focus groups and so on; rather it proposes a new ideology of doing research and of producing knowledge. All research methods can be used in participatory research provided they are used within its ideological framework.

Finn (1994) outlines three key elements that distinguish participatory research from traditional approaches to social and other sciences: *people*, *power* and *praxis*. It is people-centred (Brown 1985) in the sense that the process of critical inquiry is informed by and responds to their experiences and needs. Participatory research is about giving power to ordinary people. Power is crucial to the construction of reality, language, meanings and rituals of truth (Foucault 1973). Participatory research promotes empowerment through the development of common knowledge and critical awareness which are suppressed by the dominant knowledge system. Participatory research is also about praxis (Lather 1986, Maguire 1987). It recognizes the inseparability of theory and practice and critical awareness of the personal-political dialectic. Participatory research is grounded in an explicit political stance and clearly articulated value base of social justice and the transformation of those contemporary sociocultural structures and processes that support degeneration of participatory democracy, injustice and inequality.

One of the possible outcomes of the production of knowledge within the ideology of participatory research is the avoidance of essentialism, which assumes that there are essential cultural differences between people that always override other aspects of their being. Douglas (1998) suggested that a common essentialist practice in research is the assignment of health problems to the culture of an individual to the exclusion of other important influences, such as country of origin, area of residence, socio-economic status and gender.

Culturally competent research is research that takes into account the ideology of participatory research. The production of knowledge along these lines is still in its infancy; the approach has been and will continue to be challenged by those convinced that only the traditional methods of inquiry are 'scientific' and able to produce 'objective' and generalizable knowledge. However, health professionals must question both the validity and desirability of such claims. Guba & Lincoln (1989) – amongst many others – provide a convincing argument which concludes that the detached ('objective') posture of researcher–researched is untenable, as research is a human process, inevitably reflecting the values of human constructors. These values enter into inquiry at choice points such as the problem selection, the instruments and the analytic methods used, the interpretations, conclusions and recommendations made.

CULTURAL SENSITIVITY

People-centred research is not only a key principle when dealing with research issues around cultural knowledge. Considering research participants as true partners is an essential component of cultural sensitivity in research and a crucial element in anti-oppressive practice (Dalrymple & Burke 1995). Partnership demands that power relationships are challenged and that real choices are offered to people. These outcomes involve a process of facilitation, advocacy and negotiation that can only be achieved on a foundation of trust, respect and empathy.

Attention to researcher communication skills is a key component of cultural sensitivity. Enabling research participants to communicate in their native language, particularly when the research topic is one that will cause them distress or when the participant does not have full mastery of the primary language of the investigation, not only shows sensitivity but will provide better quality data. Of course communication is not just about language. It also includes body language, awareness of acceptable behaviours, such as appropriate ways of greeting people, being sensitive to customs and rules such as those governing status, privacy, gender, time and so on; all these sensitivities apply during all stages of the research process but are particularly important during the data collection stage. Becoming a culturally sensitive communicator is an essential skill for researchers. This has to be learned and refined in the same way that the skill of constructing a questionnaire, or the skill of analysing data has to be learned.

An example of culturally sensitive research is the matching of the ethnicity and culture of the interviewer with that of the participant whenever possible. This encourages a more equal context for interviewing which allows more sensitive and accurate information to be collected. A researcher with the same ethnic and cultural background as the participant will possess 'a rich fore understanding' (Ashworth 1986), an insider/'emic' view (Leininger 1991, Kauffman 1994) will have more favourable access conditions, the cooperation of a large number of people (Hanson 1994), and a genuine interest in the health and welfare of their community (Hillier & Rachman 1996). Care should be taken to counteract the disadvantages of ethnic/cultural matching. As far back as 1978, Kratz suggested that researchers who share the target community's culture and ethnic background may take some of what the research participant is saying for granted and are less likely to ask those naive questions which could yield useful explanations. Hammersley & Atkinson (1995) advise that in order to avoid over-identification and over-rapport with the population being studied, the researcher should aim to adopt a marginal position of simultaneous insider/outsider, and be intellectually poised between familiarity and strangeness. Although they acknowledge that this is very difficult to achieve, it is not impossible. Burman (1996), on the other hand, suggested that having easy access and cooperation may result in exploitation of the group. For this reason, culturally competent research should be underpinned by both professional ethics and internationally agreed codes of ethics and human rights.

Another example of culturally sensitive research is the notion of content equivalence. This requires the researcher to ensure that the questions asked are relevant to the target culture and that they do not include concepts that are offending, as for instance asking a devout Muslim to state how much alcohol he consumes per week, or an orthodox Jew if his newborn son will be circumcized. Naturally, if there is a strong rationale for conducting research on such culturally sensitive topics, this must be done following an extensive immersion into the particular culture and in collaboration with appropriate people from that culture, in order to prepare the data collection phase in as sensitive a way as possible.

CULTURAL COMPETENCE

This requires the synthesis and application of previously gained awareness, knowledge and sensitivity. An important component of this stage is the ability to recognize and challenge forms of racialized/discriminatory thinking such as essentialism, ethnocentricity and racism. Here I discuss how key stages of the research process can be made culturally competent, illustrating my points with examples from two of the research projects I have conducted with colleagues: (1) the EMBRACE UK (Papadopoulos & Gebrehiwot 2002, see Ch. 8), which investigated the Ethiopian refugees' beliefs, migration and adaptation processes, and their experiences with the healthcare system, and (2) the Health ASERT Programme Wales (see Ch. 11), which investigated the health promotion needs of minority ethnic groups, refugees, Gypsy Travellers and New Age Travellers.

Study design

As discussed above, the involvement of the target community is crucial at the study design stage. Such involvement will ensure that the research problem is firmly responding to the realities and perceptions of the target groups, and is sensitively articulated and presented. The Health ASERT Wales was initiated by the National Assembly for Wales, Health Promotion Division; however, my colleagues and I began by trying to understand the cultural and structural issues related to the target groups by consulting the published literature as well as numerous key individuals involved with local and national organizations dealing with the research target groups. Not only did we become more aware of the specific health promotion issues that concerned the target groups, we were also sensitized about the acceptable research methods and were questioned about our commitment to future actions which might result from the knowledge generation that we were to embark on.

Research participants

In both the Health ASERT Programme Wales, and the EMBRACE UK projects, target groups' participation was sought through their involvement in the development of the research proposal and data collection instruments, in the collection and provision of data through individual interviews, focus groups and questionnaires, in the transcription of interviews and translation of transcripts, in the validation of findings, and in the case of the EMBRACE UK project, in the dissemination of findings too.

It is essential that clear and detailed inclusion and exclusion criteria for research participants are developed in consultation with the collaborating organizations or the community representatives involved in the research design. It is important not to exclude sections of the target group because they are difficult to reach, such as refugee groups, or reluctant to participate, such as Gypsy Travellers, or even discouraged from participating, as in the case of women in some cultural groups. Nevertheless, numerous ethical dilemmas may arise so broad ethical principles, such as avoidance of actions that may violate the moral standards of the cultures involved, or avoidance of causing harm, should be upheld (see Ch. 5 for a detailed discussion on transcultural ethics). Guidance and advice from the community representatives is also crucial and the research team may have to modify their commonly used techniques, as in the case of sampling, to more unconventional ones. For example, it may be more realistic to opt for a purposive sample for a survey since a random sample would be impossible to achieve. Other examples include considerations around research variables such as age, ethnicity, education, marital status and so on, all of which must be expressed in ways that are meaningful to the communities being studied. For example, in the EMBRACE UK project, based on the advice given by our partners we used three age groups: 12–25 (adolescents and young adults), 25–59 (mid-life), and 60 + (elders).

Data collection

Culturally competent researchers realize that data collection raises numerous language issues. What language do the targeted research participants speak? Should information material and data collection tools be produced in different languages or will this be ineffective because large numbers of the target group are illiterate in their own language, or even do not have a written form of the language they speak? If interviews are to be used for collecting data, should the use of an interpreter be preferred over the use of a bi-lingual researcher? If data are collected in a language other than English how is the translation handled to assure quality and accuracy?

Birbili (2003) reports that collecting data in one language and presenting the findings in another is now increasingly common among social researchers. The factors that affect the quality of translation include the linguistic competence of the translator and the translator's knowledge of the culture of the people under study. Temple (1997) points out that the use of translators and interpreters is not merely a technical matter that has little bearing on the outcome, it has epistemological consequences as it influences what is found. Researchers need to constantly discuss and debate conceptual issues with their translators in order to ensure that conceptual equivalence has been achieved. Similarly, readers of the research report need to be informed about who those people were and what kind of role they played at all stages of the research endeavour.

In the EMBRACE UK project, the advice given by our partners was that most interviews would have to be conducted in an Ethiopian language; it was anticipated that most participants would speak the official Ethiopian language, which is the Amhara. The decision was also taken that it would be desirable to recruit bi-lingual researchers to match the characteristics of the participants. Part of the role of those conducting the interviews was to recruit participants with the help of the community organization. Further, we saw the recruitment of a number of Ethiopians for the data collection and first level analysis as capacity building for the Ethiopian community. Eight Ethiopian research assistants were recruited to work on the project on a part-time basis. They all attended a structured training programme to familiarize themselves with the aims of the project, develop and/or refine their interview skills and become fully cognizant of their role. This included: recruiting research participants, gaining consent, arranging a venue for the interview, conducting the interview in the participant's preferred language, tape recording the interview, keeping field notes, attending supervision sessions, transcribing the interviews verbatim, translating the interviews if needed, and identifying what in their views were the main issues of each interview.

During their training the research assistants helped to test the interview schedule. A verbal agreement was reached regarding the comparability of meaning of the concepts to be explored, which were written in English, and those to be used in Amharic. In order to test the accuracy of the translated concepts, the first interview of each research assistant was considered as a pilot. Conceptual comparability or equivalence needs to be taken very seriously as often concepts in one language do not exist in another. For example, Hunt & Bhopal (2003) reported that the term 'feeling blue' has different connotations in different languages, whereas the terms 'check-up' and 'Pap smear' have no conceptual equivalence in any Chinese language.

Helping the research assistants to adopt the marginal position of simultaneous insider/outsider was another topic focused on during training. Particular attention was given to ensure that researchers could follow the lead questions with relevant probing, thus avoiding taking what was said for granted. The research assistants were encouraged to become reflexive and were required during the study to record in their field notes the effect they may have had on research participants and the communication process, as well as how they dealt with a difficult situation, such as being asked to offer help or advice by the research participants during the interview, or when talking about a very sensitive topic such as depression or despair when they may have had much to identify with in that particular situation. The supervision process enabled them to discuss any problems they had encountered and to explore solutions or alternative ways. In fact the research assistants provided useful insights and made practical suggestions, which improved the data collection process.

For the Health ASERT Programme Wales, focus group facilitators who were fluent in the community language were recruited from each of the target communities, except in the case of the Gypsy Travellers' focus groups, which were conducted by two health visitors who had worked with them for a number of years and who were trusted by them. As in the case of the EMBRACE UK project, the facilitators were trained by the research team for their role.

Translating and back–translating interview transcripts

In qualitative research data may be collected through a variety of methods such as one-to-one interviews, focus group interviews, observation, self-completed questionnaires and so on. If data are not in English, written translation to English is a must, even if the research team are fluent in the language used to collect the data. Skipping the translation and back-translation process must be avoided as crucial meanings will be missed. The practice of producing only a summary of the data into English should also be avoided. A culturally competent researcher would ensure that these processes are adequately resourced within a realistic timetable.

Usunier (2003) reports that even basic concepts such as autonomy, leadership, friendliness, motivation, satisfaction, authority, well-being, shame and guilt etc. are often used in research questionnaires as if they had universal meaning. However, words often express meaning shared only in the particular cultural and language group, especially when they relate to perceptions and interactions. I recently discovered that there is no word for 'please' in Finnish. Instead the Finnish word for 'thank you' is used. If concepts are understood differently, there is a great chance that the findings will be, to a large extent, a reflection of differences in understanding.

Once the data are fully translated into English, back-translation should follow in order to assure the accuracy and quality of the translation and to eliminate any translation-related problems. Back-translation ensures that translation was not an exercise of mere lexical equivalence, but one of conceptual equivalence too. Firstly, target language transcripts are translated into English and then the English transcripts are translated back to the target language by a second bi-lingual person (not involved with the original translation efforts). The two versions of the target language transcripts are then compared to determine how closely they match. A close match indicates that the translator is competent.

As discussed above, the bi-lingual interviewers of the EMBRACE UK project also transcribed and translated the interviews into English. The project employed three Ethiopian academics to act as back-translators. At the early stage of the data collection processes, a translated transcript from each interviewer was randomly selected and submitted for back-translation. The original Ethiopian transcript and the one produced by the back-translator were then read and carefully compared by the leader of the partner organization who was also the co-director of the project. Differences in expression were identified but the reviewer was satisfied that the conceptual meaning remained true to the original transcript. This process assured the research team that the English translations were of good quality and none of the original meaning was lost or misrepresented. For, despite the training and supervision given to interviewers and the fact they are more likely to understand the meaning intended by the interviewees than an 'outsider' researcher, there is a danger of producing an edited English version of the original transcript for a number of reasons. For example, in another study conducted under my supervision, where the interview included questions on the sexual behaviour of Arab Muslim women, it was discovered through the back-translation process that the interviewer/translator had omitted or rephrased small portions of the interview which in her view were portraying these women in a negative light.

To ensure the linguistic and conceptual accuracy of the translated Health ASERT Programme Wales transcripts, a modified back-translation exercise was performed. An individual from each of the focus groups conducted in a mother tongue was asked to ensure that:

(a) the translation conveyed the correct information and meaning
(b) the translator did not alter or omit any information; and

(c) the translator had used language that accurately conveyed the emotional weight and conceptual value expressed by the original speaker.

Data analysis and validation

The methodological rigour described above prepares the way for a rigorous analysis. However, even this may not guard the researchers against unwitting ethnocentricity and cultural bias during the analysis process. This could result in the perpetuation of essentialist views and may lead to oppressive and racist attitudes amongst policy-makers and service providers. It is therefore important that various approaches are adopted to ensure that this does not happen and that the analysis is accurate, fair and sensitively presented. Validating the analysis is an important process in qualitative research. Silverman (1993) suggests that there are two forms of validation particularly appropriate for qualitative research, that of triangulation and that of respondent validation. Triangulation is the process through which different kinds of data, or data derived from different methods, are compared to see whether they corroborate one another. Researcher triangulation has also been suggested as good practice. Respondent validation occurs when the findings are taken back to the research participants in order to be verified.

The data from the Health ASERT Wales project were analysed using a constant comparative process of defining and redefining any emerging themes in the light of new data. The emerging themes were elaborated conceptually using theoretical and empirical constructs from the literature. The initial first level analysis of the focus group data was performed by the focus group facilitators. Independent analysis of a random sample of transcripts was performed by myself and a research fellow who worked on the project. It was agreed that a coding frame would be used in order to analyse the remaining transcripts using the computer package NUD*IST. As reported in Chapter 11, respondent validation was undertaken in this project. One participant from each focus group was selected by the focus group facilitators (except the Travellers, where one participant representing all the Traveller subgroups was selected). They were asked to review and validate the findings in terms of:

(a) whether the findings made sense to them
(b) whether the findings represented what they understood to be the main issues that arose in the focus groups, and
(c) whether any important issues raised in the focus groups had been left out. In addition, the focus group findings were discussed during a consultation exercise with the focus group facilitators who were also able to validate the findings.

In the EMBRACE UK project, researcher and methodological triangulation were utilized. Further, the preliminary findings were presented at two peer review conferences, which provided an opportunity for discussion, reflection and validation. The findings were also presented to the steering committee, which was constituted by community representatives (proxy respondent validation) as well as other stakeholders. Given the methodological rigour of the project, and the advantages of a research team that included both 'insiders' (Ethiopians) providing the 'emic' perspective, and 'outsiders' (non-Ethiopians) providing the 'etic' perspective, the research team was confident that the findings were free from cultural bias (non-essentialist), had truth value (credibility), were dependable (reliability) and that they could be applicable to the rest of the Ethiopian UK community (generalizability).

Reporting and disseminating the findings

Reporting the findings should be done in sensitive and inclusive ways. Firstly, it is crucial that members of the participating groups are not excluded during this stage. Secondly, the voices of the participants must be allowed to be heard. Thirdly, the report (or at the minimum its executive summary) must be translated into the community languages of the participants, and if necessary into other formats such as audio tapes, to give them easy access to the findings. Fourthly, dissemination activities such as conferences should not be the exclusivity of the academics, but should involve members of the partner organizations. Fifthly, community mass media should be used as many cultural groups now have access to these media. Sixthly, the reporting and dissemination of the findings must avoid essentialism for all the reasons given in the previous sections. Finally the research report must include an action plan for change. This is an act of respect to the participants who gave their time up, and often much more, in order to contribute to a project which they believed would benefit their community.

CONCLUDING CONSIDERATIONS

In summary, I characterize culturally competent research as:

Reflexive: begins with the attainment of high levels of cultural self-awareness and awareness of the cultures of others

Inclusive: adopts the ideology of participatory research

Relevant: produces knowledge that is relevant and accessible to ordinary people

Non-essentializing: adopts a definition of cultural competence that includes both culture and structure and pays equal attention to both

Rigorous: pays attention to the use of concepts, language, and communication

Ethical: a research model for the twenty-first century diverse world.

It could be argued that a culturally competent approach to research is unrealistic as it may be perceived as long-winded, time-consuming, resource intensive and a needlessly politically correct approach. I would argue that culturally incompetent research is wasteful, dangerous and unethical. It is true that many of the skills I described as essential for culturally competent research need time to be developed, but then competencies of any kind take time to develop. Since most of us would not accept culturally incompetent health care (even though many of us have to for lack of an alternative), why should we regard knowledge or evidence that was derived through culturally incompetent ways as acceptable? And if we believe that research should be rigorous and appropriate then we must factor into our proposals adequate funding and time, and funding bodies must support this. Culturally competent research promotes inclusivity and fairness. Further, the principles I described above are applicable to all types of research. Within the global context of today's information flows, culturally competent research can facilitate high quality cross-cultural and comparative research at national and international levels.

<table>
<tr><td>REFLECTIVE
QUESTIONS</td><td>1. Critically reflect on the importance of culturally competent research in the twenty-first century.
2. Think of a research paper you have recently read. Was the methodology used culturally competent? If it was not, do you feel that the findings are valid?
3. If you were a member of a research funding body, what would you do in order to ensure that you and your colleagues fund research that is culturally competent?</td></tr>
</table>

REFERENCES

Ashworth P (ed) 1986 Qualitative research in psychology. Duquesne University Press, Pittsburgh, PA

Birbili M 2003 Publishing on the internet. Translating from one language to another. Social Research Update 31. University of Surrey. Online. Available: http://www.soc.surrey.ac.uk/sru/SRU31.html 18 Sept 2003

Brown L D 1985 People-centered development and participatory research. Harvard Educational Review 55(1):69–75

Burman E 1996 Interviewing. In: Bannister P, Burman E, Parker I et al Qualitative methods in psychology. A research guide. Open University Press, Buckingham

Dahlgren G, Whitehead M 1991 Policies and strategies to promote equity in health. Institute for Future Studies, Stockholm

Dalrymple J, Burke B 1995 Anti-oppressive practice. Social care and the law. Open University Press, Buckingham

Douglas J 1998 Developing appropriate research methodologies with black and minority ethnic communities. Part 1: reflections on the research process. Health Education Journal 57:329–338

Finn J 1994 The promise of participatory research. Journal of Progressive Human Services 5(2):25–42

Foucault M 1973 The order of things: an archaeology of the human sciences. Vintage Books, New York

Guba E, Lincoln Y 1989 Fourth generation evaluation. Sage, London

Hammersley M, Atkinson P 1995 Ethnography. Principles in practice. 2nd edn. Routledge, London

Hanson E J 1994 Issues concerning the familiarity of researchers with the research setting. Journal of Advanced Nursing 20:940–942

Hillier S, Rachman S 1996 Childhood development and behavioural and emotional problems as perceived by Bangladeshi parents in East London. In: Kelleher D, Hillier S (eds) Researching cultural differences in health. Routledge. London

Hunt S, Bhopal R 2003 Self reports in research with non-English speakers. British Medical Journal 327:352–353

Kauffman K S 1994 The insider/outsider dilemma: Field experience of white researcher 'getting in' a poor black community. Nursing Research 43(3):179–183

Kratz C R 1978 Care of the long-term sick in the community. Churchill Livingstone, London

Lather P 1986 Research as praxis. Harvard Educational Review 56(3):257–277

Leininger M M (ed) 1991 Culture care, diversity and universality: a theory of nursing. NLN Press. New York

Leininger M M 1995 Transcultural nursing. Concepts, theories, research and practices. McGraw-Hill, New York

Maguire P 1987 Doing participatory research: a feminist approach. University of Massachusetts, Amherst

Papadopoulos I 2005 Developing culturally competent researchers: a model for its development. In: Nazroo J (ed) Methods for health and social research in multicultural societies. Taylor and Francis

Papadopoulos I, Gebrehiwot A 2002 The EMBRACE UK Project: Ethiopian migrants, their beliefs, refugeedom, adaptation, calamities, and experiences in the United Kingdom. Research Centre for Transcultural Studies in Health. Middlesex University, London

Papadopoulos I, Lees S 2002 Developing culturally competent researchers. Journal of Advanced Nursing 37(3):258–264

Papadopoulos I, Tilki M, Taylor G 1998 Transcultural care. A guide for health care professionals. Quay Books, Wiltshire

Porter C, Villarruel A 1993 Nursing research with African American and Hispanic people: guidelines for action. Nursing Outlook 41(2):59–67

Silverman D 1993 Interpreting qualitative data: methods for analysing, talk, text and interaction. Sage, London

Temple B 1997 Watch your tongue: issues in translation and cross-cultural research. Sociology 31(3):607–618

Usunier J C 2003 The use of language in investigating conceptual equivalence in cross-cultural research. Online. Available: http://marketing.byu.edu/htmlpages/ccrs/proceedings99/usunier.htm 18 Sept 2003

PART 2

Developing culture–specific competencies

PART CONTENTS

Chapter **7**

Cancer and culture: meanings and experiences

Irena Papadopoulos and Shelley Lees

LEARNING OBJECTIVES

After reading this chapter you should:
• gain understanding of the similarities and differences of cancer meanings and experiences in different cultural groups in the United Kingdom
• understand the role of the health professional in providing culturally competent care to all cancer patients.

INTRODUCTION

With the diminished threat to life from communicable diseases (with the exception of HIV/AIDS) cancer has become one of Western societies' most feared illnesses. Increased incidence of cancer over the last century has made cancer the second major cause of death in developed countries. Moreover, it will continue to be a leading cause of death throughout the world in the twenty-first century, principally due to ageing populations, more effective cures for once fatal communicable diseases, and the rising incidence of certain forms of cancer, notably lung cancer resulting from tobacco use. Parkin et al (1999) report that the most recent estimates of cancer in 1990 suggest a total of 8.1 million new cases, of which almost exactly half are found in developing countries; in the same year 5.2 million deaths occurred, of which about 55% were in developing countries.

As a life-threatening illness cancer elicits an immediate emotional response that has no relationship to rational thinking, depth of knowledge, or the individual's role in society (Slevin et al 1996, Burns 1982). In response to the struggle to express the lived experience of cancer in language, metaphors abound which reveal an understanding of the body, self, illness, life and death (Teucher 2003). The most common metaphors in the language of cancer are those of war, as noted by Lupton (1998). Cancer is perceived as 'evil', 'the scourge', 'an invisible enemy' or a contemporary 'plague' and the cancer sufferer is seen to fight a 'victorious battle', is brave and does not 'give in'. Likewise cancer has become a metaphor for all that is wrong in society – crime, drug abuse, strikes, immigration and political dissent are described as 'cancers' in society (Sontag 1989). Lupton also notes that in cancer narratives society becomes a metaphor for the body, which is peopled by 'good' and 'useful' cells with social order threatened by deviant cells that refuse to obey societal laws. Herzlich & Pierret (1986) describe cancer as fraught with phantasms of rot invading the body, or animals that gnaw and destroy.

Whilst acknowledging the common use of such metaphors, Teucher (2003) questions the universality of these metaphors and proposes that instead there are individual and culturally distinct uses of cancer metaphors to express cancer meanings and experiences. This highlights the poor understanding of cancer meanings and experiences of different cultural and ethnic groups, particularly within the United Kingdom.

Cancer research has tended to focus on the majority white population without acknowledging its significant threat to health and well-being of other ethnic communities. The data available on cancer incidence amongst different ethnic groups in the United Kingdom indicate that overall cancer incidence and mortality is low in most minority ethnic populations, with the exception of the Irish who have the highest mortality rates from cancer, particularly from lung and prostate cancer and leukaemia (Balarajan 1995, Harding & Allen 1996, Harding & Balarajan 1996, Harding & Maxwell 1997, Harding 1998, Harding & Rosato, 1999). Even with a lower incidence than the white majority, significant numbers of minority ethnic people are affected by cancer. As far back twenty years ago cancer was a common cause of death amongst migrants from the Indian subcontinent, Caribbean and African Commonwealth, such that one in ten Indian and African men aged 20–49 and one in five Caribbean men (of all ages) died from cancer in the UK, with the corresponding proportions higher among women (Bhopal & Rankin 1996). This cancer-related mortality among minority ethnic populations has likely increased over the last twenty years as a result of demographic changes such as ageing (Department of Health 1995). For example, Winter et al (1999) compared cancer incidence among south Asians living in England with Indian subcontinent rates and found the results consistent with a transition from the lower cancer risk of the country of origin to the higher risks in England. They suggest that detrimental changes in lifestyle and exposure to new environmental risk factors have occurred in the migrant south Asian population. Smith et al (2003) also conducted a study to explore trends in lung cancer incidence from 1990 to 1999 in Leicester. Although they also found lung cancer rates were lower for south Asians than non-south Asians, they found the incidence increasing among south Asian men despite falling among non-south Asians.

In an attempt to understand variations and increased incidence of cancer amongst different ethnic groups, the broad explanatory framework developed by Townsend & Davidson (1988) to explain patterns of health status in minority ethnic groups, and further developed by Smaje in 1995, is presented below.

BROAD EXPLANATORY FRAMEWORK FOR VARIATIONS IN CANCER INCIDENCE

ARTEFACT EXPLANATIONS

'Artefact explanations' for variations in health involve the use of data that are possibly misleading or inappropriate, rendering the findings of studies invalid. For instance, studies concerning cancer and ethnicity have often used different definitions of ethnicity that do not allow comparison. In particular confusion exists because researchers have tended to use country of birth as a proxy for ethnic origin. Harding & Allen (1996) warn that this obscures the heterogeneous composition of these groupings in terms of cultural differences and area of origin, as well as excluding descendants of migrants. Such heterogeneous approaches can mask different cancer incidence amongst subgroups, as McCormack et al (2004) found amongst first-generation South Asian migrant women with breast cancer. Furthermore, the quality of ethnic monitoring of cancer patients has been poor in both primary and secondary care, frustrating the collection of valid data.

MATERIAL EXPLANATIONS

'Material explanations' refer to correlations between socio-economic status and poor health; for example, the effects of being unable to afford a healthy diet, living in unsatisfactory accommodation and the stresses of unemployment, which disproportionately affect people from minority ethnic groups (Taylor 1998, Acheson 1998). On the other hand, Smaje (1995) proposes that material factors alone are insufficient to explain variations in ethnic patterns of health experience. For example, Marmot et al (1984) suggest that social class is a poorer predictor of mortality among minority ethnic groups than for the majority population; specifically they found greater mortality among Caribbean-born men of higher social class compared to those of lower class. Harding & Balarajan (1996) also found that socio-economic status alone cannot fully explain the raised incidence of cancer amongst the second-generation Irish. However, according to the American Cancer Society (2000), some of the differences in cancer incidence and screening prevalence rates among ethnic groups in the USA may be due to factors associated with social class, although with 32% of African Americans, 32% of Native Americans, 28% of Hispanics, and 12% of Asians living in poverty compared with 11% of whites in 1990, the relationship between social class and ethnicity is complex.

SOCIAL SELECTION EXPLANATION

'Social selection explanations' suggest that health variations result from social mobility; healthy people are able to find better jobs, which allows access to better housing, diet, education and so on. As Smaje (1995) suggests, it is possible that migrants will, in comparison to their peers, be either positively selected for heath – as with ambitious young people looking to improve their prospects by travelling abroad – or negatively selected, as with socially marginal people moving on from communities that cannot support them. Marmot et al (1984) suggest the existence of positive health selection for several migrant groups on the basis of a better mortality experience than that which prevails in the country of origin. Thus, positive health selection may explain the low mortality rates for people born in the Caribbean, in spite of their generally poorer socio-economic status. Although the 'social selection explanation' may complement other explanations for variations in health, Smaje (1995) warns that the available research evidence based on this approach is inconclusive. Whatever the logic of social selection, its impact seems to diminish over time.

THE EFFECTS OF MIGRATION EXPLANATION

'The effects of migration explanation' suggests that the experience of migration itself may have a direct impact on health. Smaje & Field (1997: 150) observe that 'it should not be assumed that the patterning of cancer incidence is immutable. The fact of migration considerably complicates analysis, and it cannot be assumed that disease patterns observed among the now elderly "pioneer" migrants will be replicated in more recent generations.' Over time, cancer rates of migrants appear to converge with those of host countries, suggesting that as populations age and adopt a Western lifestyle and diet, there are socio-economic and environmental links to the risk of the disease (Harding & Rosato 1999, Winter et al 1999).

THE EFFECTS OF RACISM EXPLANATION

'The effects of racism explanation' refers to the inequitable provision of services as well as their inability to provide care that is culturally competent. As Nazroo (2003) argues, it is racial abuse, discrimination and poor economic position, not ethnic origins, which cause poor health amongst minority groups. Racism may result in people from minority ethnic groups lacking awareness of existing services or having negative experiences when they do use the health services. This inevitably leads to low utilization of both preventative and curative services, which will impact on the incidence and outcomes of cancer amongst minority ethnic groups. In the USA, Meyerowitz et al (1998), in their comprehensive review of studies related to ethnicity and cancer outcomes, report that the impact of racist attitude on the part of medical staff is considerable and deserves further attention. Culley & Dyson (1993) suggest that material factors associated with social class and poor health are compounded by racism; thus it may be useful to think of racism as an important underlying cause of ethnic differences in overall health experiences and a potentially significant immediate cause of certain specific outcomes.

GENETIC EXPLANATIONS

'Genetic explanations' account for differences in health by drawing attention to inherited disorders which may impact on the health of those affected. Setting aside the political arguments surrounding genetic explanations of health differences across ethnic groups, researchers have found that when controlling for other factors, ethnic differences in cancer survival rates do exist but they have not fully succeeded in explaining this. A literature review on genetic testing by Noorani & McGahan (1999) concluded that age, ethnicity and family history (hereditary) are definite risk factors for prostate cancer.

CULTURAL EXPLANATIONS

'Cultural explanations' suggest that differences between ethnic groups in cultural values, beliefs and lifestyles may explain patterns of health status and service utilization. Helman (1994) states that each culture has its own system of health beliefs, perceptions and ideas about health and illness, which underpin health-related behaviours. Cooley & Jennings-Dozier (1998) reinforce Helman's position by proposing that culturally derived beliefs about health and illness, use of a lay referral system, use of folk treatments and the importance of family, community and spiritual support are some of the cultural concepts that must be considered. However, Smaje (1995) warns that culture is often invoked much more broadly as a convenient category of explanation to account for ethnic diversity in patterns of health experience, particularly where other explanations appear to fail. This has sometimes resulted in stereotyped assumptions, thus 'blaming the victim' and diverting attention from more pressing social factors such as material deprivation and racism. It is therefore important that cultural analyses are located within the broader social context in which both minority and majority cultural/ethnic groups exist and that a person's culture should not be used to apportion blame for his misfortunes.

There have been few UK-based studies exploring the cultural explanations about cancer held by people from different cultural groups. Those conducted internationally suggest that different cultural backgrounds do impact on cancer meanings and experiences. For instance, Nwoga (1994) observed that in Nigeria traditional healers believe that cancer can be caused by an evil curse, magic, bad blood, infection by germs, bad air, incestuous acts or adultery. Morgan et al (1995) reported that Hispanic American women believe that bumps and bruises can cause cancer and that surgery causes cancer to spread; and Granda-Cameron (1999) observed that Latin Americans (both men and women) believe that cancer may be contagious, may be due to having sex at an early age, that infections predispose a person to cancer, and that cancer may develop as a result of God's punishment. Although these studies suggest that different cultural groups hold different beliefs, a US study by Klonoff & Landrine (1994) reported no differences regarding the perceived causes of lung cancer among people from different ethnic groups, although a number of gender differences did emerge.

MEANINGS AND EXPERIENCES OF CANCER AMONGST DIFFERENT ETHNIC GROUPS

Whilst there is a small but growing body of knowledge on the impact of changing lifestyles, genetic constitution and socio-economic status on cancer incidence and outcomes of different ethnic groups, there is currently very little knowledge about the impact of culture on the meanings and experiences of cancer. Culture-based cancer beliefs could influence participation in prevention and early detection activities, decisions about treatment, as well as emotional responses to the disease. Thus, understanding culturally based responses to cancer is as important to healthcare workers as knowledge of statistical trends (Nielsen et al 1992). In the light of this the authors have conducted three studies to explore the meanings and experiences of cancer of people from different ethnic groups. These are presented below as three case studies:

- Cancer beliefs, knowledge and experiences among the Greek and Greek Cypriot community of North London (Papadopoulos 2001)
- Meanings and experiences of cancer of the Chinese community of Soho, London (Lees, Papadopoulos & Ridge 2004)
- Meanings and experiences of cancer for male cancer sufferers and their wives from six different ethnic groups (Papadopoulos & Lees 2002).

CASE STUDY ONE: CANCER BELIEFS, KNOWLEDGE AND EXPERIENCES AMONG THE GREEK AND GREEK CYPRIOT COMMUNITY OF NORTH LONDON

In 1999–2001 Papadopoulos conducted a qualitative study to investigate and describe cancer beliefs, knowledge and related behaviours among first- and second-generation Greek and Greek Cypriots living in North London. Three focus groups were conducted with 35 Greek and Greek Cypriot men and women and in-depth interviews were conducted with three cancer sufferers and their significant other. With the exception of the 'young people' focus group, all data were collected in Greek. The discussions and interviews revealed a number of important cancer beliefs, knowledge and behaviours that are meaningful within the Greek and Greek Cypriot cultural context.

Cancer beliefs and meanings

There are a range of beliefs and explanations of cancer causation by Greeks and Greek Cypriots including biomedical explanations, such as genetic, environmental and lifestyle factors (particularly smoking and exposure to the sun), stress or powerful emotions, and amongst the elderly, 'Satan'. Whatever the cause, cancer, for Greek and Greek Cypriots, is associated with negative feelings, bad things (*to kako*), sadness and fear due to their belief that cancer means suffering, agony, pain and death. In evoking such strong feelings, the word cancer (*karkinos*) is avoided, such that many fear that speaking the word in itself may cause cancer. This is illustrated by one participant who muttered '*exo abo etho*' ([cancer] get out of here) whilst sweeping the air in front of her with her hands, as though pushing the cancer away. As one elderly participant described, '*When I hear the word, I imagine an animal with eight legs and horns*', whilst another said: '*I imagine an evil animal when I hear the word, I imagine that this evil exists which goes into the body and it kills it*'. Rather than using the word cancer a number of metaphors are used, such as '*anathema*' or '*anathematismeno*' (something that is really bad and unwanted), '*aschimi arostia*' (ugly disease), or '*bojeenon*' (never mentioned). The association with evil is highlighted by the metaphor '*xorismenos*' (something that has been planted by Satan) to describe cancer. In order to counter this evil, Greek/Greek Cypriot people turn to God for help by saying '*O Theos na to xorisi*' (may God get rid of it) or '*O Theos na mas filai*' (may God look after us) whilst sometimes crossing themselves. Greek metaphors for cancer also denote gender and nature: describing malignant cancers as 'feminine' (which reproduce) and 'bad' in nature (*kakoithis*) and benign cancers as 'masculine' and 'good' in nature (*kaloithis*).

Knowledge about cancer

The Greek and Greek Cypriot participants suggested that cancer is usually caused by harmful substances such as tobacco, alcohol, chemicals and pollutants in water and foods, and harmful emotions such as stress and anxiety. In order to prevent cancer the younger participants placed particular value on screening, believing that if it is 'caught early' it is curable. Other than screening the participants accepted there was lack of knowledge about the signs and symptoms of cancer, particularly amongst elderly Greek and Greek Cypriots who avoid learning about cancer due to their fear of the disease. As one elderly woman said, '*When that comes, God forbid, (I will face it), but I don't want to learn about it from now*'. Response to the physical signs and symptoms are also hampered by shame, particularly amongst the elderly. One elderly woman believed that this shame had led to her mother's untimely death from uterine cancer because '*she was too embarrassed to tell anyone, she hid it from all of us*'. On the other hand, the participants demonstrated good knowledge about cancer treatment and curability although also suggesting such treatment can be assisted by '*having God on your side*', support from loved ones, or a positive attitude. As one elderly man suggested, '*It's all in the mind, my brother fought and he told himself he was not going to die (and) he got well. I say the mind is powerful*'.

Cancer experiences

Greek and Greek Cypriot cancer sufferers' immediate response to a cancer diagnosis are feelings of fear, anger and despair. These feelings diminish, aided by the belief in the need to *be strong in order to survive*. Coping strategies are adopted such as seeking solace in religion, which gives hope and comfort, or trying to put the disease out of their minds. As with their desire to avoid mentioning cancer, cancer sufferers avoid talking about their diagnosis. A middle-aged woman reported that *part of the reason why we avoid talking about cancer is the implicit morality behind it; we don't want to accept that something as bad as cancer has hit our families; many consider it as punishment from God*. Cancer also greatly affects immediate families and friends, with initial feelings of fear and despair on learning of their loved one's diagnosis. However, they try to overcome their initial feelings of despair, accepting that they also need to be (or at least appear to be) strong and give courage to their loved one. They see their role as protecting their loved one, particularly by filtering information between the loved one and health professionals.

CASE STUDY TWO: MEANINGS AND EXPERIENCES OF CANCER AMONG THE CHINESE COMMUNITY IN SOHO, LONDON

In 2003–2004 Lees, Papadopoulos & Ridge conducted a qualitative study to explore meanings and experiences of migrant Chinese people living and working in Soho using the focus group method. Five focus groups were conducted with 35 Chinese men and women from the following groups: (a) Chinese health and social care professionals, (b) asylum seekers, (c) migrants with unknown legal status, (d) young adults and (e) elders. All the focus groups, except the professional group, were conducted in either Mandarin or Cantonese and facilitated by a Chinese research assistant.

Cancer beliefs and meanings

For the Chinese, cancer is a 'fatal illness' (絕症 *Juezhang*), which evokes strong negative feelings of fear, anxiety, sadness and helplessness and is described as 'horrible' (可怕, *Kepa*) or 'scary'. Despite cancer evoking such strong feelings, the Chinese do not use metaphors but instead refer to the disease directly as cancer (癌症, *Aizheng*) or tumour (腫瘤, *Zhongliu*), with two types – benign cancer (慢性, *Manxing*) and malignant (惡性, *Exing*).

Knowledge about cancer causation and prevention

The Chinese have a number of explanations about cancer causation, which can broadly be grouped into internal or external causes. Internal causes are those that relate to the body and emotions such as *Zching Shui* (mood). A weakened body, usually as a consequence of poor health or genetic disposition, is unable to resist cancer. Mood, usually as a consequence of anxiety, stress or anger, also weakens the body's resistance to cancer. As one Chinese adult participant suggested, a stressed body *will manufacture poisonous elements which are harmful to health. Our own characters can also be counted as a factor, bad tempered people feel sick easily*. For the Chinese participants the most important external cause of cancer is food, especially those that are seen as unhealthy, or prepared or cooked in a particular way. Cancer-causing foods include chicken skin, old peanuts, fermented bean curd, pickled cabbage, preserved eggs ('thousand year old eggs') and mouldy food. Unhealthy foods are those high in salt, sugar and fat and 'fast foods'. Harmful food preparation includes preserving foods (usually salted or smoked) and chemically processing foods, whilst harmful cooking methods include frying in repeatedly used oil, cooking food until black or burnt and cooking in unhygienic conditions. As one Chinese health professional reported, *'I found problems of food preparation in Chinese take-aways and restaurants. They repeatedly use the same oil to fry potato chips until the oil turns black. As we know burnt food will cause cancer'*. Other external causes include environmental factors such as exposure to the sun, dust from construction, air pollution, high voltage power lines, radiation, and unhealthy lifestyles such as smoking, taking snuff and drinking alcohol.

Preventing cancer for the Chinese therefore means attending to these internal and external causes. This involves being in a 'good mood', or, as one of the asylum seekers put it, *'We should always keep our smile and live happily'*, and maintaining a healthy body through exercise, and personal hygiene, both of which were particularly emphasized. Avoiding 'cancer-causing' foods and eating healthy foods is also important for the Chinese. Healthy foods include chicken, eggs, Japanese mushroom, asparagus, garlic, green tea, and 'natural foods'. Avoiding the sun, unsanitary conditions and air pollution and not smoking are also considered important.

Knowledge and beliefs about treatments and outcomes

The Chinese participants understand that cancer can be cured by biomedicine or traditional Chinese medicine (TCM), preferably in combination. TCM treatments mentioned were herbs, food supplements and in particular, the glossy ganoderma fungus (*Lingzhi*) which grows in graveyards. Other Chinese approaches to curing include Qigong (a Chinese system of prescribed physical exercises or movements performed in a meditative state), acupuncture and 'spiritual treatment'. The participants suggested that TCM in general is a better form of treatment for cancer than biomedicine because it does not have any side effects, and is seen to 'cure' cancer as opposed to biomedicine's approach of 'controlling' cancer.

Whilst accepting that cancer should be treated by both Western medicine and TCM, the participants also suggested a number of factors that can enhance survival, which again involves countering the internal and external causes of cancer. Thus, as cancer can be caused by bad mood, for example, once a person has cancer, this 'moodiness' breaks down resistance and reduces the chances of being cured. Hope is seen as a counter to bad mood and an aid in the 'fight' against the disease. The Chinese believe that cancer sufferers need support to be in a good mood – *'tell them to be happy'*, *'not to worry'*, and *'be positive'*. Again the Chinese participants suggested that cancer curing can be aided by building up the weakened, unwell body by eating a healthy diet, being active and getting adequate rest and sleep.

Cancer experiences

Many of the Chinese participants had known someone with cancer, either a family member or a close friend. Some of the people they knew had survived cancer but others had died. In general they were positive about the treatment that the cancer sufferers had received, in terms of both biomedicine and TCM, although some were negative about the biomedical treatment: *'chemotherapy damaged the patient's balance . . . Hospital treatment is fine but he also needs Chinese herbs to balance the body's yin and yang'*. For those that knew cancer sufferers who had died there was a sense that they were shocked by their diagnosis and outcome, and some were concerned that they had not supported the cancer sufferer: *'I think I should have encouraged him more, told him he will recover soon, consoled him, told him to try everything in order to improve his chances of living'*. On the other hand, many Chinese families do not disclose the truth to cancer sufferers (particularly if they are elderly) in order to protect them from knowing that they might die soon. As one Chinese migrant suggested, *'if one of the members of the family contracted cancer, the other members of the family will not tell the whole truth to the cancer sufferer because they do not want to hurt him . . . Their body resistance slows down dramatically, I would say if they know the truth, they are unlikely to die of cancer but their own depression'*.

The participants also acknowledged that once diagnosed Chinese cancer sufferers, particularly the elderly, do not talk openly about cancer, although they are more open with family members. This is for a number of reasons: stigma, to avoid hurting family and friends, limited knowledge, to be remembered as they were before they were ill, and to avoid a 'gloomy' subject.

CASE STUDY THREE: CANCER MEANINGS AND EXPERIENCES BY CANCER SUFFERERS AND THEIR SIGNIFICANT OTHERS FROM DIFFERENT ETHNIC GROUPS

In 2000–2002 Papadopoulos and Lees conducted a study to explore the meanings and experiences of cancer for men from different ethnic groups. In-depth semi-structured individual interviews were conducted with six cancer sufferers and their significant others from the following ethnic groups: white British, Irish, Greek Cypriot, Jamaican, Montserratian, Bangladeshi. (these are self defined ethnic categories)

Cancer beliefs and meanings

Men and women from all the ethnic groups used metaphors and descriptions of cancer that indicate that it is a feared and stigmatized disease across different cultures. The Greek and Greek Cypriots, as noted in case study one, use particularly evocative metaphors to describe their feelings about cancer. Whilst the other groups described cancer in a negative way they tended to avoid referring to the disease at all. As the spouse of the Jamaican cancer sufferer put it, *'Cancer is a terrible word, [it] sounds like it will eat you out, your whole body. But a "growth", you know when you use it, it don't sound like it will destroy your body like that'* (Table 7.1).

Table 7.1   Cancer metaphors and descriptions

Ethnicity	Metaphors	Descriptions
Bangladeshi	'Ngar' (Ulcer, sore)	None
Greek Cypriot	'Argasti' (Virulent weed) 'Kako' (Badness) 'Ashimi arostia' (Ugly illness) 'Faousa' (Black death) 'Banougla' (Bubonic fever) 'Mavri arostia' (Black illness)	Dangerous Mysterious Hidden Secretive Tortuous Snake-like disease Sinful
Jamaican	Growth	Bad disease
Irish	Big C, It	None
Montserratian	–	Nasty disease
White English	Big C	Life-threatening disease

Explaining cancer causation

Explanations of cancer causation varied amongst different ethnic groups, although most participants suggested that lifestyle factors can cause certain cancers: '. . . *avoiding excessive drinking . . . Avoid certain foods, avoid smoking*' (Table 7.2). Although all the cancer sufferers suggested explanations of cancer causation, none could explain the cause of their own cancer apart from the white English man. There was little expectation that they should know; as the Greek Cypriot man argued, '*even the doctor may not know how the cancer begins*'. Some of the women, on the other hand, had their own explanations. For instance, the Greek Cypriot woman suspected that her husband's cancer might have been caused from worry about a recent family breakdown: '*his children not speaking is going to eat him up*', and the Jamaican woman wondered if smoking had caused her husband's cancer: '*they did say that smoking gives cancer right and he been smoking since very young*'.

Cancer experiences

Understanding and acknowledging symptoms of cancer varied amongst the different ethnic groups. The white English man was the only participant who reported being aware that he had symptoms and sought help immediately. The Greek Cypriot and Jamaican cancer sufferers admitted that they delayed going to the doctor whilst the Montserratian and Irish cancer sufferers only acknowledged their symptoms once they had sought medical help for another condition. The men took some time before they discussed their concerns about their symptoms with their wives and all, except the white English man, were encouraged to seek help by their wives or, in the case of the Jamaican cancer sufferer, by his daughter (who is a nurse).

Table 7.2   Knowledge of cancer causation

Cause of cancer	Quotations	Cultural group
Lifestyle		
Smoking	'*Well it's obvious that smoking is the biggest factor*' (white English woman)	Montserratian, white English, Greek Cypriot, Jamaican
Alcohol	'*Alcohol I suppose, I racked my brain and the only thing I can think of is alcohol*' (Irish man)	Montserratian, Greek Cypriot, Irish
Poverty leading to stress	'*. . . no job, gotta sign on, no money, they're poor, and that's all pressure*' (Montserratian man)	Montserratian
Work leading to stress	'*. . . you work hard, you do different hours of shift work and so on, your eating habit change, your digesting system change, one thing lead up to another*' (Montserratian man)	Montserratian
Food:		Montserratian, Greek Cypriot, Jamaican, white English
Change in diet	'*. . . because the kind of food that my body used to, it's not getting it anymore*' (Montserratian man)	
Chemicals in food	'*. . . buy organic food to be on the safe side, all the other (food) they either sprayed or something*' (Montserratian man)	
Poor food quality	'*. . . in the Caribbean they get healthy food to eat because it is fresh, you can go to the tree and pick up a fruit or mango. And the fish caught today and it fresh, the meat killed today and it fresh. Nothing frozen or on ice*' (Montserratian man)	
Unhealthy diet	'*. . . salt is a killer, sugar is not very good and using that daily and daily and daily, everything get in your blood and then it probably form something*' (Montserratian man)	
Environment		
Water	'*It could be all the water, you don't boil the water now*' (Jamaican woman)	Montserratian, Jamaican
Pollution	'*. . . you inhale the pollution*' (Montserratian man)	Montserratian
Weather	'*. . . being in a cold country you doesn't sweat*' (Montserratian man)	Montserratian
Emotions		
Worry	'*I think you get it from worry*' (Greek Cypriot woman)	Montserratian, Greek Cypriot
Not expressing feelings	'*. . . we women can talk and talk and we feel better for it but men don't talk*' (Greek Cypriot woman)	Greek Cypriot
Body		
Weak immune system	'*Your immune system might be stronger than mine and it can deal with a lot of things*' (Montserratian man)	Montserratian
Ageing	'*When you are young it's fine but you growing older and your immune system can't take all of it*' (Montserratian man)	Montserratian
Inheritance	'*. . . it goes in some families, and some it doesn't*' (Jamaican man) '*. . . it's probably passing it in the genes*' (white English man)	Montserratian, Irish, Jamaican, white English
Spiritual intervention		
God	'*I have faith in God and he is the one that gives the illnesses*' (Greek Cypriot woman)	Greek Cypriot, Bangladeshi

Communicating with health professionals

The first 'cancer' communication event that these men had with health-care professionals was with their general practitioner (GP) and involved discussing their symptoms. The subsequent contact and communication with other health professionals depended on whether their GPs actively listened and trusted what the men were telling them. The next significant communication event was at the disclosure of their diagnosis. All the men were with their wives or daughters at disclosure, except the white English man. Irrespective of how this was conducted, the disclosure elicited a negative emotional response from all the men including fear, numbness, horror, shock and distress. These responses resulted in high levels of anxiety and despair, which influenced how they made sense of their illness and how they communicated this with others. For example, the Jamaican cancer sufferer described being distressed and speechless because 'if it develops, you don't have much more to live'. He also reported to have been 'very numb, very dead'. The Greek Cypriot man felt that 'this is an illness when somebody gets it, they're finished'. The Bangladeshi man remembered that on being told that 'everything's damaged' and he was 'going to die', he and his wife were 'silent and very, very upset, we were horrified'. Where hope for the future was communicated by health professionals during disclosure of diagnosis, the men reported that this alleviated, to a varying extent, their anxiety and despair. The white English, Montserratian and Greek Cypriot men reported that being told by their doctors that they had a good chance of survival provided them with hope. On the other hand, the Irish man felt that both his GP and the hospital doctors seemed to avoid telling him his diagnosis. According to him, 'they kept dodging it all the time . . . they kept saying I don't think it is'.

Communicating with families or friends

Following disclosure of their diagnosis, the men sought support from their wives and immediate family. With the support of their wives they all told their children, all of whom were either teenagers or adults. The response of the immediate families ranged from concern to fear, possibly depending on how they were presented with the news. For example, the white English man reported that his children's response was 'concern but nothing unusual, nothing out of control'. This, he suggested, was because he had 'put it to them . . . that it's a curable situation if caught in time'. Whereas the children of the Bangladeshi couple were 'horrified, . . . scared. They prayed, and they were crying'. Despite sharing their diagnoses with their immediate family most of the men did not discuss their illness with their extended family or friends, usually because they felt it was a private matter, or that, within their culture, it is not something to be discussed. Privacy was really important for the white English and the Greek Cypriot men, although they were aware that their wives discussed their illness with others. The women were more willing to discuss their husband's cancer; the Jamaican woman suggested that men did not like discussing their condition because many of them 'have so much pride that they don't want anyone to know at all about their sickness'. The Greek Cypriot woman told other relatives because she did not want to be 'dishonest' when they had inquired about her husband. The Jamaican and Irish spouses also discussed the men's illness with their extended families, although the Irish couple reported that whilst they did talk *'openly about it'*, they did not discuss *'every last detail'*.

Another form of communication was the attention that the men received either directly or indirectly. Direct communicative attention was demonstrated by the direct support given to them by their immediate family. The wives gave daily support to their husbands through encouragement, concern and caring. The men also felt supported by their wider family. This was with the exception of the white English woman who felt that her husband did not need support because, according to her, he was *'actually very cheerful and positive'*. Indirect communicative attention was something that the men were aware of but did not occur in their presence. This took the form of relatives and friends enquiring about them and discussing their health and welfare with their immediate families. The men appeared to appreciate this attention because it made them feel valued human beings, despite their illness.

Communicating with God/Allah

The white English couple were the only ones who did not hold any religious belief and therefore did not report communicating with God. The Jamaican woman, a Christian, prayed for her husband regularly and asked God *'to heal him from the cancer'*, gaining strength from praying which in turn helped her to support him emotionally. The Montserratian man, an active church-going Christian, felt supported by the congregation at his church. He also sought solace in praying and in his belief that *'if you are a spiritual person and believe in God you shouldn't be frightened because the spirit is with you'*. The Irish couple also sought solace from their faith – the Irish woman's mother sent a Mass card every week and another relative brought him a piece of 'Padre Pio's glove' (a piece of glove from a priest who is believed to have miraculous healing powers), which *'definitely did something for me'*. The Bangladeshi couple, both Muslims, found their faith a source of comfort, reading the Qur'an, praying daily and visiting the mosque when he was well enough. Finally the Greek Cypriot woman, a Greek Orthodox Christian, prayed regularly for her husband's recovery.

DISCUSSION

The authors do not suggest that the findings presented above are generalizable but they may be transferable to similar cases and cultural groups. These studies have shown that whilst there are many similarities amongst people from different ethnic groups, there are also a number of variations in the cancer explanations and experiences.

METAPHORS AND DESCRIPTIONS

There are a number of similarities and differences in cancer metaphors across cultures, which predominantly relate cancer to morality, although these descriptions may or may not emanate from those cultures that have a strong religious basis. For example, the Greek and Greek Cypriots have a number of moral descriptions of cancer and are a strongly religious culture, whilst the Bangladeshi and Irish have no such descriptions of cancer, but are also strongly religious cultures. The physical descriptions of cancer, particularly by the Greek Cypriots, as something that invades and spreads relates to Herzlich & Pierret's (1986) description of cancer as fraught with phantasms of rot invading the body, or animals that gnaw and destroy. Moreover, the absence of metaphors by some ethnic groups can also be understood culturally; the idea that cancer is shameful and should remain nameless, or abbreviated to Big C, suggests that these cultures see cancer as something to be ashamed of. Greek Cypriots also give cancer gender – a cancer that spreads is female; a cancer that does not spread is male. The association is thus drawn with reproducing cancer cells and women's fertility. Moral associations could also be drawn – older Greeks and Greek Cypriots consider women to be like Eve (another link to religious beliefs) who tempts and sins, actions that are bad or evil just as cancer is seen to be (Papadopoulos 2001).

EXPLAINING CANCER

Given the historically poor scientific understanding of cancer, it is not surprising that cancer beliefs change over time. In nineteenth century England cancer was thought to be caused by hyperactivity and hyperintensity. One English doctor urged his patients 'to avoid overtaxing their strength, and to bear the ills of life with equanimity; above all things, not to "give way" to any grief' (Sontag 1989). By the 1980s explanations of cancer causation amongst the white English included moral wrongdoing and leading an unclean life (Box 1984). Today cancer beliefs are likely to be influenced by exposure to scientific explanations, usually filtered through the media.

Whatever their cultural background most of the participants in these studies accept that certain lifestyle activities cause cancer. Most of the groups accepted in particular that smoking causes cancer. As this is an accepted cause of cancer amongst the scientific community this indicates that this shared belief is a result of health warnings and health education messages. Food and diet as a cause of cancer is a more controversial area. Mixed messages are sent out by the scientific community about the role of different foods and diets in cancer causation. For the participants, though, food and diet are important factors in cancer causation, although their importance varied by ethnicity. The Chinese, in particular, believed 'unhealthy food' to be a very important cause of cancer. Some evidence from research in the Chinese community may support this. For instance, Yang (1997) has found that the consumption of salted fish, especially during weaning, and other preserved foods, in combination with the Epstein–Barr virus, has been shown to be a major risk factor for nasopharyngeal cancer. Yang also notes that the consumption of salty foods and infection with *Helicobacter pylori* are believed to be risk factors for stomach cancer, and consumption of mouldy food has been suspected to increase the risk of oesophageal cancer.

For all the participants in all three studies there is no one single explanation of cancer causation. Instead it is, depending on the cultural background, different combinations of factors that make the body vulnerable to the illness. For the Greeks and Greek Cypriots it is the combination of spiritual intervention, negative emotions and lifestyle factors, while for the Chinese, psychological and physical symptoms are not necessarily considered as inseparable, and there is a focus on balance or equilibrium to describe good health.

It should be acknowledged that there might exist a gap between cultural and individual beliefs regarding cancer causation. For example, a study of a Native American group found that whilst the group generally ascribes cancer to a 'weak body', individual cancer patients attribute it to heredity or God's will (Weiner 1993). Further, the American cultural view of illness as a challenge to be courageously met is not always reflected in the reactions of individual cancer patients (Navon 1999). Therefore it is important to be aware that the beliefs held by the participants may reflect their individual approaches to illness as much as their cultural beliefs.

REACTION TO DIAGNOSIS

Kagawa-Singer (1996) argues that all people face similar types of situations when confronted with cancer but each cultural group experiences them in different ways depending on its environment, resources and worldview. Fallowfield et al (1995) argue that the distress that people feel on hearing that they have a life-threatening disease, such as cancer, is due to the lay assumption that the disease has a poor outcome and involves unpleasant treatment. Kodiath & Kodiath (1995) and Ali et al (1993) have also found that reactions of anxiety and distress are similarly manifested by American, Egyptian and Indian cancer patients. What varies are the ways in which different people seek explanations and solace to overcome this despair and fear and come to terms with their illness.

HELP SEEKING

Whilst people may hold traditional beliefs, Patcher (1994) argues that people rarely hold them to the exclusion of acceptance of biomedical care but seem able to hold a plural belief system that allows for different types of intervention. The findings in case study two highlight the Chinese acceptance of a plural approach to healing. This is supported by Holroyd (2002), who has found a variety of health-seeking behaviours by elderly Chinese in Hong Kong, including religious practices, eating special foods, regular exercise and sleep, and visiting Chinese medical specialists, herbalists and biomedical doctors. The participants in case study three all sought and subsequently adhered to biomedical care. Although they all reported to be satisfied with their medical care they nonetheless all (with the exception of the white English man) used some form of alternative therapy, particularly prayer. Thus, the men from all cultural groups, except the white English, were able to embrace spiritual or alternative healing alongside biomedical care without perceiving any contradiction between the different systems.

COMMUNICATING ABOUT CANCER

One of the major issues with cancer is that it is an illness that is not talked about, either in general, or by cancer sufferers themselves. There are differences amongst different cultural groups, with the Greeks and Greek Cypriots the most reluctant to talk about it. On the other hand, there does seem to be a tendency for the elderly from all cultural backgrounds to avoid talking about cancer. Talking about cancer seems to evoke distress in many people. Fallowfield et al (1995) suggest that this distress is reinforced at diagnosis if the doctor uses euphemisms instead of the word 'cancer'. Furthermore, perhaps due to their own discomfort, doctors tend to focus the communication at disclosure on the need for further diagnostic procedures, complex therapies and an often unknown prognosis. Finally, in times of distress and illness communicating with God/Allah is a natural response by many cultural groups and is connected to their 'sense of relatedness to a transcendent dimension, or to something greater than the self' (Reed 1991).

CONCLUSION

This chapter has shown that there are a number of explanations for different cancer incidence and outcomes for people from different ethnic groups living in the UK. Whilst acknowledging the importance of socioeconomic factors in particular, this chapter has explored cultural meanings and explanations of cancer to enable understanding of their impact on the help-seeking behaviour. This exploration has highlighted the similarities of meanings and experiences of cancer amongst different cultural groups. It is a disease that evokes strong negative feelings in all cultural groups, either for those who are diagnosed with the disease or for people who have no experience of the cancer. This feeling of fear impacts on people's desire to seek both knowledge and then help, once they are concerned about possible symptoms. Again there are few cultural variations in this. Once help is sought and provided, cultural variations in meanings and experiences become important such that they impact on an individual's ability to seek support, to communicate needs and also to seek alternative care.

We hope that readers will, through the insights provided in this chapter, be able to develop their cultural competence and apply the information of this chapter to achieve a more culturally sensitive and appropriate care when assessing, and managing the cancer journeys of their patients.

REFLECTIVE QUESTION

1. Based on the information provided in this chapter, list five indicators of culturally competent health care for the following ethnic groups:
   Greek and Greek Cypriots
   Chinese.

REFERENCES

Acheson D 1998 Independent inquiry into inequalities in health report. Stationery Office, London

Ali NS, Khalil HZ, Yousef WA 1993 A comparison of American and Egyptian cancer patients' and unmet needs. Cancer Nursing 18:193–203

American Cancer Society 2000 Facts and figures: cancer in minorities. Online. Available: http://www.cancer.org/statistics/cff2000/minoritycancer.html 22 Jun 2000

Balarajan R 1995 Ethnicity and variations in the nation's health. Health Trends 27(4):114–119

Bhopal R S, Rankin J 1996 Cancer in minority ethnic populations. British Journal of Cancer 74(Suppl XXIX): S22–S32

Box V 1984 Cancer: myths and misconceptions. Journal of the Royal Society of Health 104(5):161–166, 170

Burns N 1982 Nursing and cancer. Saunders, Philadelphia

Cooley M E, Jennings-Dozier K 1998 Cultural assessment of black American men treated for prostate cancer: clinical case studies. Oncology Nursing Forum 25(10):1729–1736

Culley L, Dyson S 1993 'Race', inequality and health. Sociology Review 3(1):24–27

Department of Health 1995 Variations in health. What can the Department of Health and the NHS do? HMSO, London

Fallowfield L, Ford S, Lewis S 1995 No news is not good news: Information preferences of patients with cancer. Psycho-Oncology 4:197–202

Granda-Cameron C 1999 The experience of having cancer in Latin America. Cancer Nursing 22(1):51–57

Harding S 1998 The incidence of cancers among second-generation Irish living in England and Wales. British Journal of Cancer 78(7):958–961

Harding S, Allen E 1996 Sources and uses of data on cancer among ethnic groups. British Journal of Cancer 74(Suppl XXIX):S17–S21

Harding S, Balarajan R 1996 Patterns of mortality in second generation Irish living in England and Wales: Longitudinal study. British Medical Journal 312:1389–1392

Harding S, Maxwell R 1997 Differences in the mortality of migrants. In: Drever F, Whitehead M (eds) Health inequalities. Decennial supplement. The Stationery Office, London, p 108–121

Harding S, Rosato M 1999 Cancer incidence among first generation Scottish, Irish, West Indian and south Asian migrants living in England and Wales. Ethnicity and Health 4(1/2):83–92

Helman C G 1994 Culture, health and illness: an introduction for health professionals. 3rd edn. Butterworth-Heinemann, Oxford

Herzlich C, Pierret J 1986 Illness: from causes to meaning. In: Currer C, Stacey M (eds) Concepts of health, illness and disease: A comparative perspective. Berg Publishers, Oxford

Holroyd E 2002 Health-seeking behaviours and social change: The experience of the Hong Kong Chinese elderly. Qualitative Health Research 12(6):731–750

Kagawa-Singer M 1996 Cultural systems. In: McCorkle R et al (eds) Cancer nursing: a comprehensive textbook. 2nd edn. Saunders, Philadelphia, p 38–52

Klonoff E A, Landrine H 1994 Culture and gender diversity in commonsense beliefs about the causes of six illnesses. Journal of Behavioral Medicine 17(4):407–418

Kodiath M F, Kodiath A 1995 A comparative study of patients who experience chronic malignant pain in India and the United States. Cancer Nursing 18:189–196

Lees S, Papadopoulos I, Ridge M 2004 The CIRCLE Study: An exploration of the meanings and experiences of cancer of Chinese people living and working in Soho, London. Middlesex University, London

Lupton D 1998 Medicine as culture: illness, disease and the body in Western societies. Sage, London

McCormack V A, Mangtani P, Bhakta D et al 2004 Heterogeneity of breast cancer risk within the South Asian female population in England: a population-based case-control study of first-generation migrants. British Journal of Cancer 90:160–166

Marmot M G, Adelstein A M, Bulusu L 1984 Immigrant mortality in England and Wales 1970–78. Studies on medical and population subjects No. 47. Office of Population Censuses and Surveys, HMSO, London

Meyerowitz B E, Richardson J, Hudson S, Leedham B 1998 Ethnicity and cancer outcomes: Behavioral and psychosocial considerations. Psychological Bulletin 123(1):47–70

Morgan C, Park E, Cortes D E 1995 Beliefs, knowledge, and behaviour about cancer among urban Hispanic women. Journal of the National Cancer Institute Monographs 18:57–63

Navon L 1999 Voices from the world: cultural views of cancer around the world. Cancer Nursing 22(1):39–45

Nazroo J 2003 The structuring of ethnic inequalities in health: economic position, racial discrimination, and racism. American Journal of Public Health 93(2):277–284

Nielsen B B, McMillan S, Diaz E 1992 Instruments that measure beliefs about cancer from a cultural perspective. Cancer Nursing 15(2):109–115

Noorani H Z, McGahan L 1999 Predictive genetic testing for breast and prostate cancer. Technology Report Is, 85, Canadian Coordinating Office for Health Technology Assessment, Ottawa

Nwoga I A 1994 Traditional healers and perceptions of the causes and treatment of cancer. Cancer Nursing 17(6):470–478

Papadopoulos I 2001 Let's talk about cancer: an exploration of the impact of culture on cancer attitudes and related practices of Greek and Greek Cypriots living in North London. GGCE, London

Papadopoulos I, Lees S 2002 Cancer and culture: investigating meanings and experiences of cancer of men from different ethnic groups: a pilot study. Middlesex University, London

Parkin D, Pisani P, Ferlay J (1999) Global Cancer Statistics, CA Cancer Journal for Clinicians 49(1):33–64

Patcher L 1994 Culture and clinical care: folk illness beliefs and behaviours and their implications for health care delivery. Journal of the American Medical Association 271:690–694

Reed P G 1991 An emerging paradigm for the investigation of spirituality in nursing. Research in Nursing and Health 15:349–357

Slevin M, Nichols S E, Downer S M et al 1996 Emotional support for cancer patients: what do patients really want? British Journal of Cancer 74:1275–1279

Smaje C 1995 Health, race and ethnicity: Making sense of the evidence. King's Fund, London

Smaje C, Field D 1997 Absent minorities? Ethnicity and the use of palliative care services. In: Field D, Hockey J, Small N (eds) Death, gender and ethnicity. Routledge, London, p 147–165

Smith L K, Botha J L, Benghiat A, Steward W P 2003 Latest trends in cancer incidence among UK South Asians in Leicester. British Journal of Cancer 89(1):70–73

Sontag S 1989 Illness as metaphor/AIDS and its metaphors. Anchor, New York

Taylor G 1998 Health and citizenship. In: Papadopoulos I, Tilki M, Taylor G Transcultural care. A guide for health care professionals. Quay Books, Dinton, p 18–43

Teucher U 2003 The therapeutic psychopoetics of cancer metaphors: challenges in interdisciplinarity. History of Intellectual Culture 3(1):1–15

Townsend P, Davidson N 1988 The Black Report. In: Townsend P, Davidson N, Whitehead M (eds) Inequalities in health: the Black Report and the health divide. Penguin, London, p 31–213

Weiner D 1993 Health beliefs about cancer among the Luiseno Indians of California. Alaskan Medicine 35:285–286

Winter H, Cheng K K, Cummins C et al 1999 Cancer incidence in the south Asian population of England (1990–92). British Journal of Cancer 79(3/4):645–654

Yang C S 1997 Chinese diet in the causation and prevention of cancer. Presented at the 1997 CAMS Semi-annual Scientific Meeting. Online. Available: http://www.camsociety.org 27 Jul 2004

Chapter **8**

The health and social care needs of Ethiopian asylum seekers and refugees living in the UK

Irena Papadopoulos, Margaret Lay, Shelley Lees and Alem Gebrehiwot

CHAPTER CONTENTS

LEARNING OBJECTIVES

After reading this chapter you should:
- gain an understanding of the ethnohistory of Ethiopia
- appreciate why Ethiopians fled their country
- increase your knowledge regarding the processes of adaptation and settlement that migrants go through and how these impact on their physical and mental health
- become aware of some of the health beliefs and self-care practices of Ethiopian people
- increase your sensitivity regarding the barriers and enablers of adaptation
- be more culturally competent when caring for Ethiopian migrants.

INTRODUCTION

The experience of refugeedom by itself is a very, very shocking experience. People lose their identity, their culture and they lose everything. So, they are status-less in this country. They are nobody . . . This experience really shakes people from top to bottom. (Male Ethiopian study participant)

We live in a time of mass migration and many countries are receiving large numbers of refugees. Baker et al (1994) argue that it is essential to understand the experience of migration through the lived experience of resettlement. The experiences and process of settlement of any refugee group in the country of asylum depends on a number of factors including their cultural and religious background, their personal experiences and attributes as well as the receiving country's policies.

Providing health and social care that meets the needs of the many different ethnic groups who now live either temporarily or permanently in the United Kingdom poses major challenges to the health and welfare services. Cultural diversity within any society necessitates the adoption of an approach to health and social care that is open and questioning, and transcultural models of care need to be fully embraced. The biomedical approach to nursing and medicine dominant in Western societies may threaten to dehumanize patients less familiar with Western health beliefs and healthcare practices and to leave many of their needs unmet.

It is, of course, impossible for every health and social care worker to know the details of the culture of every ethnic group; besides, doing so makes the assumption that all people sharing an ethnic background share the same culture and beliefs. However, it is important for health and social care workers to understand the significance of the differences and similarities in health beliefs and healthcare practices between the most common ethnic groups in their constituencies, and how these are affected by migration.

There is some evidence that the physical health status of many asylum seekers on arrival to the UK is often good compared to the general population (Wolhuter 2003, Haringey Council 1997). As discussed in Chapter 7, Smaje (1995) proposed that positive selection may take place whereby those who are healthy, younger and more able are more likely to leave their country than those who are elderly or sick. However, some refugees' health may be compromised before they arrive due to imprisonment and torture. Even healthy asylum seekers report deterioration in their health status in the first two or three years after arrival in the UK, mainly due to poverty, social exclusion, poor accommodation and poor nutrition (Gammell et al 1993, Wolhuter 2003, Vallely et al 1999). Barriers to health care have also been reported to exacerbate their health problems (Vallely et al 1999). Immigration policy can also impact on the health and well-being of asylum seekers.

BRITISH IMMIGRATION LEGISLATION

Numerous changes have been made to British immigration legislation in response to increased worldwide political unrest and war leading to a rise in asylum applications and calls from the British public for greater control of immigration. During the time span of the study (1999–2001) there were two ways to apply for asylum in the UK: (a) to the immigration officer on arriving at the port of entry, and (b) to the Home Office after entering the country either as a student or as a visitor. Others entered using illegal means such as being smuggled in by traffickers. In 1999 the Immigration and Asylum Act was introduced which included the dispersal policy. This entailed asylum seekers and refugees being allocated to centres throughout the country, often to areas that lacked experience of receiving and providing services for asylum seekers. It also introduced the food voucher system which, many campaigners argued, resulted in asylum seekers becoming readily identifiable and vulnerable to discrimination.

In 2002 the Nationality, Immigration and Asylum Act 2002 came into effect. The key provisions of this Act in respect of asylum seekers were the establishment of accommodation centres; the curtailment of access to support for those who did not claim asylum at the earliest opportunity (immediately upon arrival) or did not provide a full and accurate account of their circumstances. The Act also removed the right of asylum seekers to work or undertake vocational training until a positive decision on their asylum application was given, irrespective of how long they had waited for a decision. Prior to 2002, asylum applicants could apply to the Home Office to work provided they had waited at least two years for a decision. A positive change brought by the new Act was the abolition of the much reviled food voucher system, which was replaced by a cash voucher system.

ETHNOHISTORY OF ETHIOPIA

LOCATION AND GEOGRAPHICAL FEATURES OF ETHIOPIA

The Federal Democratic Republic of Ethiopia has an area of just over one million square kilometres and lies in north-eastern Africa otherwise known as the Horn of Africa. It is bordered by Eritrea and Djibouti to the north, Somalia to the east, Kenya to the south and Sudan to the west. The largest city is the federal capital Addis Ababa (population 2 112 737 in 1994).

POPULATION

At the beginning of 2004 Ethiopia had approximately 68 million people, making it the third most populous country in Africa after Nigeria and Egypt. Forty-six per cent (46%) of the population were between 0 and 14 years of age, 52% were aged 15–64 years and only 3% were aged over 65 years. The average life expectancy for Ethiopians was 41 years. The net migration rate in 1997 was estimated to be 1.32 migrants per 1000 population (World Factbook 2004).

There are over 80 different ethnic groups in Ethiopia, the Oromo being the largest group comprising over one-third of the total population (40%). The Amhara and Tigre make up almost another third (32%), Sidamo 9%, Shankella (6%), Afar (4%), Gurage 2%, and other (1%).

Around half the population in 2004 was Muslim (45–50%), Ethiopian Christian Orthodox constituted 35–40%, animist 12%, and other 3–8%. Languages are also diverse with Amharic, Tigrigna, Oromiffa, Guaragigna, Somali, Arabic, other local languages and English being spoken. Amharic is the official language and English the main foreign language taught in schools and also widely used in official and business circles.

ETHIOPIA'S HISTORY OF REFUGEEDOM

Ethiopia has generated waves of refugees for several decades, most of whom fled to neighbouring African countries. The reasons for people fleeing include drought and famine, civil war and most recently human rights abuses. In 1974 a military junta, the Derg regime, deposed Emperor Haile Selassie and established a socialist state. Torn by violent coups, uprisings, wide-scale drought and massive refugee problems, the regime was finally toppled by a coalition of rebel forces, the Ethiopian People's Revolutionary Democratic Front (EPRDF), in 1991. A new government was established which created the Federal Democratic Republic of Ethiopia.

The long history of political oppression and war in Ethiopia has led several researchers to highlight the need to understand the effects of trauma and exile on Ethiopian refugees in the UK (Gamaledin-Ashami 1993, Huka 1996, Bariso 1997). Burnett & Fassil (2002) maintain that some effects can be positive in that refugees making the often arduous journey into exile are courageous, resourceful and resilient and these qualities can assist them to rebuild their lives.

THE EMBRACE UK STUDY

The data on which this chapter is based were derived from the EMBRACE UK study (Papadopoulos & Gebrehiwot 2002). This study explored the following:

- events motivating Ethiopians to seek asylum
- how they gained entry to the UK
- their experiences of adaptation and settlement in the UK
- their social networks
- their lifestyles
- their health and sickness beliefs
- their mental and physical health in the UK
- their health-seeking behaviours in Ethiopia and the UK
- their self-care practices in Ethiopia and the UK.

As the determinants of health are embedded in many of the above aspects of refugees' lives, this chapter will attempt to synthesize these aspects to provide as complete a picture as possible of the complex nature

Figure 8.1   A conceptual representation of the study.

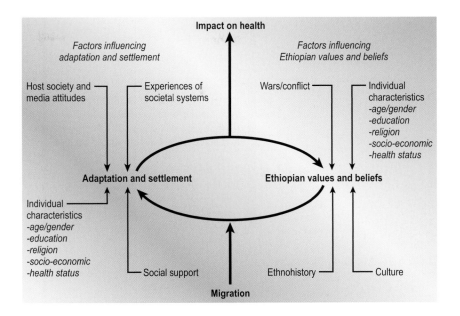

of their health and social care needs and the impact of refugeedom on these. A conceptual representation of the study is given in Figure 8.1.

METHODOLOGY

The EMBRACE UK study was conducted during 1999–2001. It used a multi-method participatory model whereby members of the Ethiopian community worked closely with the researchers at Middlesex University and were involved in every stage of the research process, including proposal writing, identifying participants, interviewing, transcribing taped interviews, translating to English, back-translation, data validation, report writing and dissemination.

Sampling and data collection

Qualitative data were collected through *semi-structured depth interviews* with 106 Ethiopians: 98 lay participants, 5 of whom had a history of diagnosed mental illness, and 8 'expert' participants (Ethiopians providing professional services to Ethiopian refugees). Box 8.1 provides the interview guide used.

Eight Ethiopian research assistants were recruited and trained in interviewing techniques and conducted all of the interviews, mainly in Amharic. In order to collect quantifiable and supplementary data relating to personal details, housing, employment, education and training, benefits, use of health and social services, health status, lifestyles, culture and religion, each interviewee was also asked to complete a semi-structured questionnaire. A combination of quota and snowball sampling (where study participants are asked to nominate other potential participants) was used to identify participants through personal contacts,

Box 8.1   Depth interview questions

What does it mean to you to be healthy?

Can you think of someone who is healthy? Explain why you think this person is healthy.

If there is sickness in the family who is the person who has the main caring role?

Why do you think people get sick?

If you become ill what sort of things do you do to get better?

Is this different from what you would have done if you were in Ethiopia? How and why?

How does life in Ethiopia differ from the life you have in the UK?

Tell me why you left Ethiopia and how?

How are you settling in the UK?

Tell me about any contact you have had with Ethiopian organizations?

Table 8.1   Ethiopian life cycle

Stage	Age (years)	Key markers
Adolescents and young adults	12–25	School/early adulthood, normally a time of entering work and forming adult relationships
Mid-life	26–59	Consolidation of significant adult relationship, development of own family, consolidation and development of career
Elders	60 plus	Finishing paid work, second generation of own family (grandparent)

through their contact with the Ethiopian Community Centre in the UK (ECCUK) and through advertisements on an Ethiopian radio station. An equal number of Ethiopians of all age groups over 12 years (relevant to the Ethiopian life cycle), and an equal number of women and men, were aimed for. The Ethiopian life cycle categories were identified by the Ethiopian staff at the ECCUK as potential key markers of different experiences amongst the Ethiopian refugee community (Table 8.1).

Transcribing, translating and back–translating the interview data

Part of the research assistants' role was to transcribe the interviews. Where the interviews were conducted in Amharic the researchers also translated and transcribed them in English. In order to assure the quality of translations, a randomly selected translated transcript from each research assistant was back-translated to Amharic by a different research assistant. The Ethiopian study director compared the two Amharic versions of each research assistant and confirmed their accuracy. It was found that although some expressions differed, the conceptual meaning remained true to the original transcript.

Data analysis and validation

An initial analysis of the qualitative data was performed by the Ethiopian interviewers in order to elicit the main issues from their perspective. Further analysis was conducted using the constant comparative process of defining and redefining emerging themes in the light of new data. The emerging themes were then elaborated conceptually both from the data and by using theoretical and empirical constructs from the literature (Patton 1990). The validity of the qualitative analysis was achieved through researcher triangulation, and through comparisons with published literature. Given the methodological rigour and the advantages of a research team which included both 'insiders' (Ethiopians) and 'outsiders' (non-Ethiopians), the authors are confident that the qualitative findings have truth value, are dependable and are applicable to the rest of the Ethiopian UK community. Quantitative analysis was conducted using SPSS for Windows. Simple descriptive statistical analysis was performed and where possible relationships and associations were explored. Only those that were found to be statistically significant have been reported.

Strengths and limitations of the methodology

The strength of the methodological approach was that it enabled access to Ethiopian asylum seekers and refugees and provided 'insider' knowledge (the 'emic' perspective). Further, the use of Ethiopian interviews enabled the collection of culturally sensitive and accurate information in the participants' preferred language. The study's participatory research model also provided capacity building for Ethiopian individuals and their community. The limitations to the methodological approach include the possibility that the interviewers, as 'insiders', may have taken some information for granted without adequate probing, which an 'outsider' interviewer may have pursued. Furthermore, as they may have identified with the participants, it is possible that in some cases they did not ask about, or probe into, any trauma suffered. Another limitation is that the quantitative findings are not representative of the whole Ethiopian refugee community in the UK due to the sampling approach.

THE SAMPLE

Tables 8.2 and 8.3 outline the characteristics of the participants. Almost equal numbers of females and males participated in the study. Age groups were broken down by stages of life relevant to the Ethiopian life cycle. There were very few in the youngest and oldest age groups.

Table 8.2 Age group of participants

Age group	Number	%
12–15	10	9.4
16–25	34	32.1
26–59	60	56.6
60+	2	1.9
Total	106	100.0

Table 8.3   Gender, marital status, ethnicity, religion and immigration status

Gender	52% female, 48% male
Marital status	75% single, 25% married
Self-defined ethnicity	37% Amhara, 23% black African, 18% other African, 12% Amhara and other Ethiopian, 10% Oromo
Religion[a]	55% Orthodox Christian, 35% other Christian, 8% Muslim, 2% Jehovah's Witness
Immigration status[b]	40% ILR, 36% temporary admission, 12% ELR, 7% refugee status, 5% other

[a]Data from 63 participants.
[b]Data from 94 participants.

Box 8.2   Definitions

Asylum seeker: 'An asylum seeker is a person who has left their country of origin, has applied for recognition as a refugee in another country, and is awaiting a decision on their application.' (UNHCR 2005)

Refugee: A refugee is a person who 'owing to a well-founded fear of being persecuted for reasons of race, religion, nationality, membership of a particular social group, or political opinion, is outside the country of his nationality, and is unable to or, owing to such fear, is unwilling to avail himself of the protection of that country'. (UNHCR, citing Article 1, 1951 Convention Relating to the Status of Refugees)

Temporary admission: (Asylum seeker) given to a person who has lodged a claim for asylum with the Immigration and Nationality Directorate.

Indefinite leave to remain: (ILR): Granted 'refugee status' and a right to permanent residency in the UK. Has the same rights as a UK citizen.

Exceptional leave to remain: (ELR): Asylum claim did not fully satisfy criteria but applicant can stay on humanitarian or compassionate grounds. Granted ELR for 4 years, then can apply again for ILR. (Refugee Council 2000)

Since 1 April 2003 the Home Office no longer grants ELR, but will consider granting either 'Humanitarian Protection' or 'Discretionary Leave'.

For practical reasons the terms 'asylum seeker' and 'refugee' will be used interchangeably in this chapter.

Most participants were single, one-quarter were married, and none reported being widowed. There was little gender difference in marital status. Just over a quarter had children or spouse dependants.

Of the 63 (59%) participants who stated their religion, most ($n = 57$: 90%) were Christians; of these some specified that they were either Orthodox Christian ($n = 35$) or Protestant ($n = 6$). Others stated they were Muslim ($n = 5$) or Jehovah's Witness ($n = 1$).

One-quarter (24%) reported living in the UK less than a year, 11% between 1 and 5 years, whilst 65% reported living in the UK for over 5 years. Of those who answered the question regarding their immigration status ($n = 94$), 40% had indefinite leave to remain (ILR), 36% reported that they had temporary admission, and 12% had exceptional leave to remain (ELR). Those with refugee status constituted the smallest group (7%) (see Box 8.2 for definitions). The rest (5%) had British citizenship, were awaiting deportation, or their status was unspecified.

Over one-third (37%) described themselves as Amhara; 12% were of mixed ethnic origin of Amhara and another ethnicity, principally Oromo; 23% described themselves as 'black African' (even though they were born and brought up in Ethiopia); and 10% Oromo. Others included Gurage, Tigre and 'Ethiopian'.

Amharic was the mother tongue of 82% of the participants, whilst for 10% Oromiffa was. Others reported Tigrigna, Guaragigna, Wolaitgna and English as being their mother tongue.

Of 76 participants who responded regarding their occupation in Ethiopia, almost half ($n = 37$: 49%) reported that they had been students (including at school). The remainder (51%) had been employed or self-employed, often as professionals such as lawyers and accountants. However, many ($n = 21$) did not respond to this question and for others ($n = 9$) it was not applicable. Regarding their current occupation in the UK, of 105 who were not new arrivals, one-third (33%) reported that they were employed or self-employed, around a quarter (27%) unemployed, and 41% were students, some of whom were also working. Six (6%) were doing voluntary work, sometimes whilst studying or during unemployment.

Of the 84 participants who responded regarding their educational level on arrival in the UK, 10% reported that they had 'diplomas', mostly in vocational subjects, and 19% reported that they had a Bachelor degree or higher degree. Several others (7%) stated what their professional status was without giving their qualifications; and 24% said they had 'secondary school' level qualifications; 15% had none; and the remainder had other types of qualifications.

REASONS FOR FLEEING AND MODES OF ESCAPE

Reasons for leaving Ethiopia

Over half ($n = 50$) of the lay participants reported that they had left Ethiopia for 'political' reasons such as lack of freedom to express their opinions, harassment, coercion into joining allegiance with the ruling political party, and corruption. Many were professionals who were accused of, or suspected of, having links with or supporting dissident groups. A male participant described his situation thus:

> *The reason why I left my country was that I wrote papers critical to the Government. As it was part of my career, I used to write papers. As a result of my writing in the papers, I was denied freedom of speech and writing. Above all I was kept behind bars and beaten up.*

Some left or were sent away by parents to avoid being conscripted into the army or to escape the consequences of war. Nineteen interviewees ($n = 19$) reported leaving Ethiopia because they or family members had been imprisoned or because they feared being imprisoned. Some of those who had been political prisoners said that they had been detained in dark, overcrowded and suffocating conditions or had been beaten and/or tortured. Others said that their family and friends had been killed and they feared the same fate. Economic reasons for coming to the UK were given by six interviewees.

The participants described the Ethiopia they fled from, using the following terms:

- oppressive
- undemocratic
- corrupt
- poor human rights/little freedom of expression
- divided on ethnic lines
- chaotic
- no peace.

Means of escape

The means used to escape from Ethiopia varied but commonly included using false travel documents and overstaying on a valid visa. Getting to the UK was invariably expensive, and the financial support of family and friends was often necessary. Illegal travel documents were said to be very costly and usually obtained by bribing officials or paying a 'middle man'. Fifteen participants reported that they had come to the UK via another country, most commonly via Bulgaria.

Experiences with the UK immigration department

In 1999, it took an average of 18 months for the Home Office to process applications for asylum. Some of the participants said they had been waiting for a decision for over 5 years and they reported that this caused them considerable stress:

The most important thing that stresses me is my immigration case. I sometimes have nightmares about it. I wonder if they are going to reject me. (Female participant)

The psychological consequences of political persecution in Ethiopia were reported to create emotional insecurity and a fear of authority. This had the capacity to diminish their ability to convince the immigration department that their application for asylum was genuine. Ethiopians tend to avoid eye contact as an expression of respect for and deference to people in authority, which in the UK is more likely to be interpreted as a sign of lying and therefore a reason for deportation.

ADAPTING TO THE UK CULTURE

Acculturation

Although some participants had explicit aims to integrate by learning about British culture, adaptation was recognized by many as being difficult. Trying to adapt to the British culture was said by some participants to be a cause of stress, depression and poor health, as described by a male participant:

I had a nice life in Ethiopia. I am not saying everybody was like me. For the last twenty years I had a happy life. In that country [Ethiopia] when I was working as a journalist, I had a good life. Of course I had a rough ride too. I was in jail. However, at times I prefer prison to life in exile. . . . I am trying to overcome the sequel of life in exile such as loneliness, lack of partner and family separation.

One of the 'expert' participants explained the difficulties experienced by Ethiopian refugees in this way:

> *Ethiopian refugees who come from the traditional society where social relationship and family bondage is very strong, find it difficult to integrate, to communicate with the British society, where they do not know the system, where they do not speak the language, where the sense of privacy is highly valued.*

The factors that were reported to assist them to adapt to UK society included:

- information about the health and social systems
- material and emotional support
- opportunities for development, such as English language classes
- help finding jobs or starting businesses
- the freedom and democracy in the UK

For many, their religious belief and practice gave them hope, guidance, continuity, familiarity and spiritual support during their struggle to adapt to British culture.

Factors causing variance in acculturation and adaptation

Gender

Women were reported to adapt better to life in the UK. Conversely, men were said to be more likely to experience difficulties adapting as many of them could not maintain their social status and position in the family. One of the 'expert' participants reported that:

> *The male refugees find it difficult to accept the reality of being a resource, being unemployed, and loathe the idea of doing the 'dirty jobs' that denies their traditional role as breadwinners . . . man of the 'adebabai'. They consider themselves as failures and become demoralized, leading to depression and self-neglect. On the other hand, relatively speaking, women adjust better and faster to the life of exile or asylum. . . . Adebabai is an Amharic word. It means 'outside of home' [public arena]. Men argue, litigate or discourse among themselves to show that someone is a man, a strong man, a wise man, an influential person. Whereas, domestic affairs such as cooking, cleaning and other aspects are left to women.*

Age

Variation in adaptation among different age groups was also found, with some young participants believing that they could adapt more quickly and being able to learn the language better than older people. On the other hand, young refugees found it difficult to live independently of their parents as they reported lack of relevant skills. In Ethiopia the family carries responsibility for children until they get married. Leaving home suddenly and prematurely meant they quickly needed to learn to budget, cook, clean and make decisions for themselves as well as having to cope with separation from their family.

Urban versus rural living

Adaptation was also found to be dependent on whether the participant originated from a rural or urban location. Many of our study participants were well-educated individuals who had lived in urban areas in Ethiopia such as Addis Ababa; this made their living in a large city like London a little easier. However, many described marked cultural differences between urban life in Ethiopia and urban life in the UK that caused them significant stress. These differences included the tendency of people in the UK to live very private lives and to be too busy working.

Time

Length of time in the UK appeared to correlate with their level of adaptation; the longer they were in the UK the better they appeared to be adapted, although some participants did not feel a sense of belonging despite many years in the UK.

Downward social mobility and adapting to a new identity

Most study participants had to adapt to belonging to a different social class, usually lower, with depressed economic circumstances.

Another major life change reported by the participants on arrival to the UK was their loss of status as citizens and the acquisition of a new and negatively construed tag of 'foreigner' and 'asylum seeker', as a male participant described:

> *Living in exile in a foreign country has repercussions. There is what is called 'status'. Status means to be a refugee and to be called 'a refugee'. This has a big psychological impact on refugees. When I was in Ethiopia whether I was working or not, to be an Ethiopian was enough for me.*

The stigma of the tag 'asylum seeker' was compounded by the food voucher system (since abolished) which was publicly visible when shopping in supermarkets. The decreased social standing they experienced in the UK was compounded by the prejudices and discrimination against them whipped up by certain sections of the media which portrayed them as 'spongers' and flagrant abusers of the British welfare system. Being portrayed in negative terms added to their sense of alienation and hampered their attempts to settle and integrate.

Employment

At the time of the study those seeking asylum were not allowed to do paid work in the UK unless they made an application to the Home Office and had been waiting for a decision for 2 years or more. Thirty-three per cent (33%) of the participants reported that they were employed, 27% were unemployed, and 41% were students. As might be expected, employment status was associated with the length of stay in the UK and immigration status. Participants reported a multitude of barriers to employment in the UK:

- lack of work experience in the UK (40%)
- lack of appropriate qualifications (38%)
- lack of UK recognized qualifications (27%)
- their immigration status (29%)
- lack of English language skills (27%)
- discrimination (27%).

Other factors that prevented them from finding employment included: lack of money to travel to interviews or to look for work, health problems, lack of affordable childcare, and poor understanding of the employment system. A major problem for many of the participants was finding an occupation that was comparable to their occupation in Ethiopia, as many of the participants had been professionals such as lawyers and accountants. A participant described vividly the impact that downward social mobility had on him thus:

> *Back home I was a university lecturer . . . [this] puts people in a special position in the society. I used to meet my ex-students working for different organizations. . . . They would wish me health and peace, with respect. In this country however, I am nothing. I am nothing at all.*

On the other hand, employment was reported to help them to settle in the UK and to gain a sense of belonging and citizenship.

Many of the participants were, or had been working towards, removing the barriers to suitable employment through English language and vocational courses. However, financial hardship and housing issues created barriers to some taking up or completing their studies; for example, living in half-board accommodation when set meal times coincided with the times of courses meant that some had to chose between having a meal or attending a class. Some were disappointed that despite gaining extra qualifications they still could not find appropriate work.

Experiences with housing

Most participants lived in Greater London, mainly in Haringey, Islington and Westminster. Liverpool and Leeds hosted the remainder. Almost a third (30%) were housing association tenants, 22% were council tenants (all of whom had been in the country for 5 or more years) and 12% lived in bed and breakfast accommodation. Thirty-six per cent lived in one room only.

Dissatisfaction with their current accommodation was common (48%), mainly among those who were homeless, living with friends, private tenants or living in bed and breakfast accommodation. Lack of space and privacy were the most common housing problems, in particular having to share a kitchen and bathroom with several other people especially when they were of a different ethnic group or gender. Other problems included the poor condition of the buildings, noisy or hostile neighbours, insecurity of tenancy and problems with the location. Lack of safety was also a problem for some, particularly women, some of whom reported being afraid of unannounced visits from their landlords and men sharing their accommodation.

Material security

During the interview, financial difficulties were reported by one-third of participants (33%); one-fifth (19%) described being at least reasonably well off and these were generally in employment, although others in employment reported financial difficulties. One-third of the participants (33%) reported that they received income support, usually accompanied by housing benefit, and a few participants (8%) received unemployment benefit or food vouchers. Some (15%) reported experiencing difficulties claiming benefits, including not being entitled, delays in processing claims, and protracted and complicated claiming procedures. As reported above, low income prevented many participants from finding work as they could not afford the bus or train fares to travel to find work or to attend courses.

Experiences with statutory social welfare services

Eighteen per cent of the participants were in contact with a social worker whereas 25% had been in contact with an Ethiopian community organization. Thirty-eight per cent had sought help from a solicitor or from other professional services, and 24% had sought help from interpreting services. Housing services were also frequently used, particularly the Homeless Persons Unit (used by 24% of the participants). Half of those who had used housing services reported having had a negative experience, describing them as *'daunting'*, or as having *'unhelpful staff'*, being a *'poor service'*, and having *'long waiting lists'*. The participants were infrequent users of day services such as nurseries and day centres.

Social support

Social isolation and loneliness were identified by participants as causes of stress and barriers to their acculturation. Over a quarter (27%) of the participants spontaneously reported that their social life was better in Ethiopia than in the UK. In Ethiopia family, friends and neighbours were reported to be very important. Neighbours were frequently described as being like *'one big family'*. This was in contrast to the UK, which was seen as *'private'* and *'individualistic'*. Attempts to recreate neighbourliness in the UK were often thwarted by a fear of being misunderstood and resulted in some participants isolating themselves. Despite this, many of the participants (60%) said their friends were the main source of support when feeling unhappy and many (66%) would also often look to friends for help with health or social welfare problems, before turning to a partner.

Finding friends was difficult in the UK, particularly those who shared the same culture. Ethiopians who had lived in the UK for several years were perceived by some of our participants differently insofar as they had acculturated and ceased to be 'Ethiopian'. Staying in contact with friends was also found to be hard in the UK as they often lived at some distance from each other and the cost of travel was prohibitive. Another barrier to sustaining supportive friendship was the pace of life in the UK and people being too preoccupied with their jobs.

HEALTH AND SICKNESS BELIEFS AND PRACTICES

Health beliefs

The participants were asked what it means to them to be healthy, to describe someone who is healthy and explain why they considered that person as healthy. The most prevalent belief of the participants was that healthiness *is* happiness and happiness *is* healthiness. For the participants happiness both contributes to health and is an indication of it. Happiness ('Desta') to them means fulfilling dreams, ambitions and basic needs; having harmonious relationships; not being depressed, stressed or worried; being physically fit and not suffering from illness and being mentally well. This is how some of the participants expressed the meanings of happiness:

When you are healthy, you feel happy. You would chat and have fun with people. You have a happy life with your family. In general you would have a happy relationship with people. (Female participant)

A male participant added:

If your dreams are fulfilled according to your wish without worries it means that you have succeeded in achieving something. This means that you have fed your mental well-being with happiness . . . The food to our mental well-being is success, bright future, satisfaction and happiness in life.

The participants were aware that being a refugee had had a negative impact on their happiness.

In this country, if I laugh once in a month it is great. I mean if I laugh from the bottom of my heart – true laughter once a month. Back home I used to laugh every day. I was happy all the time. I was happy, even when I had no money. I was happy, in spite of not wearing good shoes. I was happy, I had friends, I had a family. There are many things that were making me happy. (Male participant)

Our evidence suggests that if refugeedom denies happiness, it also denies health.

As well as the above meanings of health and happiness, healthiness was also described as having 'positive' personal capabilities and attributes (such as independence, motivation, self-confidence and hopefulness), spiritual well-being and a healthy environment. The relationship between health and happiness and all these concepts is illustrated in Figure 8.2.

Beliefs about sickness causation

The participants held a number of beliefs about sickness causation which were influenced by their experiences both in Ethiopia and in the UK. Whilst for them happiness was viewed as the primary 'cause' of health, disease was seen as the primary 'cause' of sickness. Beliefs about the causes of sickness included:

Figure 8.2   Conceptual model of Ethiopian migrants' health beliefs.

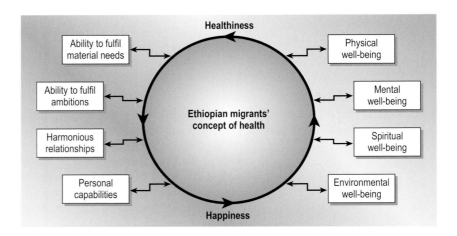

- disease (germs and viruses spread through blood, air, food and water, poor cleanliness and sanitation)
- food (eating the wrong foods, eating contaminated food)
- climate and environment (pollution, flooding, swamps with malarial mosquitoes, weather changes, cold weather, too much sun)
- accidents
- poor socio-economic conditions (inability to afford to eat a balanced diet, keep clean, pay bills, and find suitable shelter)
- depression and stress
- unhealthy behaviours (unprotected sex, alcohol/drugs, smoking cigarettes, lack of exercise)
- social isolation/loneliness
- supernatural causes (God, Satan or evil spirits, magic, the evil eye)
- other causes (included self-neglect, inherited disease and iatrogenic causes such as the bad effects of traditional medicines)

Of note in the list above is their recognition of the negative impact of depression and stress, loneliness and social isolation on health. They were acutely aware of the threat to their health as a consequence of their social circumstances.

Their belief in supernatural causes of illness was held sometimes simultaneously with a belief in natural causes such as germs, heredity and the climate, and social causes such as poverty and pollution.

One of the male participants portrayed the complexity of health beliefs held by Ethiopians when he said:

The reason why I am healthy is because of the will of God. God gave us health, which is very important. I am healthy. On top of that I look after my cleanliness and myself. I also keep my house clean. I also look for the cleanliness of my environment. I am free from addictions and alcohol consumption. I look after my health not to be ill.

Both younger and older people and people who had been in the UK for short and long periods held beliefs about supernatural causes. As one of the male participants said:

In our country they strongly believe in this illness (caused by 'Buda') from one end of the country to the other.

Beliefs related to mental health and mental illness

Mental health tended to be described in behavioural terms, such as *'responding sensibly'*, *'communicating well'* and *'being able to handle a crisis'*, and as subjective experiences, such as *'being free of stress'*, *'being confident'* and *'being able to know right and wrong'*.

Whilst the five participants with mental health problems were specifically asked about the meaning of mental health most of the other participants, as well as the 'expert' informants, emphasized the importance of mental well-being to the whole health and happiness of the individual. Boxes 8.3 and 8.4 represent their beliefs about mental health and well-being.

Box 8.3   Mental health in behavioural terms

- Responding sensibly
- Being reasonable
- Not imposing one's ideas on others
- Communicating well
- Interacting with others
- Integrating and adapting
- Fulfilling one's needs or desires
- Taking responsibility
- Being independent
- Overcoming problems
- Being able to handle a crisis
- Being able to analyse situations

Box 8.4   Mental health as a subjective state

- Not having mental illness
- Avoiding and being free of stress
- Having a clear bright mental state
- Having mental strength
- Knowing right and wrong
- Viewing things in a balanced way
- Thinking about one's health and well-being
- Having mental satisfaction
- Not having a trauma
- Being confident
- Being mentally active

Mental illness or 'madness' carries a stigma in Ethiopian culture. It is believed to be the work of the devil and a punishment for the sins of the patient or a person close to them. Madness is also thought to be due to spirit possession such as by 'Zar' spirits. 'Buda' (evil eye) is also believed to cause mental illness. Depression is perceived as having both natural and supernatural causation and remedies. The stigma of madness was reported to lead to people being secretive about mental health problems, thus making them less likely to utilize mental health facilities:

Late presentation is one of the problems. The reason is that we Ethiopians are accustomed to keeping our problems to our families and ourselves. . . . Especially, if the problem is associated with psychological/mental illness, it is considered as a serious illness and people do not seek consultation because of the stigma attached to this. . . . I would not go to the psychiatrist for counselling. I do not think the psychiatrist is useful in our situation. (Male participant)

An 'expert' participant explained:

Anyone that has mental illness is regarded as a mad person. So, no one wants to admit. No one wants to be branded as a mad person. So, everyone with any symptoms of depression and some kind of mental illness would like to avoid being seen as one of the mad people back home. So, they would be forced to be secretive to their friends, relatives, even to the professionals when they suffer from that type of illness.

Psychosocial explanations were also given such as responses to traumatic events in Ethiopia, for example persecution, having to endure many losses on migrating to the UK, and loneliness. Loneliness was seen to be a major cause of depression and stress, and these were in turn reported to be major causes of ill health.

When we were back home . . . we had no knowledge about depression. However, when we see refugees who came to this country . . . [and] leave their families or parents behind, they experience a lonely life here. They have no one to turn to for advice, they have no one to share ideas with, they have no one to consult. (Female participant)

EXPERIENCES OF ILL HEALTH

When asked how their health had been in the past year most participants described their health as 'very good' or 'good' in the last year. Half of them reported experiencing a physical health problem since arriving in the UK, such as headaches, migraine or colds. However, when asked what made them feel ill, 61% of the participants reported that unhappiness caused by stress or worry did. Stress was caused by loneliness, housing problems, boredom, family problems, unemployment, a lack of spiritual life, uncertainty about their asylum decision and problems communicating in English.

Forty-eight per cent also reported that their low income or lack of money was a cause of illness through, for example, not being able to afford nutritious or culturally appropriate food, or to afford accommodation with adequate cooking facilities. Those living in half-board accommodation were often given little choice about what food they ate; this particularly created difficulties for the Christian Orthodox and Muslim participants who do not eat pork or who fast.

The most common type of health problems reported to have been experienced since arrival in the UK were mental health related. Fifteen participants (including five who were known to have had a diagnosed mental illness) said they had suffered either from depression, stress or 'mental illness'. Most of these participants were men (12 /15), eight were employed, five unemployed and two were students. Most had been in the UK for over 5 years. Furthermore, 45% of all the participants agreed to the question asking if they felt sad or unhappy for long periods of time.

HELP SEEKING AND COPING WITH ILL HEALTH

The health care sought by the participants in the UK depended on the type or seriousness of the illness but commonly included a GP ($n = 74$) and hospital services. Some said they had consulted friends or family often as a first resort and used over-the-counter medicines and ate 'good' or traditional foods. There appeared to be a high level of knowledge about how to access primary and secondary health services. Nearly all the participants (97%) were registered with a GP and 78% found the UK health services easy to use. On the other hand, only 36% of the participants had reported that they used dental services.

Some participants did not understand the primary care system or method of referral and were often stunned at the long waiting times. Difficulty communicating with healthcare practitioners due to a lack of interpreters was another problem. Others said they had experienced poor or inappropriate treatment. A female participant described her negative experience thus:

> *Throughout the five years, he [the GP] examined me and prescribed the medicine . . . He never sought an interpreter . . . It was with my kidney performing only three per cent that I finally reached the doctors.*

Western medicines were sometimes combined with traditional remedies. However, many were cautious about some traditional remedies as they had not been researched. Religious practices such as praying or drinking 'Tsebele' (holy water) were also seen to be important healing acts.

Ethiopian people were reported to be shy of discussing their illness with doctors, as an 'expert' participant described:

> *Most of the time they don't go [to the doctor] even if they do, they cannot explain what their illness is. Never mind in this country even in our country if the doctor asks what the problem is, they can't say it, especially if the doctor is an older person. This is because in our culture you respect your elders, as a result they get very shy, and because of their shyness they leave the doctors without saying what they want.*

Cultural factors such as deference to specific types of people, therefore, can be seen to have a significant potential impact on health, insofar as illnesses could be neglected.

COPING WITH MENTAL HEALTH PROBLEMS

The participants reported that due to the stigma of 'madness' Ethiopians are secretive about mental health problems and are likely to under-utilize mental health facilities. Instead political and social solutions for problems that caused stress were seen to be the answer for some, such as reducing social isolation. Drinking or bathing in holy water (Tsebele) and prayer were reported as cures for madness when it was believed to have been caused by supernatural forces.

Ethiopians also believe that laughter and happiness is good therapy and important to maintaining mental health, but some said having fun and laughter was difficult in the UK. Self-help for emotional problems was common. Very few mentioned seeing a counsellor or their GP. However, of the 45% of participants who said they felt sad or unhappy for long periods of time three-quarters said they would like to talk to someone trained in working with refugees about their feelings.

Most participants acknowledged that although the UK provided better health services than Ethiopia, the unavailability of family, friends and neighbours to give informal support and care, and the lack of traditional Ethiopian remedies were negative aspects of dealing with sickness in the UK.

DISCUSSION

THE IMPACT OF MIGRATION, ADAPTATION AND SETTLEMENT ON HEALTH

The accounts of the participants showed a variation of migration, adaptation and settlement experiences all of which impact upon their health in a number of ways. Furnham & Bochner (1986) argue that the experience of migration affects mental health and leads to greater levels of stress and mental illness. However, even though the refugees' health may be compromised before they arrive in their host country, due to imprisonment and torture, Smaje (1995) proposes that positive selection may take place whereby the healthy, younger and more able people are more likely to leave their country than those who are elderly or sick. The latter is possibly the case as there is some evidence that the physical health status of many asylum seekers on arrival to the UK is often good compared to the UK population (Wolhuter 2003, Haringey Council 1997). However, their health status may not be maintained as the health of many refugees declines in the first two or three years after arrival in the UK, mainly due to poverty, social exclusion, poor accommodation and poor nutrition (Gammell et al 1993, Wolhuter 2003, Vallely et al 1999). Barriers to health care for refugees also exacerbate their health problems (Vallely et al 1999).

BARRIERS AND ENABLERS TO ADAPTATION AND SETTLEMENT

Whilst the majority of the participants reported feeling marginalized and excluded by British society, a few suggested that they were beginning to settle and integrate into the wider society. The findings of this study indicate that positive settlement experiences were not dependent on length of stay, as some participants did not feel a sense of belonging despite many years in the UK, but on both personal and societal factors. This is echoed by Bloch (2000), who maintains that the settlement of refugees and asylum seekers depends on a range of factors including the policies of the country of asylum as well as the experiences and attitudes of individuals to exile.

BARRIERS TO SUCCESSFUL ADAPTATION AND SETTLEMENT

This study has highlighted a number of barriers to the successful adaptation and settlement of Ethiopian refugees in the UK including the stigma of being a refugee, difficulties in finding employment, living in poverty, living in poor accommodation, feeling socially excluded and isolated, having a poor command of English, and experiencing difficulties in understanding the host culture. These barriers have also been found by researchers in other countries; for example, an investigation into the initial settlement experiences of Ethiopian and Somali refugees in Toronto, Canada, revealed that these refugees faced social exclusion and multiple forms of disadvantage, including high unemployment, underemployment and overcrowded living conditions. These resulted in frustration and despair, which led some individuals, particularly young men, to exhibit suicidal behaviours (Danso 2002).

On arrival in the UK, refugees face a number of prejudices and hostile attitudes, not least perpetuated by the popular media. Indeed, a survey of public opinion on attitudes to refugees and asylum seekers (MORI 2002) stated that an increasing number of people (11% in 1997, 43% in 2000) polled about why people seek asylum in the UK said it was due to economic reasons. Many had a grossly inflated idea of the percentage of the world's refugees and asylum seekers who live in the UK. These views, often fuelled by the media, hamper refugees' attempts to integrate and make a useful contribution to the host country. Sales (2002) proposes that the social exclusion and stigmatization to which refugees are exposed damages their chances of settling, whilst racist discourse against asylum seekers impacts on everyone from these communities, whatever their legal status.

This study confirms findings from other studies that asylum seekers and refugees share the problems of many other marginalized groups in British society, such as high levels of unemployment, poor housing and racism (Bloch 2000, Carey-Wood et al 1995, Woodhead 2000). Ethiopian refugees' experiences of racism is not unique to the UK, as Danso (2002) has also found that institutional and everyday racism towards Ethiopian and Somali refugees in Toronto created formidable barriers to integration into their new country.

As well as the problems refugees share with other marginalized groups, this study has found that Ethiopian refugees, like other refugees, also suffer the additional stress caused by their asylum status, separation from family, uncertainties about their future, and the need to adapt to a new culture.

ENABLERS TO SUCCESSFUL ADAPTATION AND SETTLEMENT

It is clear from this study that the reasons for leaving Ethiopia were compelling, and the cost was high, both financially and in human terms. The resourcefulness and resilience expressed by the participants in the face of their experiences reflects that seen in other refugees (Burnett & Fassil 2002). This study has highlighted a number of other factors that enable adaptation and settlement. Personal factors include a desire for integration and a belief in the benefits of this, positive socio-economic circumstances, achieving refugee status or British citizenship, access to training and education and proficiency in English. Societal factors include the ease of access to health and social services, availability of social support, the democracy and freedom of the UK compared to Ethiopia, and the multicultural nature of British society.

This study has also highlighted the importance of age and gender for adaptation and settlement. In addition, religious belief and practice by the participants appears to have played a positive role in easing them through the process of adaptation to life in the UK.

HEALTH AND ILLNESS BELIEFS AND PRACTICES

This study has shown that the impact of refugeedom on the health beliefs and practices of Ethiopian refugees is variable and complex. In Ethiopia people have both traditional and biomedical health beliefs and health-care systems, although the latter is mediated through ideological and cultural factors. Young (1986) described a theory of health beliefs that is based on a dichotomy: *externalizing medical belief systems* (due to outside factors emanating from the social, natural and supernatural world) found in tribal societies, and *internalizing medical belief systems* (inside factors emphasizing the physiological and pathological) found in more complex societies. The Ethiopian system, Young proposes, falls some-where in between these two. This is borne out by our findings; for example, external factors mentioned include loneliness, poverty, evil spirits, the evil eye, magic, climate and environmental changes, and internal factors mentioned include germs and viruses, accidents, taking drugs, smoking and inherited diseases, with almost equal weight being given to both.

Ethiopians describe health holistically, and do not separate concepts of physical health from those of mental and spiritual health. Although they hold a strong belief in God and 'God's will' they believe in the need to live harmoniously within their community, free from stress and worries, as well as placing emphasis on the individual's responsibility for their own health.

The degree to which the Ethiopian migrants' health beliefs had been modified due to the effects of migration are difficult to ascertain but Berhane et al (2001) found that women in Ethiopia had a very broad understanding of health although for most rural women health is a disease-free state. This would indicate that Ethiopian migrants in the UK place a stronger emphasis on externalized factors (such as happiness) than they did at home. Furthermore, they have moved to a society where the healthcare system places emphasis on internal factors.

Another way the effects of migration on Ethiopians' health beliefs can be shown is by their changing healthcare practices between Ethiopia and the UK, as decisions about healthcare seeking for all individuals, what-ever their culture, are influenced to some extent by health beliefs. For example, Ethiopians are less likely to seek the help of a psychiatrist if the symptoms are believed to be caused by spirit possession. Ethiopian healthcare practices have changed to differing degrees after migration – in most cases traditional remedies were more likely to be sought in Ethiopia whilst Western medicine is more likely to be sought in the UK. This probably reflects both acculturation and differences in health resources (traditional remedies and practitioners are hard to come by in the UK whereas Western medicine is freely available). The degree to which acculturation has taken place and the consequent acceptance of Western medical beliefs is unclear but there is some evidence (Spector 1991) that it can take three generations before migrants fully acculturate. Even if acculturation does occur there is often a movement towards reviving lost beliefs and practices and a desire to take on the identities of the homeland. This is of particular importance to health policy-makers and practitioners.

Refugees' experiences with the healthcare system in the host country will also impact on their practices. For example, a negative experience may deter them from seeking help from a particular source again. Negative experiences may be a result of problems with communication, racism, poor provision of information or culturally inappropriate care. Culturally inappropriate care is ethnocentric and does not acknowledge the individual's needs in terms of religion, diet, language, beliefs, family support which differ from those of the majority, usually white, culture.

Finally, the effects of migration are more than moving from one culture to another, or one healthcare system to another. Reasons for flight such as oppression, violence, fear and poverty are factors that impact on the health of refugees. Furthermore, their experiences in the host country such as poor housing, unemployment, racism and isolation also impact on their health. It is difficult to ascertain how these factors affect health beliefs but as Ethiopian refugees see happiness and healthiness as insepa-rable, it is probable that these negative experiences and the consequent unhappiness they have caused have highlighted to them the relationship between health and subjective well-being.

CONCLUSION

It is particularly important that health and social care providers under-stand that Ethiopian beliefs have evolved within a complex society over thousands of years, and are unlikely to disappear, even after a number of generations. They should understand that many refugees have had traumatic experiences and continue to live in desperate circumstances. Finally, whilst it would be impossible for health and social care profes-sionals to understand the needs of every refugee culture, they should address their own cultural competence, in order to ensure that care is based on cultural awareness, knowledge and sensitivity which takes into consideration Ethiopian people's health beliefs, practices and needs.

REFLECTIVE QUESTIONS

1. How useful did you find the ethnohistorical information provided in the chapter in terms of helping you understand the findings of the EMBRACE UK study?
2. The EMBRACE UK study provided research-evidenced knowledge to help underpin the health and social care of Ethiopian refugees and asylum seekers. Reflect on the importance of evidenced-based cultur-ally competent care.
3. The EMBRACE UK study clearly illustrated that both culture and structure must be taken into consideration when caring for Ethiopian refugees and asylum seekers. Reflect on the reasons why it may be dangerous to consider only the cultural background of the people we care for.

Acknowledgement

We wish to thank all those who took part in this study and the National Lottery Charities Board for funding it.

REFERENCES

Baker C, Arseneault A, Gallant G 1994 Resettlement without the support of an ethnocultural community. Journal of Advanced Nursing, 20:1064–1072

Bariso E U 1997 The Horn of Africa health project. North Thames Regional Health Authority. London

Berhane Y, Gossaye Y, Emmelin M, Hogberg U 2001 Women's health in rural settings in social transition in Ethiopia. Social Science and Medicine 53:1525–1539

Bloch A 2000 Refugee settlement in Britain: the impact of policy on participation. Journal of Ethnic and Migration Studies 26(1):75–88

Burnett A, Fassil Y 2002 Meeting the health needs of refugee and asylum seekers in the UK: an information and resource pack for health workers. Department of Health, London

Carey-Wood J, Duke K, Kam V, Marshall T 1995 The settlement of refugees in Britain. Home Office Research Study 141. HMSO, London

Danso R 2002 From 'There' to 'Here': An investigation of the initial settlement experiences of Ethiopian and Somali refugees in Toronto. GeoJournal 56(1):3–14

Furnham A, Bochner S 1986 Culture shock: Psychological reactions to unfamiliar environments. Routledge. London

Gamaledin-Ashami M 1993 A report on the study of homelessness among young people from the Horn of Africa in selected areas of London. Charity Projects, London

Gammell H, Ndahiro A, Nichola N, Windsor J 1993 Refugees (political asylum seekers) service provision and access to the NHS. College of Health, London

Haringey Council 1997 Refugees and asylum seekers in Haringey. Research project report. Haringey Council, London

Huka G 1996 Ethiopian Health Support (EHS): service provisions and organisational strategy. EHS Group, London

Market and Opinion Research International (MORI) 2002 Attitudes towards refugees and asylum seekers for Refugee Week. MORI, London

Nationality, Immigration and Asylum Act 2002 Her Majesty's Stationery Office, London

Papadopoulos I, Gebrehiwot A 2002 The EMBRACE UK project: The Ethiopian migrants, their beliefs, refugeedom, adaptation, calamities, and experiences in the United Kingdom. Middlesex University, London

Patton M Q 1990 Qualitative evaluation and research methods. Sage, New York

Refugee Council 2000 Information for asylum seekers. Refugee Council, London

Sales R 2002 The deserving and the undeserving? Refugees, asylum seekers and welfare in Britain. Critical Social Policy 22(3):456–478

Smaje C 1995 Health, race, and ethnicity: making sense of the evidence. King's Fund, London

Spector R 1991 Cultural diversity in health and illness. 3rd edn. Appleton and Lange, East Norwalk

UNHCR 2005 UNHCR in the UK. Basic definitions. Online. Available: http://www.unhcr.org.uk/info/briefings/basic_facts/definitions.html 30 Mar 2005

Vallely A, Scott C, Hallums J 1999 The health needs of refugees: using rapid appraisal to assess needs and identify priority areas for public health action. Public Health Medicine 1(3):103–107

Wolhuter J 2003 Alien nation. The Parliamentary Health Magazine 5:34–35

Woodhead D 2000 The health and well-being of asylum seekers and refugees. King's Fund, London

World Factbook 2004 Online. Available: http://www.odci.gov/cia/publications/factbook/geos/et.html 14 Jul 2004

Young A 1986 Internalising and externalizing medical belief systems: an Ethiopian example. In: Currer C, Stacey M (eds) Concepts of health, illness and disease: A comparative perspective. Berg Publishers, Oxford

Chapter **9**

Notions of motherhood and the maternity needs of Arab Muslim women

Myfanwy Davies and Irena Papadopoulos

LEARNING OBJECTIVES

After reading this chapter you should be able to:
- understand that cultural beliefs and norms mould physical experiences of maternity and inform the maternity needs of individual women
- appreciate that the maternal body may serve among women as a symbol of cultural integrity.
- obtain an overview of the potential of narrative approaches to studying culture
- appreciate broad factors that may inform the maternal identities of Arab Muslim women as users of NHS maternity services

- be aware of cultural and institutional factors that may condition perceptions of the body, of individual agency and of the use of maternity information among practitioners
- obtain an overview of diverse maternal identities adopted among groups of Arab Muslim women and appreciate how individual perceptions of the maternity encounter with health practitioners may be conditioned by notions of the homeland, Islam and regional and class identities
- appreciate that perceptions of the preferences, needs and merits of users of maternity services among health practitioners may be informed by institutional and cultural models of white and non-white women
- question the basis of one's own views of women's needs as users of maternity services as these may relate to negative perceptions of other cultures and to stereotypes of feminine identity and the body
- question the bases of institutional practices and beliefs concerning information, motherhood and non-white cultures.

INTRODUCTION

This chapter is founded on a doctoral study that explored patterns of communication between maternity practitioners and Arab Muslim users of the United Kingdom (UK) National Health Service (NHS) maternity care. It describes aspects of the relationship between culture and the body for Arab Muslim women and among UK health practitioners and outlines some issues of identification and difference within the practitioner–patient encounter.

By describing the cultural dimensions of the needs experienced by women as users of NHS maternity services and those outlined by health practitioners, the chapter aims to add to a foundation of cultural knowledge of diverse groups of Arab Muslim women in the UK and of NHS health practitioners. Findings reported here illustrate how individual Arab Muslim women and health practitioners experience encounters in maternity services through cultural frames of reference that they themselves construct. Accordingly, findings relating to the cultural values attached to labour pain, to 'dangers' associated with acceptance of medical advice about decisions to undergo intervention are described to illustrate the individual basis on which cultural beliefs and practices are established. These findings also relate to issues of migration and identity. A further pattern relates to the use of scans and information about the effects of potentially hazardous behaviours on the child, and these forms of information may be used to construct maternal identities. Through considering questions of class and medical knowledge, the ways in which these patterns relate to perceptions of belonging to urban Arab centres is considered. The discussion of findings produced from the accounts of health professional participants seeks to suggest ways in which the articulation of professional identities may rest on the construction of gender and racial difference. Beliefs concerning individual actions and the status of the feminine body among non-white groups that are referenced in the accounts of practitioners are discussed as these enable practitioners to differentiate from non-white patients and to withdraw from responsibilities to communicate with individual non-white women.

Finally, by outlining the cultural and institutional frames through which such identities are produced, the chapter seeks to promote awareness among practitioners and policy-makers of the cultural environment of maternity services. Through identifying the processes of producing difference and identification within individual encounters with Arab Muslim women, it is hoped that policies and individual practices may be developed to support the delivery of equitable maternity care to these groups. As the analysis focuses on the means by which non-white women are represented as a single group among health practitioners, it is also hoped that the discussion may contribute to improving practices of communication with diverse groups of non-white women using UK maternity services.

MOTHERHOOD AND SELF-IDENTITY

The project adopted an approach to identity that was based on the understanding that a consistent self is formed by individuals through accounts of themselves and their actions (Ricouer 1990). Similarly, the identities of groups were understood to be established through individual accounts of interaction with symbols of cultural difference (Barth 1998). The project focused on the relation of 'natural' experiences of maternal embodiment (pregnancy, birthing, nurturing) to cultural understandings of the maternal body. Nonetheless, the experience of the body is unavoidably informed by cultural constructions through which the body symbolizes the social group (Douglas 2003). In this way, points of entry into the body such as the mouth come to represent ways through which the identity of the group might be compromised. As such, these openings are protected by specific practices such as avoiding certain foods and engaging in ritual washing (Douglas 2004). As women may bear the children of men from outside a group without the knowledge of others, female reproductive bodies symbolize a source of danger and are protected by cultural norms restricting the sexual and social behaviour of women (Douglas 2004).

Studies of the ways in which women experience their bodies in relation to cultural representations have divided into two main approaches. An approach that emphasizes cultural and historical processes of representing the feminine body has suggested that the experience of sexual difference is itself cultural (de Beauvoir 1997, Butler 1999). In contrast, a second approach has explored the ways in which individual women perceive their bodies in relation to cultural notions of femininity and the reproductive body. The study that is discussed here adopted the second position outlined, and as such it considered that 'natural' experiences of the body exist through cultural notions of society, femininity and mother-hood (Bigwood 1999).

ARAB MUSLIM WOMEN AND CULTURAL VIEWS OF MOTHERHOOD

As has been suggested above, the construction of symbolic bodies informs women's individual experiences of motherhood across societies (Douglas 2003). Nonetheless, among migrant and non-white women, maternal identity may be negotiated with a number of symbolic bodies reflecting various cultural systems, having differing degrees of influence on the woman. Cultural systems that are likely to frame experiences of mother-hood among Arab Muslim women in the UK are those of colonialism, contemporary racism, political Islam and Arab Nationalism. Additionally, Arab Muslim women may adopt practices of reinterpreting tradition in order to claim a larger cultural scope to express their individual selves.

In order to justify the exploitation of colonized groups, black, South Asian and Muslim women were depicted in European travel literature and administrative reports, from the eighteenth century to the middle of the twentieth century, as being oppressed and silenced by their own societies. As such, projects for the colonization of these societies were represented as serving to liberate 'native' women. In addition to failing to reflect the diverse conditions of women's lives, through systematically failing to attend to the voices of individual Arab Muslim women, these representations also contributed to traditions of erotic writing which depicted Arab Muslim women as the willing and ignorant victims of sexual and social humiliation (Lowe 1991, Mabro 1996).

Similarly, during the late nineteenth and early twentieth centuries, feminist periodicals calling for women's rights to vote presented the improvement of the condition of Muslim women – through British women's suffrage – as a means through which British women could play their part in the mission of the British Empire to improve non-white societies. Hence, just as depictions of Muslim and non-white men served to suggest the superiority of the European colonizer, who alone was represented as offering civilization to 'native' societies, so these depic-tions of the condition of Muslim women served to suggest notions of enlightenment, power and patriotism among British feminists. In contrast, by associating domestic and maternal roles among Muslim women with a degraded social and personal condition, these British feminist periodicals appear to have assigned to Muslim women identifi-cations with the maternal body that British feminists sought to shed (Burton 1994). Through representations of contemporary Muslim women – notably of Afghan women under the rule of the Taliban – these colonial practices of assigning to Muslim women identities that deny individual difference appear to continue in Western feminist practice (Volpp 2003).

Islamism, also known as Islamic fundamentalism, is a term used to describe political movements that seek to establish Islamic states. As colonialism represented the relations of Islam and Western societies as ones of essential difference, so Islamism draws on the same notion of irreducible divide that opposes Islam to 'Western' traditions of secularism and democracy (Al-Azmeh 1993). Similarly, as colonialism sought to represent Muslim societies as being free of social and historical complexity, so Islamism has also sought to deny diversity within the Muslim world (Al-Azmeh 1993). Islamist representations of Muslim women appear to draw on colonial notions of the 'cultural' role of Muslim women within the domestic sphere. Accordingly, within Islamist opinion women have become represented as contributing to the Islamist cause by bearing children and through instructing them in Islamist values (Afshar 1998). Opposition to this system of representing Muslim women solely as symbols of cultural difference has drawn on Islamic sacred texts and on the Muslim legal tradition. Described as 'Islamic feminism', these approaches have developed new models of gender relations in Muslim societies from prescriptions to social equality attributed to early Islamic teaching and law (Mernissi 1991).

Following independence, Arab Nationalist movements established secular states in Egypt, Iraq, Syria and Yemen. In contrast to systems of representing women used within Islamism and colonialism, Arab Nationalist movements tended to use depictions of working women to suggest social and economic progress (Ahmed 1992, Joseph 2000). Nonetheless, elsewhere in the Arab world, maternity and the maternal body were used by governments as symbols of identity and difference to notions of Western societies (Bodran 1995, Larcin 1999). Similarly, in situations of conflict within the Arab world, women are portrayed as the producers of soldiers and martyrs (Sayigh 1993). Such practices of representing mothers have been reinforced where Arab Nationalism has become influenced by Islamism, as has been the case within Palestinian communities through the influence of the Iranian-backed Hamas (Hammami 1996).

While possibilities for expanding cultural models of motherhood exist within Islamic scholarship and within Arab Nationalist movements, the greatest potentials for Arab Muslim women to express individual maternal selves lie in practices of reinterpreting tradition. While the cultural imperative to cover women's bodies may be associated with the symbolic protection of the boundaries of the group, acts of veiling among Muslim women in Europe have been suggested to serve to establish the difference of the migrant community in migration and may represent a protective response to racism (Amir-Moazami & Salvatore 2003). Similarly, veiling may serve to establish links to the Arab world and to other Arab Muslim communities in migration. While such practices appear to accept the passive symbolic role of the feminine body, through suggesting women's religious commitment, covering the body may also serve to negotiate increased freedom of movement and extended rights to education (Amir-Moazami & Salvatore 2003). Hence, where Islam is perceived as being taught to children by their mothers and as being exemplified by their mothers' actions, young Muslim women who demonstrate their religious commitment through their dress draw on considerable support for their educational and professional projects. Education and professional activity may thus be seen among Muslim communities to contribute to the maternal capacities of women who are visibly devout.

HEALTH PRACTITIONERS AND CULTURAL VIEWS OF THE MATERNITY PATIENT

Just as national and religious cultures limit the abilities of women to express maternal identities through the symbolic construction of the maternal body, so medical institutions reflect similar cultural patterns of representing the body. As such, the patient–practitioner encounter may serve to impose wider relations of power on the bodies of individual women (Foucault 1995, 2003). Accordingly, through institutional practices of obstetric examination, the patient is obliged to submit to incursion on – and in – the body. Medical practices of questioning may not only oblige the patient to give up embodied knowledge of the self but would also appear to emphasize the 'confession' of unhealthy behaviours. Similarly, practices of providing information on risk-related behaviour to maternity patients would appear to serve to encourage women to regulate their pregnant embodiment according to (ever-narrowing) medical perceptions of the normal progress of pregnancy.

Additionally, depictions of the maternal body in French and British obstetric literature that represented conception, pregnancy and birth as processes that occur without the mother's effort have been suggested to function to remove women's own agency in becoming mothers (Moscucci 1990). Such constructions of the maternal body as the location in which processes of generation take place appear to coexist with important philosophical movements in Europe that have constructed agency as the property of the active mind and have opposed agency to the (feminine) body (Bordo 1987). Appearing to reflect aspects of this European model of agency and its conflictual relationship to the feminine body are constructions of patient decision-making that emphasize the desirability of exercising individual agency over the body during pregnancy, labour and birth. As Arab Muslim women have been suggested to be represented in British and Western media as identifying particularly strongly with maternity and with private domestic roles, such constructions of the body and of agency within the medical encounter may serve to reinforce cultural stereotypes of these groups, their needs and merits.

METHODOLOGY

SAMPLE GROUPS AND METHODS

The project used a combined focus group and individual interview approach with Arab Muslim participants. Accordingly, focus groups were conducted with 24 Arab Muslim women (6 of these being Iraqis, 10 Moroccan, and 8 Yemeni) with individual interviews having been held with 6 Iraqis, 10 Moroccans and 6 Yemenis. All participants in these groups were Sunni Muslims and were recruited through community associations. The practitioner sample consisted of general practitioners

(GPs) (4), midwives (4) and obstetricians (5). These groups were recruited through GP surgeries, through a midwife contact in a large maternity hospital in West London and through direct contact with obstetricians. While the largest group of health practitioners was white British and had no religious affiliations (4), other cultural and religious groups were Catholics (2 of these being Irish and 1 Spanish) and Hindus (2). The remaining participants were a black African atheist, a second-generation Jamaican Anglican, a Jamaican Muslim and a white English lapsed Catholic.

DATA COLLECTION, ANALYSIS AND VERIFICATION

A variant of the narrative inquiry approach was used to plan procedures used in interviewing study participants and in the interpretation of the data produced. Reconstructed 'stories' drawing on published work on experiences of maternity care and on fragments of accounts previously given to the researcher were used to prompt Arab Muslim participants' accounts during focus groups and individual interviews (Papadopoulos et al 2001). Reflecting a strong preference among health professional participants, direct questions were used to invite responses among these groups (see the section below on shortcomings in the study design). Practices of interpreting the data produced from both main participant groups involved identifying 'stories' with recognizable events and characters within each interview transcript and analysing these as individual accounts (McCormack 2000a, 2000b). Further steps undertaken in the interpretation of the accounts included repeated listening to tapes, followed by the production of notes on the multiple contexts in which the encounter occurred. Patterns in the use of language and narrative in each story were examined. Finally, attention was given to points in the story at which the speaker modified or clarified the account as these might relate to changes in relation to cultural constructions of the medical encounter and the feminine body. Sample participants from each participant group were sent reconstructed stories illustrating themes taken from their interview accounts in order to validate the findings produced through this process.

Material produced to publicize the study and that subsequently used in interviews with Arab Muslim women participants was translated into the Arabic dialects spoken among these national groups. As has been recommended by Papadopoulos & Lees (2002), all material used by participants was back-translated into English by a second translator. Similarly, interview guides were discussed at length with interpreters from each group. English transcripts produced for interviews conducted in Arabic dialects were back-translated to verify the quality of the translation.

ETHICAL ISSUES

Ethical approval for interviews and focus groups with Iraqi, Moroccan and Yemeni participants was obtained from an internal university ethics committee while approval for interviews with health professional participants was obtained from the Primary Health Care Trust by whom these participants were employed. The three dimensions of beneficence, dignity and justice described in the Belmont Report (National Commission for the Protection of Human Subjects of Biomedical and Behavioural Research 1978) structured interactions with participants and the use of the data throughout the project.

SHORTCOMINGS OF THE PROJECT

Despite the overall success of the methodology used, a number of short-comings were identified and were addressed during the interpretation of the study data.

Following a pilot interview with a health practitioner participant, during which the participant questioned the transparency of the use of reconstructed stories as prompts, this method was not used to prompt participant accounts during interviews with the health practitioner group. While it would have been preferable to use the narrative approach throughout each stage of data collection, interpretation and presentation, the difficulty encountered by the participant during the pilot interview served to suggest issues of authority and control within the interview encounter that emerged more fully through the interpretation of the interview accounts of other health practitioner participants.

A complication that arose in the interviews with Arab Muslim partici-pants related to issues of privacy. A set of interviews was conducted at a social gathering at which the interpreter was also the host and would come and go out of the interview room as she was needed. In one case, where a participant was discussing changes in her sexual orientation following the birth of her first child, the interpreter intervened to warn that the participant's account was not to be taken literally. Following the correction of the account – which was not contradicted by the participant – the context of the comments became difficult to establish. Nonetheless, this incident – together with other participants' practice of discussing the interview with those who had not yet been interviewed – appears to have entailed that the data collected reflected a consensus among the group that reflected how the group preferred to be seen. In this way, the poten-tial for participants to tailor accounts to perceptions of the researcher's views and interests was minimized. Similarly, these practices of interven-tion, prior discussion and the presence of the interpreter offered a 'public' context for accounts that might be contrasted with those recounted during individual interviews in participants' homes.

RESULTS

MATERNITY NEEDS: THE WOMEN'S PERSPECTIVE

The preferences and needs of Arab Muslim participants as users of maternity care related to cultural perceptions of motherhood, the mater-nal body and the uses of information about the body. These perceptions appear to have reflected patterns of imagining homelands, regions, localities and homes in the Arab world, and also appear to have reflected their relation with sections of British society. Two major perspectives on motherhood, cultural belonging and experiences of NHS maternity care, emerged among the study participants. The families of most Moroccan participants had migrated from villages in the interior, and these participants recounted similar maternity needs and experiences to Yemeni participants who had themselves migrated from villages or from poorer neighbourhoods of the capital. Given the influence of village origins and local customs on these accounts, participants in these groups were termed 'rural'. A divergent pattern of representing motherhood, the NHS and links to the homeland emerged among Iraqi women, all of whom were from middle-class neighbourhoods of Baghdad. In order to highlight the distinction between the model of motherhood outlined in this group and that suggested by 'rural' participants, participants in the Iraqi group were termed 'urban'.

EMBODIED AGENCY AS A LINK TO CULTURAL ORIGINS

Yemeni migrant participants together with first- and second-generation Moroccan participants emphasized their pride in their physical strength and in their ability to remain calm during pregnancy, labour and birth. Among second-generation Moroccan participants, in particular, stories told by their own mothers or by friends were perceived to enable the pregnant women to take on an adult role among women belonging to the national group. Among both Yemeni and Moroccan participants, stories tended to emphasize the mother's strength and to praise her ability to tolerate labour pain. The ability to give birth without pain relief was suggested by Moroccan participants as representing a national virtue that was also associated with family origins in rural areas of Morocco.

The value of labour pain as proof of cultural belonging did not lie in a notion of maternal suffering as a virtue in itself. Rather, maintaining sensation during labour and birth was perceived to serve to provide the mother with knowledge of her progress, without which she was perceived as being unable to take on responsibility for her child. Where women did not maintain sensation during birth, their behaviour in labour was recalled as having been inappropriate (talking and laughing). Such behaviour was also suggested to have entailed that women were not considered as having become adults in entering motherhood.

Pain was perceived across all three Arab Muslim participant groups to initiate women into the cultural roles of motherhood. Through reducing birthing women to a state of dependence similar to that of the child, labour pain was perceived among the 'urban' group to serve as a bond with the child and with other women in the family. Among 'rural' participants, labour and birthing pain was associated with the loss of a sense of self and with a metaphoric death and rebirth through which women adopted their identities as mothers. For participants across 'urban' and 'rural' groups, the entry into motherhood was perceived to claim all their resources and to oblige them to abandon their previous identities and social behaviour. This perception of motherhood was reported to lead some Arab Muslim women to seek to abort the fetus. Reactions of panic and depression in early pregnancy were recounted to have been faced by many 'rural' participants and were perceived to be overcome through the stories of friends and family, and through adopting regional and nationalist notions of the value of embodied agency in birth. Similarly, among 'urban' participants, experiences of sadness or panic in early pregnancy were alleviated by the accounts of friends or relatives that emphasized the key instructive role of the Muslim mother in the family and society.

MATERNITY CARE AS A DANGER TO NATURAL-CULTURAL IDENTITY

Among Yemeni, and particularly among Moroccan participants, the mother's emotional state was perceived as directly affecting the well-being of the fetus. As such, practices of protecting oneself from distress during pregnancy were seen as being crucial to the safety of the fetus. A cause of distress that was perceived as difficult to avoid was information provided by health practitioners. Information concerning screening, risks to the child and particularly reports that the fetus might be diseased were perceived to pose a real danger to the pregnancy. Accordingly, some older migrant women described how they would systematically ignore all medical advice on potential hazards to themselves and the fetus. Nonetheless, the majority of 'rural' participants were torn between the imperative to avoid worry and the desire for medical knowledge that might offer reassurance. Among this group, a pattern of accounts described the effects of incorrect or exaggerated information on medical assessments of hazards to the pregnancy. Practices of using such information were recounted with considerable regret due to perceptions of the potential harm caused to the fetus by the mother's worry. Hence, where it led to distress, the use of such information during pregnancy was also viewed as limiting women's abilities to maintain embodied agency.

Given the perception of a symbolic maternal body that was founded primarily on practices of embodied agency, a similar difficulty among 'rural' participants using NHS maternity services related to accepting pain relief or obstetric intervention. Widespread perceptions that health practitioners exaggerated dangers to the baby contributed to the regret that consent was given for intervention among this group. The reported preponderance of practices of obstetric intervention within the NHS and perceptions of the reduced significance of motherhood within British society were reported among this group as a major sign of cultural difference. Such perceptions of difference and the associated perceptions of alienation from NHS health practitioners appear to have contributed to giving a psychic dimension to experiences of physical transgression during intervention. In this way, where participants recalled acts of intervention, they tended to describe themselves as being outside their bodies. Within such accounts, references to the uterus and to the birth canal seldom used the personal pronoun ('*my* uterus'). Having emphasized the universal nature of the experience of birth, these accounts also further emphasized participants' lack of embodied agency in the process.

While the disruptive effects of intervention on 'rural' participants were suggested through accounts in which they appear to have exteriorized themselves from the process of birth, experiences of fear and vulnerability were also associated with undergoing obstetric intervention. Among this group which associated embodied agency with symbolic notions of motherhood, the actions of obstetricians, who may have been conducting entirely necessary interventions, appear to have been perceived by the participants as compromising their personal identities. Accordingly, experiences of intervention were described in terms of being 'flat out on a table' and were considered to be 'violent and not easy to think about afterwards'. Further suggesting the relation of intervention and incursion into the sense of self, practices of examination considered unnecessary by a participant were described as 'fondling'.

INFORMATION AND WILLED AGENCY

In contrast to those examples discussed above, in which embodied maternal agency was a central characteristic of the symbolic body constructed by women in the 'rural' group, among the 'urban' group, the symbolic body was constructed around notions of the control of sensation through acts of willed agency. For this group, maternity information was a culturally legitimate means through which to adopt a maternal role. Medical information on potential dangers to the fetus was used to modify behaviours during pregnancy and was discussed through reference to maternal 'responsibilities' to respect the 'right' attributed to the fetus. Just as references to 'rights' appear to have suggested the separate status of the fetus, so visual images obtained from the first scan were valued among this group, for appearing to represent the fetus as having an existence independent from that of the mother. Such representations were recalled to have a profound effect on pregnant women in the 'urban' group through providing the means to project forward into a relationship with an individual child. The notion of the separate nature of the fetus was perceived among the 'urban' group to be fundamental to 'Islamic' maternal duties of social and religious instruction.

Islam represented an identity that was often cited by participants in this group in order to distinguish themselves from models of motherhood considered to be characteristically British or English. Nonetheless, the symbolic maternal body constructed by this group appears to have been largely determined by class and regional identities. As such, descriptions of labour pain, were criticized by participants in the 'urban' group who imagined that such accounts were used among working-class and rural Iraqi women in the UK as a means of maintaining links to villages and to areas of Baghdad. By emphasizing the physicality of birth, such accounts of 'blood, sweat and being like an animal' were perceived as being 'insulting to all women'. Hence, such descriptions of pain and of the open maternal body that were attributed to working-class and rural Iraqi women appear to have been imagined among participants in the 'urban' group to pose a threat to their cultural perception of themselves through a symbolic body that was regulated by acts of willed agency.

Despite the positive perception of information provided by health practitioners among the 'urban' group, as the use of maternity information to modify behaviour and to make decisions was considered to initiate women into maternal identities, an important criticism of communication with health practitioners among this group related to perceptions of the reduced importance of motherhood in the NHS. Such perceptions referred particularly to relationships with midwives, who were perceived to use negative stereotypes regarding the intelligence of this group in order to distance themselves from requests for support or information during labour.

MATERNITY NEEDS: THE HEALTH PRACTITIONERS' PERSPECTIVE

Perceptions of the needs of Arab Muslim women among the three occupational groups of health professional participants (midwives, obstetricians and GPs) were largely determined by cultural views of the feminine or maternal body and the functions of maternity information in serving such models. An important pattern among the majority of participants in these groups related to the relationship of these models of gender and individual agency to constructions of 'cultural' difference. A further pattern related to the construction of 'culture' as a characteristic belonging only to non-white groups. In this way, the professional identities of health practitioner participants appear to have been set in opposition to 'cultural' identifications. As experiences of 'culture' were perceived to be substantially similar across non-white groups, the notion of 'culture' appears to have served to justify claims about the defining role of racial difference in determining the appropriate use of NHS maternity services. Where 'culture' was held responsible for the perceived failure of non-white women to display appropriate behaviours, the construction of 'culture' appears to have been used to suggest (white) racial superiority. Through perceptions that the needs of non-white women were determined solely by (inferior) 'cultural' beliefs, duties to respect the individual dignity of women in these groups and to provide them with individual support appear to have been obscured.

INFORMATION, CONTROL AND THE FEMININE BODY

Models of the appropriate use of maternity information centred on the imperative to regulate the experiences of the body. As such, pregnant, labouring or birthing women were imagined to control their bodies through making decisions on their maternity care. Such perceptions were associated with gendered behaviour such as dieting, exercise and birth control that was perceived as desirable among male and female health practitioner participants. In contrast, in the case of African, Asian and Arab Muslim women, such practices of controlling (and commodifying) the feminine body were not perceived to be the norm. Women within these highly divergent groups were perceived to fail to use family planning, to passively accept pregnancy owing to beliefs in fate, and to fail to exercise a profession or to control their finances. Nonetheless, the most virulent stereotypes were used to describe Arab Muslim women. These related to highly negative perceptions that Arab Muslim women were ashamed of their bodies and that these groups consequently overate. Arab Muslim mothers were criticized for their perceived acceptance of the signs of premature ageing and for their perceived tendency to suffer from avoidable physical disease and mental disorder due to the disproportionate importance perceived to be attached to motherhood among these groups.

CULTURE AND THE ABSENCE OF INDIVIDUAL NEEDS

As the behaviour of non-white women was perceived to represent the opposite of norms of successful femininity, so the actions of these groups were described in terms of their conformance to a single 'culture', which was imagined to function to disable individual choice and hence was seen to involve the inability of these groups to use maternity information to make decisions regarding their care. In this way, 'cultural' beliefs concerning the need to suffer during labour and birth were considered to universally lead non-white women to refuse pain relief and to delay their acceptance of obstetric intervention. Similarly, informal sources of knowledge of pregnancy, labour and birth within Arab Muslim, African and North Asian Muslim groups were perceived to serve to enforce expectations that women should suffer in giving birth. Within North Asian Muslim families, accounts of childbirth were also seen as offering means by which older women sought to dominate younger family members and daughters-in-law.

The contrast between the perceived role of 'culture' among non-white groups and perceptions of individual agency among white patients was suggested by two accounts offered by health practitioner participants. Where a Somali woman's refusal of intervention led to stillbirth, the woman was perceived to have acted in conformance with cultural pressures. In contrast, in describing a similar case in which the decision of a French woman led to the birth of a severely handicapped child, another participant did not hesitate to ascribe the mother's action to her individual choice.

Many health practitioner participants explained their perceptions of non-white 'culture' in relation to notions of education, as 'educated' non-white women were perceived to be no different to other patients. White middle-class groups were perceived to see maternity services in terms of consumerist notions of choices between services and care options. Non-white women were perceived as being 'educated' where their views matched those of the white middle-class group. A further characteristic of women described as 'educated' was that of seeking the best maternity treatment – which tended to be private. As such, the ascription of 'educated' or 'international' identifications to non-white women – particularly to Arab Muslim women from Gulf states – appears to have related to their having considerable financial means with which to negotiate with the maternity care system. Notably, the category of 'education' was used most widely among health practitioner participants who were themselves migrants to the UK. Among this group, it appears to have served to justify racial characterizations while obscuring the racial and ethnic difference they might themselves represent.

The role of a racist white/non-white hierarchy in constructing models of appropriate behaviour in NHS maternity services was further suggested by the health practitioner participants' attitudes to the natural childbirth movement. Across health practitioner groups, practices of using the literature of the Natural Childbirth Trust (NCT) together with practices of attending classes organized by this group were associated with white, middle-class women. Among obstetricians and GP participants, in particular, the emphasis perceived to be placed on the value of physical suffering among women influenced by this group was criticized for appearing to relate 'real' womanhood to the ability to choose to suffer pain when other options were available. Additionally, in the case of a minority of accounts, such as that describing the birth of a handicapped child to a French woman (that is discussed above), the result of the high value placed on individual autonomy and control within the natural birth movement was suggested to have directly harmed the child.

Despite having indicated that the behaviour of this white, middle-class group within maternity services might relate to cultural constructions of femininity (through notions of the control of the feminine body and the virtue of imposing suffering on it), health practitioner participants drew on these same notions of choice and control as proof of the individual basis of preferences for unassisted delivery among this group.

PRIVATE PREFERENCES AND APPROPRIATE NEEDS

As the cultural division between body and mind was used to suggest the underdeveloped agency of non-white women and thus to exclude these groups from perceptions of the appropriate uses of maternity information, so the division between public and private (personal) spheres was used to cast doubt on equal rights to NHS maternity care. Where non-white women carrying potentially difficult pregnancies refused early intervention and returned to the 'community' where their actions were supported, their return to the hospital later in pregnancy with more complex requirements for care were perceived as exercising an unjustifiable pressure on health practitioners. Similarly, preferences for treatment by female health practitioners were perceived as belonging to the private sphere. Where preferences for treatment by female health practitioners among Arab Muslim patients were reported to have led to their avoidance of care provided by a male participant, the participant referred to the provision of free NHS care as a circumstance aggravating the perceived inappropriateness of drawing on such preferences. In this way, given the public and publicly funded basis of NHS care, rights to receive care that correspond to individual needs among non-white users appear to be made conditional on adopting behaviour that is not considered as being 'cultural' or as belonging to the 'private' sphere. In order to receive care of an equal quality to that perceived to be merited by white women, non-white users of maternity services thus appear to be expected to present themselves as near as possible to the white, middle-class or 'educated' models of femininity around which notions of the appropriate needs of the uses of NHS maternity services have been constructed by health practitioners who provide their care.

CONCLUSION

Among both groups of study participants, the relationship of preferences for maternity care to participants' own symbolic notion of the maternal body determined whether the transcultural encounters described above were seen as a source of danger to personal identity – or were seen as affirming a sense of self.

As such, symbolic notions of the maternal body were suggested to mould the affective and physical needs of Arab Muslim women as users of NHS maternity services. Among Arab Muslim participants characterized as 'rural', the symbolic maternal body was constructed around notions of embodied agency. Accordingly, experiences of intervention, pain relief and the use of some forms of information were recalled to lead to the loss of identification with this symbolic body. Such experiences were associated with physical and cultural vulnerability, and tended to be regretted in retrospect. Islamist and nationalist constructions of the maternal body also appear to have served to protect rural Arab Muslim women through providing a frame within which to understand their fears of labour pain and of motherhood. While aspects of these beliefs may be alien to health practitioners, through offering recognition of the fears surrounding motherhood and the loss of embodied agency, health practitioners may aid women in these groups to maintain their individual and cultural identities during pregnancy, labour and birth. Arab Muslim participants in the group characterized as 'urban' were suggested to emphasize a division between the body and individual agency as a characteristic of 'Islamic' motherhood. Participants within this group sought maternity information on risks during pregnancy and on the processes of labour as a means of identifying with this cultural model that defined motherhood in terms of acts of willed agency. While the needs of this 'urban' group for information appear to have been consistent with models of patient decision-making in the NHS, both 'rural' and 'urban' participants reported that their needs for information and for reassurance during labour were not met. Patterns of withdrawing from demands for support among the 'urban' group were perceived to be justified by health practitioners through the use of stereotypes of the limited intelligence of migrant women. Practices of reassuring Arab Muslim women that their needs for support will be met might minimize additional experiences of vulnerability during labour and birth. Through these interactions, health practitioners might assess women's background and preferences on an individual level and might challenge stereotypes that limit their ability to provide care to women from all migrant groups.

Among health practitioner participants, cultural notions of femininity constructed through the opposition of the body to the mind and of public and private contexts were used to justify racist perceptions of (non-white) 'cultural' inferiority that determined perceptions of the appropriate needs of white and non-white women as users of NHS maternity services. A characteristic that appears to have informed perceptions of individual merit to receive care and support was that of individual agency. Non-white users of maternity services, represented through their preferences for natural birth and their perceived failure to control their weight, health and attractiveness, were suggested to have underdeveloped capacities for individual agency – and thus for choice. As such, health practitioners are advised to consider how their perceptions of the maternal body and notions of control might relate to a cultural division between body and mind. Where certain groups are characterized through behaviour seen as contrary to norms of feminine behaviour, care should be taken to explore health practitioners' attitudes to the care entitlements of these groups. Among non-white groups – and particularly among African and Arab groups – decisions on maternity care were perceived to be determined by 'culture'. Where the use of the notion of 'culture' relates to negative evaluations of the ability of certain groups to use maternity care, practitioners should consider how this notion may be used to deny the individual status of women and to withhold recognition of their needs. A criterion that was used to compensate against the effects of 'culture' was that of education. However, given that the needs and priorities of 'educated' non-white maternity users were perceived as being no different to those of British maternity users, this criterion appears to relate to the suppression of 'non-white' identifications. Finally, where the needs of non-white women were considered as 'cultural', these were also represented as belonging to the 'private' (personal) sphere. As such, given the public – and publicly funded – status of NHS maternity services, the rights of non-white women to have their needs met within maternity care appear to have been retracted. Accordingly, where the public basis of maternity care is used to question the rights of ethnic or cultural groups to appropriate care, practitioners should reflect that 'public' and 'private' – no less than 'cultural' – are not neutral terms. Rather, they are connected to British and European cultural systems of representing non-white women – that justify relations of power and that deny these groups equal treatment.

By recognizing the ways in which various symbolic bodies are constituted among Arab Muslim women, the relationship of culture to perceptions of maternity needs in individual women's experience may be appreciated by NHS health practitioners. Similarly, by becoming aware of the ways in which they themselves construct symbolic maternal bodies and the purpose these serve in interacting with patients and in identifying with institutional practices, health practitioners can guard against exclusionary practices.

REFLECTIVE QUESTIONS

1. Does the notion of cultural competence offer challenges for me and my work?
2. What are the cultural dimensions of the experience of using maternity services among women from various cultural groups?
3. How does culture affect perceptions of maternity information and knowledge among various groups of women?
4. How does culture shape practices of information giving in maternity institutions?

REFERENCES

Afshar H 1998 Islam and feminism. Macmillan, Basingstoke

Ahmed L 1992 Women and gender in Islam. Yale University Press, New Haven, CT

Al-Azmeh A 1993 Islam and modernities. Verso, London

Amir-Moazami S, Salvatore A 2003 Gender, generation, and the reform of tradition: from Muslim majority societies to western Europe. In: Allievi S, Nielsen J S (eds) Muslim networks and transnational communities in and across Europe (Muslim minorities series, 1). Brill, Leiden, p 52–77

Barth F 1998. Introduction. In: Barth F (ed) Ethnic groups and boundaries: the social organisation of culture difference. Waveland Press, Prospect Heights, IL, p 9–38

Bigwood C 1999 Renaturalizing the body (with the help of Merleau-Ponty). In: Whelton D (ed) Body and flesh a philosophical reader. Blackwells, Malden, MA, p 99–114

Bodran M 1995 Feminism, Islam and nation: gender and the making of modern Egypt. Princeton University Press, Princeton, NJ

Bordo S 1987 The flight to objectivity. SUNY Press, Albany, NY

Bordo S 2004 Unbearable weight: feminism, western culture, and the body. University of California Press, Berkeley, CA

Burton A 1994 Burdens of history. University of North Carolina Press, Chapel Hill, NC

Butler J 1999 Gender trouble: feminism and the subversion of identity. Routledge, New York

De Beauvoir S, 1997 The second sex (H M Parshley, transl). Vintage, London

Douglas M 2003 Natural symbols: explorations in cosmology. 2nd edn. Routledge, London

Douglas M 2004 Purity and danger: an analysis of concepts of pollution and taboo. Routledge, London

Foucault M 1995 *Discipline and punish* (A M Sheridan Smith, transl). Vintage, New York

Foucault M 2003 *The birth of the clinic* (A M Sheridan Smith, transl). Routledge, London

Hammami R 1996 From immodesty to collaboration: Hamas, the women's movement, and national identity in the intifada. In: Beinin J, Stork J (eds) Political Islam. Taurus, London, p 194–210

Joseph S 2000 Gender and citizenship in the Middle East. Syracuse University Press, Syracuse, NY

Larcin P 1999 Imperial identities: stereotyping, prejudice and race in colonial Algeria. Taurus, London

Lowe L 1991 Critical terrains: French and British orientalisms. Cornell University Press, Ithaca, NY

Mabro J 1996 Veiled half-truths: western travellers' perceptions of Middle Eastern women. Taurus, London

McCormack C 2000a From interview transcript to interpretative story – part 1: viewing the transcript through multiple lenses. Field Methods 12(3):282–297

McCormack C 2000b From interview transcript to interpretative story – part 2: developing an interpretative story. Field Methods 12(4):298–315

Mernissi F 1991 Women and Islam. Basil Blackwell, Oxford

Moscucci O 1990 The science of woman: gynecology and gender in England 1800–1929. Cambridge University Press, Cambridge

National Commission for the Protection Of Human Subjects of Biomedical and Behavioural Research 1978 The Belmont report: ethical principles and guidelines for the protection of human subjects of research, US Government Printing Office, Washington

Papadopoulos I, Lees S 2002 Developing culturally competent researchers. Journal of Advanced Nursing 37(3):258–264

Papadopoulos I, Scanlon K, Lees S 2001 Reporting and validating research findings through reconstructed stories. Disability and Society 17(3):269–281

Ricoeur P 1990 Time and narrative, vol 1 (K McLaughlin, D Pellauer, transl). University of Chicago Press, Chicago

Sayigh R 1993 Palestinian women and politics in Lebanon. In: Tucker J E (ed) Arab women: old boundaries, new frontiers. Indiana University Press, Bloomington, p 175–192

Volpp L 2003 Moving beyond the culture/rights debate. Paper given at: Conference on gendered bodies, transnational politics: modernities reconsidered. 12–14 December 2003, Cairo, Egypt

Chapter **10**

Illegal drugs: knowledge, attitudes and drug habits of the Greek and Greek Cypriot youth living in London

Irena Papadopoulos and Chris Papadopoulos

LEARNING OBJECTIVES

After reading this chapter you should be able to:
- outline the main issues relating to the knowledge, attitudes and drug habits of Greek and Greek Cypriot adolescents and young people living in London
- locate the above within a broader knowledge of drug policy in the UK
- gain insight into how the issues affect Greek and Greek Cypriot youths, in comparison to other young people and adults from black and ethnic minorities.

BACKGROUND

The UK government's 10-year strategy on drugs (Department of Health 1998) aims to:

- help young people resist drug misuse
- protect communities from drug-related antisocial and criminal behaviour

- provide treatment to enable people with drug problems to overcome them
- stifle the availability of illegal drugs.

The UK government has been working in partnership with other organizations aimed at reducing the number of young people under 25 using drugs by taking actions to ensure that:

- young people, parents, and those working and advising young people are informed of the risks and consequences of drug misuse
- young people from 5 years old, both inside and outside of formal education, acquire the skills to resist the pressure to misuse drugs
- healthy lifestyles and alternative activities are promoted
- young people from all backgrounds have appropriate access to help and advice.

In 1999, the substance misuse review to support the development of the London Health Strategy (Marshall et al 1999) reported the following:

- nearly half of the UK's black and minority ethnic (BME) groups live in London
- BME groups are heterogeneous with varying values, attitudes, religious beliefs and customs that affect the patterns of substance misuse
- existing services need to be transculturally appropriate, i.e. recognize diversity and shared values
- ethnic-specific services may have a valuable role to play in working with disenfranchised communities
- there is an assumption that BME groups under-utilize substance misuse services
- ethnic monitoring in service utilization should be encouraged
- ongoing cross-cultural training should be implemented
- there should be further research into the needs of refugees with regard to substance misuse services.

The same report stated that there is evidence of increased drug use and misuse nationally among young people. It suggested that highly specialist services may be needed for young people in London. It referred to the Drug Misuse Database report (Sondhi et al 1999), which found that London drug users under the age of 20 had increased by 35% between 1995 and 1998.

In 2000, the UK's Department of Health commissioned the Ethnicity and Health Unit at the University of Central Lancashire to administer and support the 'Black and Minority Ethnic Drug Misuse Needs Assessment' initiative (Bashford et al 2004). The initiative aimed to get local BME community groups across England to conduct their own needs assessments in relation to drugs education, prevention, and treatment services. Forty-seven community groups took part in this initiative, one of them being the Greek and Greek Cypriot Community of Enfield

(GGCCE). Some of the data used in this chapter were derived from this involvement (Papadopoulos 2001).

DEFINITIONS

The definitions below are based on those provided in the report *Young People and Drugs: Policy Guidance for Drug Interventions* (Standing Conference on Drug Abuse 1999).

Drug misuse   Drug taking which harms health or social functioning is described as 'drug misuse'. This may be dependency (physical or psychological) or drug taking that is part of a wider spectrum of problematic or harmful behaviour. Drug misuse requires treatment.

Drug use   Drug use is drug taking which requires a lower level of intervention than treatment. Harm may still occur through drug use, whether through intoxication, illegality or health problems, even though it may not be immediately apparent. Drug use will require the appropriate provision of interventions such as education, advice and information, to reduce the potential for harm.

Evans & Alade (2000) stated that the fact that a young person has taken a drug should not lead to the automatic conclusion that there is a problem or condition to be treated although it is essential to recognize that all drug taking by young people carries potential harm.

In this chapter the term 'drug' will mean illegal drugs referred to in the Misuse of Drugs Act 1971, as well as those illegal substances such as unprepared magic mushrooms, new derivatives of ecstasy, and any new substances that are continually becoming available. The study presented in this chapter did not deal with smoking, or alcohol misuse; it also excluded the misuse of steroidal drugs.

In this chapter, the terms 'boy' and 'girl' are used in the presentation of the focus group findings as these terms were actually used by the participants of the study that is discussed below.

The 2001 Government Census is the best indicator of population sizes of ethnic groups in London. However, as the census categories did not include a specific category for the Greek/Greek Cypriot ethnicity, it is difficult to be precise when reporting this group's population size. The London Greek and Greek Cypriot community was estimated to be in excess of 250 000 (Papadopoulos 1999). The majority of this population live in North London.

THE STUDY

This chapter presents selected quantitative and qualitative findings of a study conducted in 2000–2002. The study aimed to explore the knowledge, attitudes and drug habits of young Greek and Greek Cypriots living in one North London borough. Although the findings were originally reported in two separate reports (Papadopoulos 2001, Papadopoulos & Worrall 2003), here they have been combined in order to present a fuller picture on the topic, making this the only investigation thus far to be carried out on drugs within the Greek/Greek Cypriot community in London.

Quantitative data were collected using a self-completed questionnaire from a convenient sample of 52 participants aged 15 to 18 years in May 2001. Questionnaires were also distributed to a convenient sample of 38 adolescents/young adults, aged 9 to 18 years (median 13 years), in June 2002. The total sample size was 90, of whom 39 were males and 51 were females.

Qualitative data were collected from four focus groups involving 36 young people aged between 14 and 18 years. Specifically the focus groups were as follows:

- one mixed group (7 boys and 5 girls, aged 14–16, attending secondary school)
- one female group (8 girls, aged 14–16, attending secondary school)
- one male group (12 boys aged 14–16, attending secondary school)
- one mixed group (2 boys and 2 girls aged 17–18, attending a college for further education).

All the focus groups were conducted by peers (2 female and 1 male, second-generation Greek Cypriots, aged 16–18 years), who were also involved in the production of information leaflets about the study, and were consulted in the development of the questionnaire and focus group topic guide. Prior to conducting the focus groups the peer interviewers were provided with training which involved an introduction to the government's drugs strategy, an introduction to commonly used drugs and how to run a focus group.

FINDINGS

SURVEY

Participants were asked to list the drugs they had heard of. The most frequently cited drugs were cannabis and ecstasy, with cocaine and heroin following closely. Next came LSD, whilst the use of solvents (such as glue) was almost missing from their responses, indicating that glue sniffing may not be a habit of young Greek/Greek Cypriots.

Twenty-two participants stated that they had taken drugs (10 males and 12 females), while 65 stated they had never taken drugs, and 3 participants failed to answer the question. The most commonly used drug was cannabis, followed by ecstasy, cocaine and heroin. The majority of those taking drugs reported to be doing so on an occasional basis. Only one 16-year-old male reported taking either cannabis or ecstasy on a daily basis. Half of those taking drugs reported that their parents knew about it. The parents' response was a mixture of anger, denial and shame whilst at the same time trying to be supportive.

Participants were asked to list the reasons why they took drugs. Multiple responses were allowed. Twelve of the replies referred to taking drugs in search of a 'buzz', four replies referred to peer pressure, three to seeing drug taking as a challenge, one due to depression, and one participant stated that 'I had to try'.

When asked to list the side effects or problems caused by drugs (multiple responses were allowed) the majority of the responses given referred to physical problems (73) such as dizziness, heart failure, palpitations, liver damage, cancer, changes in physical appearance, weight loss, vomiting, dehydration, drowsiness, hot and cold flushes, hunger, tiredness, brain damage, addiction, blood disorders, HIV/AIDS, and general deterioration of health. A smaller number of responses (38) referred to psychological problems such as depression, hallucinations, mental breakdown, memory loss, mental illness, madness, alteration of mind functions, and emotional instability. Almost equal responses (36) referred to behavioural problems such as lack of control, change in attitude, change in character/personality, feeling 'high' and behaving lively, 'superman' effect, slow reactions, mood swings, suicidal behaviour, inability to respond appropriately, aggressiveness/abusive behaviour, loss of willpower and living, and sexual aggressiveness leading to violence. A sizeable number of responses (24) cited death as a problem caused by drugs. Finally social problems were referred to twice, citing antisocial behaviour, anarchy, violence, family problems, break-up of families, financial problems, promiscuity and crime; it was stated that drug addicts engaged in criminal activities in order to obtain money to feed their habit.

Participants were asked to list the sources they had used to gain information about drugs. The most frequent response (15) was school, followed by mass media such as TV/radio/newspapers (12). It was rather surprising to find that the drug advisory teams were being used (5), and that friends were not a common source of information (4).

When asked to report their parents' level of knowledge about drugs, 16 participants reported that their parents knew 'enough' whilst eight reported that their parents knew 'quite a lot'. Eight reported that their parents knew 'very little' or 'nothing'.

Twenty-one adolescents/young people knew a young Greek and Greek Cypriot person who took drugs. Forty-seven reported that in their opinion there was a drug problem amongst young people in the Greek and Greek Cypriot community, citing the use of too much 'weed' by young males.

FOCUS GROUPS

The following themes emerged from the analysis of the data collected during the four focus groups:

'We associate drugs with . . .'
'Young Greek and Greek Cypriot people take drugs because . . .'
'I have been offered drugs but . . .'
'My strategy for avoiding drugs is . . .'

'If my friend was taking drugs I would . . .'
'Role models and scary Greek parents'
'Yes, I have tried drugs'
'Many Greek/Greek Cypriot young people use drugs'
'Greek parents and drugs'.

'We associate drugs with . . .'

Most focus group participants irrespective of their age and gender responded that they associate drugs with badness and danger. They all thought that drugs are bad for people because they can harm their health or even kill those who take them. There was a certain level of fear associated with the fact that drugs can be addictive, and can have detrimental and long-lasting effects.

'Young Greek and Greek Cypriot people take drugs because . . .'

Most participants identified family conflicts as one of the main reasons for drug misuse. They cited arguments between young people and their parents, family breakdowns, and the loss of family member or a friend. Curiosity was another reason cited by many. However, an interesting theory that seemed to emerge was that Greek/Greek Cypriot youth take drugs in order to '*look hard*'. Many of the participants in the boys' focus group described this phenomenon thus: '*A lot of them* [Greek youths who take drugs] *think they are "black". They try to act "black"; they try to portray the image of the black man in an American ghetto. They walk funny, they have their trousers all the way down their knees, they imitate black people by kissing their teeth and by having a bad attitude. Some of them think they are really flash. They have about 50 rings on their fingers and 20 chains on their neck.*'

The girls' focus group explained this in terms of pride. They reported that Greek people have a lot of pride and attempt to appear as 'hard' so that other people will not '*mess about with them*'. The girls reported that the Greek/Greek Cypriot boys want to be the best by providing examples such as: '*they want to be ruling the school*'. Peer pressure was mentioned by some as another reason for taking drugs. Participants who attended further education (17–18-year-olds) also referred to the notion of '*looking hard*' but they added that Greek/Greek Cypriot boys take drugs to '*show off*'. Other factors they cited were boredom and '*getting a buzz*'.

'I have been offered drugs but . . .'

Many of those attending secondary school replied that they were offered drugs but not inside their school. Those attending further education reported that they were offered drugs inside their college. Those offering drugs were mainly friends, but on one occasion, drugs were offered by a member of the family. The boys reported that they are frequently offered drugs when they go out, especially in snooker halls. The mixed focus group also reported that they were offered drugs when they were on a school trip to France.

A few boys, but no girls, admitted to trying out drugs, mainly cannabis. One of the boys reported that he was very tempted, not because of peer pressure or any other reason but because he liked the smell of the cannabis smoke. Most girls reported that although they had been tempted, they had refused because they were scared of the consequences. *'What if I like it and want to continue?'* asked one of the girls. *'Just the thought of becoming addicted puts me off completely.'*

'My strategy for avoiding drugs is . . .'

The main strategy cited by girls was self-assertion. One of them said *'I just said no and that was it and they walked off, because I showed them that I meant it they left it like that'*. Another said *'If you sound unsure then they can persuade you to come around but if you make it blatant that you don't want it they leave you alone'*. Another girl explained how her mother and grand-mother would demand that she never left her drink out of her sight in bars and night-clubs, or that she always had her palm over the drink to prevent the drink getting spiked. Saying 'no' and meaning 'no' also seemed to be the main strategy used by the boys.

'If my friend was taking drugs I would . . .'

Both boys and girls suggested that, to begin with, they would not tell anyone if their friend was taking something 'light' such as cannabis. Rather, they would talk to their friend to remind them of the dangers and would ask them to stop. They would also inform their friend that if they did not stop they would be forced to tell the friend's parents. Both boys and girls showed great sensitivity to the need to help their friend but also to the implications of telling their friend's family. Several of them mentioned that such news *'could ruin the family'* or *'could break up the family'*. One of the girls mentioned that in a case of a relative taking drugs she would not share this information with her friends as she would not want people outside the family to know. She said that if the relative was a boy then, *'I would tell my brother so he could have a word with him; I think if my brother said something then it would get through to him because he is a boy . . . if they were both boys I think it is easier to talk because they are more aggressive and they can push you to stop'*. Some girls stated that they would not tell anyone if a friend confided in them because this would betray the trust their friend placed on them; they reported that if they could not help them they would encourage them to go and see a counsellor. The majority of both boys and girls stated that they would tell their friend's parents if he or she was taking heroin or ecstasy because both drugs kill. Boys thought that it would be better for their friend to *'get a couple of slaps'* rather than die from a drug overdose. Several boys indicated that they would not be able to cope with the death of a friend knowing they did not inform the friend's parents, who although they might get very angry at first would, in their view, try to help their son or daughter. Boys stated that they would not tell the police about their friend.

'Role models and scary Greek parents'

Both boys and girls agreed that probably the strongest incentive to stop taking drugs is seeing someone close to you dying from them. Boys emphasized that the drug user must want to stop or else any help they may get will fail. Several boys also mentioned the need for good role models such as older brothers or cousins. Having *'scary Greek parents'* who are strict and administer *'batsous'* (slaps) was also suggested as an effective deterrent.

'Yes, I have tried drugs'

Three of the participants who were attending further education admitted trying drugs. They had all used only cannabis. One of them said: *'I was 13 years old and it was offered free'*. Another reported that he was 15 when he tried it out of curiosity. The third reported that he smoked a joint as a birthday treat. They all reported that the first time they took it, it was good. However, subsequent use did not seem to make them feel good. One of them said: *'I went home and it made me feel funny. I ate so much. My mouth was just open and I couldn't feel anything. I felt deformed. I felt out of order because I kept feeling funny and I was scared I was going to get addicted'*. Another reported that the second time he took cannabis he felt tired, lazy, and had a nasty taste in his mouth. He did not like these effects so he never took it again. The third said: *'The reason why I stopped was because I felt like a hypocrite; I am always telling my parents to stop smoking, when I was smoking drugs myself'*. Only one of the participants in the secondary school boys' focus group admitted to having tried cannabis. Another secondary school boy in the mixed focus group admitted smoking cannabis once when he was at a party and someone offered it. He explained that he took it because he was drunk but has not taken any since. None of the female participants in the secondary school focus groups admitted to taking drugs.

'Many Greek/Greek Cypriot young people use drugs'

Despite the fact that only 5 of the 36 young people who took part in the focus groups reported having taken drugs, the majority were of the opinion that many young Greek/Greek Cypriot people use drugs. Most reported that more boys than girls take drugs and mainly when they go out. One participant from the boys' focus group said: *'I know loads of Greek people that are on drugs but not from the school, but their parents think that they are innocent'*.

'Greek parents and drugs'

There was a general consensus that Greek and Greek Cypriot parents are not well informed about drugs. Some young people reported that Greek parents do not want to acknowledge that their child may be taking drugs. One person said *'parents have too much faith in their children and don't believe they will go anywhere near drugs'*. Another reported that when visiting a Greek friend, the friend's brother walked in and began to behave oddly. *'He was getting happy over a new broom but his parents didn't think anything of it; they didn't notice his red eyes.'* There were a few exceptions; one of the participants in the boys' focus group mentioned that his mother, who was brought up in London, *'knows what there is to know about drugs'*. Another participant in the same group reported that his father was honest with him and told him that he had tried drugs and he told him *'that it was nothing special; if you want to go out and have a good time do it without drugs'.*

DISCUSSION

The young people who took part in this study expressed the view that all drugs are dangerous and can therefore harm not only one's health but one's relationships with family and friends. Whilst a few admitted trying drugs and even fewer that they took them on a regular basis, they all appear to be concerned about the consequences of drug taking, particularly death and addiction. It appears that the recent reports in the media of deaths as a result mainly of taking ecstasy have raised the participants' awareness that death, something that is not immediately associated with youth, is a real possibility.

The focus groups revealed that apart from family problems, the main reasons for drug taking seem to be curiosity, boredom/search for a buzz, a desire to appear tough, or an identity crisis. On the other hand, a small number of the survey respondents cited the need for a challenge and peer pressure as contributing factors. The large project referred to at the beginning of this chapter, which was coordinated by the Ethnicity and Health Unit of the University of Central Lancashire (Bashford et al 2004), reported that increased availability of drugs are perceived as a factor in why people start to use them. The prevailing view amongst their respondents (which were adults of all ages) is that drugs are easily obtainable and many described dramatic increases in drug use. Taken together, peer influence, experimentation and pleasure seeking accounted for 74% of respondents' reported reasons for starting to use drugs. Some 30% cited their reasons for drug use as being to avoid or help deal with problems.

Young Greek and Greek Cypriot participants of this study appear to have a good general knowledge about drugs and their side effects. It could, however, be argued that much of this knowledge is superficial. This is indicated by the fact that various synonyms of cannabis were listed as separate drugs, and that many common side effects were cited by fewer participants than expected. On the other hand, Bashford et al (2004) reported that there are very low levels of awareness and knowledge about drugs across all of the BME communities which took part in their study.

All the focus group participants in this study exhibited caring and thoughtful attitudes towards their friends who are taking drugs, or those who may in the future do so. Although they reported that they would try and persuade their friends to give up drugs and would even resort to telling their friend's parents if they thought that their friend was doing hard drugs, none of them mentioned that they would use their local drugs advisory service, the national drugs helpline, or the available leaflets. This finding must be of concern to those responsible for drugs campaigns, as clearly in the case of these young people, the message is not getting through. Bashford et al (2004) also reported that the majority of their respondents (80%) lacked awareness about what options there are for help with drug problems.

The response of the young Greek and Greek Cypriot participants, that their friends would not be one of their main sources for gaining information about drugs, confirms that the use of drugs is severely frowned upon within the Greek/Greek Cypriot community. Seeking information from friends who come from the same community may cause them to suspect that the seeker has a drug problem; therefore this strategy is avoided, in order to prevent such information being passed to other members of the community. It is, however, encouraging that many young people feel safe enough to approach the school for information and help. The fact that many young people obtain drugs-related information from the mass media is perhaps a sign of the times. Young people are very familiar with information technology, something which could be further exploited by health promoters and service providers. Bashford et al (2004) also found that their respondents get their information about drugs predominantly from the media. However, contrary to the findings from our study, their respondents reported that they obtain information from their friends rather than drug services or schools.

The results of the focus groups seem to suggest that either Greek/Greek Cypriot parents tend to deny that their children would or could take drugs, or that some of them are so strict that the young people would not take drugs for fear of having to face their wrath. On the other hand, the findings of the survey indicate that when parents find out that their children are taking drugs, some are angry and ashamed, but they are also supportive. It would be interesting to know how they are being supportive, and how they deal with their anger, denial, embarrassment, and so on. Bashford et al (2004) reported that the impact of drug use on families is varied. In their study this was described in terms of stress, worry, financial burdens, health and mental health problems, tensions, arguments and even violence. For many families, it is not a subject that can be discussed and families experience shame and isolation from the wider community. Family responses to drug use include sending the user to the country of origin of the family or attempting to confine them so that other people in the community do not find out. They concluded that families are coping with both the fears and the realities of drug use in relative isolation.

In our study, the majority of the participants, in both the focus groups and the survey, were of the view that the Greek/Greek Cypriot community has a drugs problem despite the fact that of the total of 90 young people who took part in the survey, only 22 admitted to having taken drugs; furthermore the findings seem to indicate that most of them have only tried drugs (mainly cannabis) on a very small number of occasions. It would be interesting to explore further the reasons for this variance between perception and practice. Bashford et al (2004) reported that 18% of their sample reported using a wide variety of drugs. Nearly one in five of them reported using cocaine and one in ten had used heroin.

CONCLUSIONS AND REFLECTIONS

Any conclusions drawn from this study must be viewed with caution for the following reasons:

- the use of a convenient survey sample
- the fact that most of the focus group participants came from one school which is located in an affluent part of North London and has an excellent academic record.

Nevertheless, the findings provide for the first time important information about drug use amongst Greek/Greek Cypriot adolescents and young adults.

This chapter has provided culturally specific information, which in our view forms a flexible knowledge tool that can be located within the broader cultural knowledge provided by the national study we used for comparison (Bashford et al 2004). We believe that such cultural knowledge and understanding will not lead to stereotyping of all young Greek and Greek Cypriots, but on the contrary, it will provide essential insights for service providers.

The study presented here is also an illustration of culturally competent research. The motivation to undertake the study arose from members of the Greek and Greek Cypriot community who were involved in all the stages of the study from the design to the dissemination of the findings. The participation of three young second-generation Greek Cypriots was crucial. As representatives of the age and ethnicity group, they provided useful insights about the topic and the language used by their age group; they also did an excellent job in conducting the focus groups. Informing the parents was paramount and was done through leaflets prepared by the young researchers, and through the London Greek Radio which interviewed the three young researchers. The young researchers verified the analysis of the focus groups and contributed a short piece on their reflections, which was included in the first report (Papadopoulos 2001).

The following recommendations are made:

- To conduct a larger and more representative survey of 15- to 18-year-old Greek and Greek Cypriots within the whole of London.
- To investigate further the very low drug use amongst the 15- to 17-year-olds found in this study. This finding may be due to a reluctance amongst the Greek and Greek Cypriot youth to report their drug taking in case they were 'found out' (even though the survey was completely anonymous). Drug taking remains highly stigmatized within the Greek community; it is considered an act of shaming the family of the user and thus every effort is made to keep it within the family walls. It is therefore recommended that the Greek and Greek Cypriot community should be encouraged to debate more openly the issues of drug use/misuse/abuse, and that community organizations, the church, and the community mass media should put this on top of their agendas.

Finally, to return to the aims of the UK government's 10-year strategy, it would appear from the findings of our study and of the national study cited above that there is still plenty to be done. On the positive side, Drug Action Teams are now established in every part of the country. They are working hard to tackle both national and local priorities. A quick internet search reveals numerous drug-related projects aimed at BME groups and young people. They appear to include culturally appropriate services such as the production of information in different community languages, the involvement of the local BME communities, and so on. On the negative side, the findings reported in this chapter reveal lack of awareness of these resources. Bashford et al (2004) also reported that there is a high level of dissatisfaction amongst those who used the available services, something which questions their cultural appropriateness. Finally, despite the government's aims to reduce access to drugs among young people this, according to the evidence presented in this chapter, has not been achieved.

REFLECTIVE EXERCISES

1. Outline three ways in which the information you have read in this chapter about the young Greek and Greek Cypriots living in London will be of use in your work.
2. Think of two cultural groups you regularly come in contact with in your workplace. Outline what you know regarding their drug knowledge, attitudes and habits.
3. How has this chapter helped you in your endeavours to become a culturally competent practitioner?

Acknowledgements

The authors would like to thank all the young people who took part in this study. Particular thanks go to the three young peer researchers Era Philippou, Maria Agathocleous and Costaki Costi. Finally, we wish to acknowledge the contribution and support of Litsa Worrall, Manager of the Greek and Greek Cypriot Community of Enfield.

REFERENCES

Bashford J, Buffin J, Patel K 2004 Black and minority ethnic drug misuse needs assessment project. Community Engagement. Report 2, The Findings. Centre for Ethnicity & Health, University of Central Lancashire, Preston

Department of Health 1998 Tackling drugs to build a better Britain (Cm 3945). The Stationery Office, London

Evans K, Alade S 2000 Vulnerable young people and drugs. Opportunities to tackle inequalities. DrugScope, London

Marshall F, Keating A, Annan J et al 1999 The substance misuse review to support the development of the London Health Strategy. ARAC, London

Misuse of Drugs Act 1971 HMSO, London

Papadopoulos I 1999 The health needs of the Greek Cypriot people living in London. Unpublished PhD thesis. University of North London (now London Metropolitan University)

Papadopoulos I 2001 HELP US CRACK IT! An investigation into the knowledge, attitudes and drug habits of Greek and Greek Cypriot adolescents living in Enfield. GGCCE, London

Papadopoulos I, Worrall L 2003 HELP US CRACK IT 2 A report on parents' and children's drug education amongst the Greek and Greek Cypriot community of North London. GGCCE, London

Sondhi A, Hickman M, Madden P et al 1999 Annual report. Data presented from 1992 to end of 1998. Thames Drug Misuse Database, London

Standing Conference on Drug Abuse (SCODA) and Children's Legal Centre 1999 Young people and drugs: policy guidance for drug interventions. SCODA and Children's Legal Centre, London

Chapter 11

Culturally competent health promotion for minority ethnic groups, refugees, Gypsy Travellers and New Age Travellers in the UK

Irena Papadopoulos and Margaret Lay

LEARNING OBJECTIVES

After reading this chapter you should be able to:
- list the principles of culturally competent research
- outline the common health promotion needs and problems identified by all the groups who took part in the study
- outline the specific health promotion needs and problems identified by each of the groups who took part in the study
- define culturally competent health promotion
- list the indicators of culturally competent health-promoting organizations.

INTRODUCTION

Minority ethnic groups in the UK (including refugees, asylum seekers and Gypsy Travellers) are diverse in terms of their socio-economic status, language, culture and lifestyles; so too are their health status, disease patterns and health behaviour (Nazroo 1997). Overall, people from ethnic minorities in the UK today have an increased risk of chronic illness including diabetes, coronary heart disease and stroke relative to the white majority population. Mortality rates from all causes are higher than average for nearly all migrant groups (Acheson 1998); there are also higher incidences of acute illness amongst some minority ethnic groups, such as tuberculosis (TB) in new entrants from the Indian subcontinent (Rawaf & Bahl 1998). A study of Gypsy Travellers' health status indicated that it is poorer than that of comparable subjects matched by age and sex (Parry et al 2004), whilst a study of Irish Travellers by Barry et al (1987) showed that their life expectancy was considerably lower than that of the rest of the Irish population.

It is now well recognized that socio-economic determinants have a major impact on health (Acheson 1998, Raphael 2004) and it follows therefore that health promotion needs will vary with differences in socio-economic conditions. Racial harassment and perceptions of racial discrimination have also been shown to have a significant impact on health (Nazroo & Karlsen 2001), as do lifestyle and health behaviours such as poor diet, lack of exercise and smoking, which are the three most important and preventable causes of ill health and premature death (Viner & Booy 2005, Doll et al 2004, Bahr 2001).

In the UK measures to counter poor access to services and healthcare inequalities are addressed in policy documents such as the Department of Health's equality framework, which states that it is:

> . . . committed to improving the health and well-being of the population through a health and social care system which is provided equally to those who need it, free at the point of need; offers a personal service which is truly patient-centred; has sufficiently increased capacity to enable choice and diversity to be offered to patients; and is fair and provides equity of access to care. (Department of Health 2003: 2)

The government White Paper *Choosing Health: Making Healthier Choices Easier* (Department of Health 2004: 3) proposed a new approach to the health of the public whereby the public sets the agenda. The Paper states that:

> To be effective in tackling health inequalities, support has to be tailored to the realities of individual lives, with services and support personalised sensitively and provided flexibly and conveniently.

Equal access to health has been defined as meaning that:

> . . . no one receives less favourable treatment because of their ethnicity, colour, creed, national origin, gender, marital status, class, disability or

sexuality. It means that everyone has equal and full access to the health care that is available. (Henley & Schott 1999: 55)

Although there is growing evidence about health and healthcare inequalities among minority ethnic people in the UK, there is little knowledge of their specific health promotion needs. In the light of this, the authors were commissioned to undertake the Health ASERT Programme Wales (2005a, 2005b, 2005c) study from which data for this chapter are derived.

THE HEALTH ASERT PROGRAMME WALES

The National Assembly for Wales, Health Promotion Division, commissioned Middlesex University to undertake the Health ASERT Programme Wales study (the acronym stands for: Asylum Seekers, Ethnic minorities, Refugees and Travellers). The study commenced in February 2003 and was completed in March 2004.

AIMS OF THE HEALTH ASERT WALES STUDY

The overall aim of the study was to enhance the evidence base on health promotion issues relating to minority ethnic groups, refugees and Traveller communities in Wales in order to inform policy and programme development in the Welsh Assembly Government's Health Promotion Division, Office of the Chief Medical Officer as well as other Welsh Assembly Government departments.

The specific aims identified by the commissioner were to:

- identify gaps in the existing evidence base of health needs and health promotion issues of the three study groups
- identify existing good practice of health promotion in relation to the three study groups
- explore ways of delivering health promotion policy/programmes targeting these groups in a culturally and socially sensitive manner
- identify issues for further research.

In addition to the primary research whereby data regarding the views of service users and service providers were obtained, reviews of the literature relating to the three groups were undertaken by Aspinall (2005a, 2005b, 2005c, 2005d) of the University of Kent. These reviews focused specifically on the gaps in the existing evidence base whilst the primary research provided rich evidence of the health promotion needs of the groups under investigation.

THE MINORITY ETHNIC POPULATIONS OF WALES

Cardiff Bay, formerly known as 'Tiger Bay', was the first multicultural society in Britain (Cardiff Tourist Information 2005). However, Wales still has a relatively small (albeit growing) proportion of minority ethnic groups compared to England. According to the 2001 Census, in Wales almost 98% of the population identified themselves as 'white', compared with 91% in England (National Statistics 2004). The largest minority ethnic group in Wales were the Irish at 0.6%, whilst 'other white' minority groups accounted for 1.3%. Only 2.1% of its residents were recorded as being non-white. The largest non-white minority ethnic groups were Pakistanis (0.3%) and Indians (0.3%). Most non-white minority ethnic groups reside in the south, in the cities of Swansea, Cardiff and Newport. The exact number of Gypsy Travellers in Wales is unknown because of their nomadic lifestyle and the lack of systematic ethnic monitoring (Commission for Racial Equality 2004). The refugee and asylum seeker population in England and Wales is in constant state of flux due to the dispersal policy (Immigration and Asylum Act 1999), so only estimates of their number can be made. According to the Refugee Council, the majority of asylum seekers in the UK in 2001 were from Iran, Afghanistan and Somalia.

THE USE OF TERMS

We use the following terms to distinguish the groups who participated in the study: (a) 'minority ethnic groups' refers to people who have migrated to the UK, who are legally resident, and their British born descendants; (b) the term 'refugees' includes asylum seekers. (c) 'gypsy Travellers' refers to all Travellers who identified themselves as an ethnic grouping irrespective of their specific ethnic origin, and excludes New Age Travellers.

METHODOLOGY

THEORETICAL UNDERPINNINGS

Health promotion

Theories and models of health promotion were explored to identify those that could helpfully guide the study. The Tannahill (1985) model was selected because of its clarity and comprehensiveness. This model consists of three interrelated and overlapping constructs: health education, health protection and disease prevention (Fig. 11.1). The model also works on different levels such as individual (micro), community (meso) and governmental (macro).

The term 'health promotion' is defined by Downie, Tannahill & Tannahill (1996: 60) as follows:

Figure 11.1   The Tannahill model of health promotion. Source: Downie, Tannahill & Tannahill (1996).

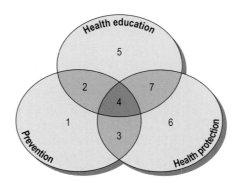

Health promotion comprises efforts to enhance positive health and reduce the risk of ill-health, through the overlapping spheres of health education, prevention, and health protection.

Seven domains (numbered in Figure 11.1) may be distinguished within health promotion, as follows:

1. Preventative measures such as immunization and cervical screening.
2. Educational efforts to influence lifestyles and to encourage the uptake of preventive services; emphasizes the importance of a two-way communication process.
3. Policy commitment to the provision of preventive measures.
4. Efforts to stimulate a social environment which demands or accepts preventive health protection measures such as in the case of seat-belts. Includes education of policy-makers and legislation.
5. The promotion of positive health education resulting in positive changes in attitudes and behaviour.
6. The promotion of a positive dimension to health protection such as the implementation of workplace smoking policy.
7. This domain embraces raising awareness of and securing support for positive health protection measures among the public and policy-makers.

Health for All (HFA) in the twenty-first century (WHO 1998)

The principles enshrined in the World Health Organization (WHO) HFA strategy also influenced the methodological approach of this study:

- health is a fundamental human right
- ethics should guide health policy, research and service provision
- equity-oriented policies and strategies should be implemented
- a gender perspective should be incorporated into health policies and strategies.

Target 6 of HFA refers specifically to measures of health promotion and recommends that monitoring should be focused on changes in:

- health behaviour (e.g. smoking)
- health determinants (e.g. social isolation)
- regulatory, fiscal and environmental policy (e.g. alcohol restriction)
- capacity-building programmes (e.g. leadership development)
- participation (e.g. communities)

Target 10 emphasizes the importance of strengthening health information systems.

Cultural competence

The study sought to identify the indicators of culturally competent health promotion from the perspective of both service users and service providers. Only the views of service users are presented in this chapter. Cultural competence in nursing has been developed over the last two decades or so since the concept was first promoted by Madeline Leininger (1995). Papadopoulos et al (1998) developed a model of cultural competence which consists of *cultural awareness, cultural sensitivity* and *cultural knowledge*; this is described fully in Chapter 2.

Participatory approach

Fundamental to the study were also the principles of participation and empowerment of those being researched (Papadopoulos 2005). In this study service users' and service providers' participation was sought through their involvement in the following aspects of the research process: development of the research proposal and data collection instruments; provision of data; focus group facilitation; transcription and translation of focus groups; validation of findings; advisory group membership; dissemination of findings.

The researchers used and further refined the participatory approach which forms an essential component of their model for developing culturally competent research and researchers discussed in Chapter 6 (Papadopoulos & Lees 2002, Papadopoulos & Gebrehiwot 2002). These principles are also fundamental to health promotion, as described by Downie et al (1996: 60):

> *The cardinal principle of health promotion thus defined is empowerment. Health education seeks to empower by providing necessary information and helping people to develop skills and a healthy level of self-esteem, so that they come to feel that significant control resides within themselves, rather than feeling buffeted about by external forces outside their sphere of influence.*

ETHICAL CONSIDERATIONS

The study gained ethical approval from the ethics committee of the School of Health and Social Sciences, Middlesex University, as well as the appropriate Welsh local research and ethics committees.

The participants of this study were provided with written information about the study in English and verbal information in their mother tongue as required and their consent was sought. Participants were assured of their anonymity and of the confidentiality of any information they provided. The emphasis on confidentiality may be particularly important for asylum seekers and refugees who report fearing deportation.

DATA COLLECTION METHODS

To elicit the views of the main minority ethnic groups, refugees, asylum seekers and Gypsy Traveller communities in Wales, focus groups were conducted with members of the following communities/groups:

- African Caribbean
- Indian
- Pakistani
- Chinese
- Somali asylum seekers
- Iranian asylum seekers

- Gypsy Travellers
- New Age Travellers.

Additional focus groups with women from the refugee, minority ethnic groups and Gypsy Traveller communities were also undertaken to ensure their views were adequately represented and to provide an opportunity for more open expression.

Focus groups were conducted with each individual community to help ensure culturally specific views would be elicited. All focus groups were tape recorded with the consent of the participants.

A topic list was developed to elicit participants' views on the following aspects of health promotion for their community: their health promotion needs; how they access health information; the health promotion and information materials available to them; health promotion and information approaches; who should conduct health promotion within their communities; problems with communicating information; venues and activities for health promotion; and suggestions/recommendations for culturally and linguistically appropriate health promotion.

Focus group facilitators who were fluent in the community language were recruited from each community, except in the case of the Gypsy Travellers' groups which were conducted by two health visitors who had worked with them for a number of years and who were trusted by them.

The facilitators were trained by the research team for their role, which was to: recruit participants; arrange the venues and refreshments; arrange child care; facilitate the focus groups; keep field notes; obtain consent from participants; transcribe and translate (when necessary) the focus group discussions; identify back-translators and individuals for the validation exercises.

A networking/snowball approach to recruitment was taken with participants being contacted by the group facilitators through link workers, interpreters, health access workers and community organizations. Participants were paid expenses and were provided with child care if needed. A total of 14 focus groups were conducted.

SEMI-STRUCTURED INTERVIEWS WITH LOCAL AND NATIONAL KEY STAKEHOLDERS

To elicit the views of 'key stakeholders' on strategy in relation to health promotion with the three study groups, a selection of key stakeholders in Wales, England, Scotland and Northern Ireland (national key stakeholders) were sent a semi-structured questionnaire for self-completion. Questions relating to the same issues were posed to nine local key stakeholders during semi-structured face-to-face depth interviews. The local key stakeholders were senior members of statutory and voluntary organizations involved with health promotion in Wales. However, this chapter presents and discusses findings from the primary research relating to the health promotion needs and preferences of minority ethnic groups (including Gypsy Travellers) from the viewpoint of the service users only.

CONSULTATION EXERCISE WITH FOCUS GROUP FACILITATORS

The focus group facilitators attended a consultation meeting when they were asked to give their views relating to health promotion for the groups in question. The consultation exercise was tape recorded with the consent of the participants.

CHARACTERISTICS OF FOCUS GROUP PARTICIPANTS

A total of 96 'service users' from the selected community groups took part in the focus groups. They were asked to give details of their gender, age group, ethnicity (self-defined), occupation, education, country of birth, mother tongue, religion and area of residence (Table 11.1). The first column in the table gives the group ID code, which is used to identify the source of each quotation in the findings section.

Although all age groups were represented in the focus groups overall, most participants were aged between 25 and 65, with the largest single group being in the 35 to 45 age group. Data are not available for three participants (Table 11.2).

Seven of the 13 who described themselves as 'Chinese' were born in Malaysia or Hong Kong.

The participants worked in a wide range of occupational groups from professional to unskilled manual jobs. Eight participants were retired and 17 described themselves as 'unemployed' or 'not working' (this

Table 11.1   Details of focus group participants

Group ID code	Focus groups	No.	Language of focus group	Main area of residence
C	Chinese	12	Cantonese	Swansea
I	Indian	10	Gujarati	Cardiff
P	Pakistani	9	Urdu	Cardiff
IRW	Iranian refugee women	10	Farsi	Cardiff
IR	Iranian refugees (mixed gender)	7	Farsi	Cardiff
MEW	Minority ethnic women	9	English	Cardiff
S	Somali refugees	9	Somali	Cardiff
AC	African Caribbean	7	English	Cardiff
WT	Welsh Travellers	6	English	Wrexham
NAT	New Age Travellers	5	English	West Midlands, England
IT	Irish Travellers	4	English	Queensferry, (Flintshire)
WET2	Welsh/English Gypsy (mixed gender)	3	English	Pontypool
ET	English Travellers	3	English	Newport
WET1	Welsh/English Gypsy women	2	English	Pontypool
	Total participants	96		

Table 11.2 Age groups of focus group participants

Age group	Number
18–25	12
25–35	21
35–45	35
45–65	20
65+	5
Not known	3
Total	96

excludes those who described themselves as housewives). Data on occupation were missing for nine participants.

DATA ANALYSIS

Audiotapes were transcribed in full and translated into English where applicable. All transcripts were entered into NUD*IST 5.0 and each was read by two researchers who agreed a coding frame for themes and sub-themes.

VERIFICATION OF TRANSLATED TRANSCRIPTS

To ensure the linguistic and conceptual accuracy of the translated transcripts, a modified back-translation exercise was performed. An individual from each of the focus groups conducted in a mother tongue was asked to ensure that:

(a) the translation conveyed the correct information and meaning
(b) the translator did not alter or omit any information
(c) the translator had used language that accurately conveyed the emotional weight and conceptual value expressed by the original speaker.

VALIDATION OF FOCUS GROUPS' FINDINGS

Respondent validation was undertaken (Silverman 1993). One participant from each focus group was selected (except the Travellers whereby one participant representing all the Traveller subgroups was selected) by the focus group facilitators. They reviewed and validated the findings in terms of:

(a) whether the findings made sense
(b) whether they represented what they understood to be the main issues that arose in the focus groups
(c) whether all important issues raised in the focus groups had been included.

In addition, the focus group findings were discussed during the consultation exercise with the focus group facilitators who were also able to validate the findings.

FINDINGS

The findings from the focus groups are presented under the five main themes listed below:

1. Main health problems
2. Health promotion activities accessed by the participant groups
3. Problems accessing health promotion services
4. Culturally and linguistically appropriate health information and advice
5. Actions required to improve health.

Direct quotes are given as illustrations and examples of the participants' views (the source of each quote is given in the abbreviated form detailed in Table 11.1). Many of the issues that are presented under the thematic headings are similar for most groups. Any variations are illustrated through the use of examples or specific quotes.

THEME 1: MAIN HEALTH PROBLEMS

The main health problems identified related to a number of diverse factors ranging from cultural, environmental and economic issues through to behavioural factors.

Cultural factors

Participants reported that migration causes stress because of cultural differences, as described by an African Caribbean participant:

I am of the opinion that to come from one culture to the other and the stress of that transition can affect you mentally. (AC)

Participants also reported that cultural factors impacted on health indirectly because health care was not always culturally appropriate. This was said to lead to lack of appropriate health promotion information, misdiagnosis, late diagnosis, late treatment and non-adherence to treatment.

Paan and khat were also thought to be causes of ill health, such as oral disease. Paan is a mixture of tobacco, betel nut, lime paste and 'perfume' wrapped in a leaf and is commonly chewed by Bangladeshis. In addition to the nicotine in tobacco, there is a stimulant (arakene) in the betel nut, related to cocaine. Khat is a green-leafed shrub that is chewed by people who live in the Horn of Africa and the Arabian peninsula. It has stimulant effects similar to amphetamine and can cause psychological dependence (Drugscope 2004).

Stress and other negative impacts on mental health were ascribed by women to their social isolation, a consequence of their oppression. An Indian woman described it thus:

There's not a mental understanding. At my age, I'm 23, being stuck at home twenty-four seven, it's just stress. I feel like sometimes that I suffer from depression. (I)

Socio-economic factors

Several participants reported that discrimination, social exclusion, uncertainty about immigration status, social isolation and difficulties finding suitable employment led to them living in relative poverty. All these factors had a detrimental effect on their psychological as well as physical well-being:

> *It is the pressure the men are under, isn't it, they go for the jobs and they are competing with the Europeans and they probably won't get the job. They are probably skilled, trained, got the qualifications and still don't get the jobs . . .? (AC)*

Environmental factors

Ill health was perceived to be related to environmental factors, such as air and environmental pollution and accidents caused by a poor environment. Gypsy Travellers particularly complained of unsafe living environments on encampments. Living on sites that were not lit and not having safe access to amenities and facilities such as shops also meant being at risk from road accidents and assault; as one of the Irish Travellers said, '*I drive a car so I don't walk, it's not safe*' (IT). Lack of money to buy household amenities or to keep the home in a good state of repair was also reported to be a risk to health and safety.

The New Age Travellers voiced concerns about the quality of the water they sourced from wells they dig themselves: '*We drink well water here; it would be interesting to get it tested. . . . When it's dry here the water gets sulphurous*' (NAT).

Age related

Participants described health problems related to age, such as childhood infectious diseases, and joint degeneration in the elderly. Lifestyle factors such as diet, smoking, alcohol misuse and lack of exercise were also understood to contribute to ill health. Their concerns about diet included additives in food; food production and preparation methods; unhealthy foods; and reactions to foods, such as hypersensitivity. The African Caribbean group was particularly concerned about school meals not being very nutritious. The Gypsy Travellers blamed their tendency to die young on their poor diet, which was said to be high in fat.

THEME 2: HEALTH PROMOTION ACTIVITIES ACCESSED BY THE PARTICIPANT GROUPS

Participants reported accessing the NHS and other governmental services which all groups reported using to varying degrees. Non-governmental sources of health promotion were also accessed including pharmacies, health food shops, outreach charity workers, and herbalists. These were most commonly mentioned by minority ethnic groups and mentioned least by refugees. The African Caribbean, Indian, Pakistani, Bangladeshi and Chinese participants collectively reported using the largest and most diverse sources of health promotion. Personal and informal sources of health promotion, such as friends and family, were used by all groups, but appeared to be particularly important for the Gypsy Travellers. Health promotion via the mass media was used by all groups;

however, the Gypsy Travellers did not tend to read magazines or use technology, such as the internet, or to attend cinemas. New Age Travellers believed their knowledge about health was good and they often accessed health information from books. They felt health promotion was improving as, 'It is taking on some homeopathic ideas', and that, 'It's also promoting good nutrition, and prevention rather than cure' (NAT).

THEME 3: PROBLEMS ACCESSING HEALTH PROMOTION

The causes of poor access to health promotion services and activities broadly fell into two main categories:

(a) those related to service provision and
(b) those related to the service users.

Barriers to health promotion related to service provision

The issue of racial discrimination was raised in almost all of the focus groups. It was seen as a barrier to getting health promotion and other healthcare services. Social exclusion was also described by several groups, such as the Irish Gypsy Travellers:

Discrimination

> . . . the government don't care about Travellers. We wish they would care . . . Travellers are like black-listed. Nobody wants to know them. Nobody wants to deal with them. (IT)

An African Caribbean described their invisibility in government policy:

> . . . there was nothing mentioned about us [in a White Paper], how they are going to change . . . very rarely do you see black and minority people specifically mentioned, whether it's in education, health . . . (AC)

Gypsy Travellers felt that discrimination explained why they were given unsuitable sites distant from facilities and services resulting in difficulties accessing health care, education and other services, such as shops and public transport. Accessing primary health care was particularly difficult for refugees and Gypsy Travellers, as the Irish Traveller group described:

> It would be good if we could get a doctor, but they are not interested. I tried from Queensferry to Liverpool but I can't get a doctor.

> . . . because they don't like Travellers. When I was in a house it was easier for me to get a doctor and now I'm not it's hard, I can't get one.

> Yes when you tell them you live on the site they don't want to know you because nobody wants to come onto the site. (IT)

Frequent eviction of Gypsy Travellers from unofficial sites (where increasing numbers have had to resort to living since the Criminal Justice and Public Order Act 1994 removed local authorities' obligation to provide legal sites) reduces continuity of care and results in missed opportunities for health promotion, such as vaccination:

> . . . sometimes you get the injections as well. Sometimes they go on in the clinic and sometimes [name of Health Visitor] comes here, but if you're travelling you miss them. (IT)

Stereotyping was also felt to be a barrier to appropriate health promotion. For example, an Iranian refugee reported that health workers assumed she was poor because she was a refugee (although many are) and consequently she was offered a free toothbrush, something which offended her. It was also reported that Muslims were assumed to be at low risk of HIV because chastity and faithfulness are required by their religion:

One of the vaccines [she probably meant blood test] that I ticked 'Yes' was HIV. Suddenly the interpreter told me you do not need this vaccine. You Muslims do not have any relation with others. I said that is right, but this disease can be caught from a dentist or a hairdresser. (IRW)

Language and communication problems

Many participants described experiencing communication problems, particularly those new to the country and the elders in some communities. Lack of properly trained interpreters was said to lead to inappropriate care, unmet needs and an undue burden on informal interpreters:

I had to go the hospital to translate for a friend of mine . . . We went there 4.00 p.m. and had to wait until 2.00 a.m. in the morning, I was there to interpret for her. The next day I couldn't go to my college because I went to bed late. (IR)

Culturally inappropriate health promotion

A Somali participant reported that health promotion leaflets may not be read not only because they are usually written in English but also because Somalis are not accustomed to this method of health promotion. Images in health promotion materials were reported to sometimes be out of date, racially stereotypical, unrepresentative, or insensitive to their culture or religion. The lack of cultural sensitivity was reported to be a factor which deterred some from accessing written health information.

Some health professionals were thought not only to have negative attitudes about people from minority ethnic groups, but also to have gaps in their knowledge relating to culture and ethnicity. For example, lack of cultural understanding was said to lead to African Caribbeans being misdiagnosed, and being unnecessarily hospitalized and sectioned under the Mental Health Act. Some doctors were reported to have difficulties recognizing signs of disease on dark skin.

Some felt there was a lack of community-based health education and other health promotion activities, such as health days or events directed specifically at their needs. Lack of publicity was also frequently mentioned.

The event in [name of place] was for all the refugees. It was not only for Iranian community. Very few people were informed about the event also. (IRW)

The Pakistani group raised the same issues:

We did not know when it happened. If it were organized by and for our community, we probably would have gone. (P)

Barriers to health promotion related to service users

Socio-economic factors

Some Gypsy Travellers reported that lack of relevant technology, such as computers and having to run electricity from generators, were barriers to accessing health promotion, as was lack of child care whilst they attended health promotion activities. Poverty was also reported to be a barrier to health promotion as it resulted in living in poorer, more polluted environments, lack of household amenities, such as a washing machine and inability to afford household repairs, resulting in safety hazards and general poor health. Further socio-economic factors such as their inability to afford transport to health services and their difficulties in obtaining NHS dental care compounded by the prohibitive cost of private dental care resulted in their exclusion from beneficial health promotion activities.

Cultural factors

Beliefs relating to health and life, such as the idea that *'you've got to die of something'* (ET) appear to prevent some Gypsy Travellers from wanting to access health promotion services or events. Another said she was *'too old to change'* (ET) but would be happy for health promotion to be given to the children. However, their desire to teach their children *'Gypsy ways'* may preclude this, particularly in relation to sex education.

Having a physical or mental illness was seen as stigmatizing by some participants and this impacted on help and advice seeking. A Pakistani participant said:

> *We feel embarrassed and shy in going to the surgery and discussing the problem. (P)*

Regarding mental health, another said:

> *Pakistan community don't acknowledge if suffering from stress. If they have a problem, don't talk about it and do not seek help. (P)*

Disapproval of health promotion activities also acted as a barrier to accessing such activities, for example vaccinations. Although some Gypsy Travellers accepted them, others disapproved of them:

> *I didn't have none of mine [vaccinations]. Anyway me mammy doesn't agree with injections. I'm scared of them. (IT)*

New Age Travellers also often disagree with vaccinations:

> *I don't mind them taking blood out but not putting anything back in. (NAT)*

Oppression of women by men was also seen to be a barrier to health promotion by the minority ethnic women's group, as women may not feel able to express their true needs during health promotion consultations when their husband is present:

> *If my husband was in front of me I wouldn't be able to say anything, in case I hurt his feelings about anything. . . . Most people are afraid or oppressed by their other half or too much worried about what they are going to think. (MEW)*

Perceptions of discrimination and intimidation

Feeling intimidated by health professionals was also described and was thought to be more common among the elderly, who consequently would not fully express their needs, and would comply without question. They also felt GPs were impatient with them if they had difficulty expressing themselves. A Pakistani participant explained these issues thus:

> *Doctors show more interest and give more attention to white people than our community people. There seems to be discrimination. . . . That's why our community people don't go back again, or ask any questions because they feel intimidated. They find it hard and difficult to express themselves and shy away. (P)*

The African Caribbean group described how they felt that health-care professionals particularly dislike black and minority ethnic people asserting themselves:

> *And I think when it's a black person standing up and asking them, there is a resistance to respond and to be answerable to a minority person. You know, they think that, 'I'm the one with the power, how dare you come in here!' (AC)*

Having to wait for appointments was felt by some to be due to discrimination, as an Iranian woman indicated:

> *If an English person goes to the doctor I don't think he would be refused medicine he wants. Or if they want to see a specialist surely they get referred to him/her straight away. (IRW)*

Gender issues

The Indian women's group suggested that there should be sex segregation in health promotion activities for Muslims. They also felt that local people should decide what health promotion should be provided rather than male religious leaders who may not reflect the best interests of women.

Sexual purity of unmarried females in Gypsy Traveller communities was said to be important. Young women are protected from knowledge about reproduction until after they are married:

> *Travelling girls from the age of nine learn to be a housewife, they cook, they clean, look after kids and be as pure as you can possibly be. You have to be pure to get married and we're not allowed to know anything. I knew nothing 'til I got married, I didn't know about virgins . . . We don't talk about pregnancy . . . (IT)*

Conversely, the males in this group were said to be allowed sexual freedom before marriage.

Literacy, language and communication issues

Language and communication issues were the most frequently reported barrier to health promotion. Low levels of literacy, particularly within the Gypsy Traveller communities and older people in some of the other communities, make it difficult for them to get information about services or to access written materials. For others, communication was problematic because they were not provided with the services of a professional interpreter when needed. A Chinese participant described the impact of this:

Especially our poor command of English, they are very impatient with us. When one is unwell, that makes us feel worse. This really needs to be improved. I know my English is not good, but I wouldn't go to them if I'm well. (C)

There were reports of children, husbands and other lay interpreters being used in health consultations, which was said to cause considerable distress to the patient and the 'interpreter'. It was also said to lead to poor quality or inappropriate advice or care, particularly for women when husbands or other male family members are used for interpreting discussion on reproduction and women's health problems, which may be difficult to discuss at the best of times:

Women problems need more promotion. Problem grows due to limited command in English. Shyness and hesitation prevents them to use the services available. They need more interpreters to express themselves fully. (P)

Lack of information about services and how to access them

Most of the groups discussed the issue of poor access to health promotion services being due to a lack of information about them and how to access them. The GP service was the only service some knew about, particularly the refugees. A lack of appropriate publicity about health events and other health promotion activities was complained of and it was reported that people seemed more aware of services and events organized by community organizations than 'mainstream' ones.

Poor transport

Difficulties accessing health promotion services because of poor access to transport, the cost of transport, and to facilities being too far away to walk to, were complained of by most participants but particularly by Gypsy Travellers as the following conversation illustrates:

They're in Newport and suchlike and if you ain't got a motor you can't get there.

I don't drive, so I'd have to get somebody to take me.

I can't catch the bus with the children. By the time I gets there it's all over and besides it costs too much on the bus. (WET2)

Getting to venues was also felt by most participants to be particularly problematic for older people and for parents struggling with several young children.

THEME 4: CULTURALLY AND LINGUISTICALLY APPROPRIATE HEALTH PROMOTION INFORMATION AND ADVICE

We were asked to explore ways of how health promotion could be made more culturally and linguistically appropriate in order to provide an impetus to move forward and make improvements. The participants gave their views on the following aspects of health promotion:

- venues for health promotion
- information needed
- formats of health promotion information

- preferred information providers
- preferred modes of receiving health promotion information
- benefits of advice and information

Venues for health promotion

The Somali and Welsh Traveller groups said they would like to see health centres or community centres specifically for their community within their locality, run by community members:

> *The way that the community could control and improve their health is by having a health centre that is in the community and run by the community members. . . . Some members of the community should be trained in health matters and those people will help the rest of the community to control their health. . . . health professionals who know and understand community health problems which are specific to the community should be employed. (S)*

The Welsh Traveller group visualized their community centre as being multifunctional, housing a school, a Sunday school, a health department and somewhere for adults to learn to read and fill in forms. A 'health bus' was also thought to be a good means of bringing health promotion to them.

The minority ethnic women's group suggested having 'health clubs' set up within the communities where health professionals could come and do health check-ups and where discussions and talks on health topics could occur. They also suggested health information on diseases affecting their community could be available at festivals and 'Melas'. Some of the community groups, such as the Indian participants, reported already having community centres that could be utilized for regular health information sessions. They said that it was important that they are accessible, particularly for the elderly, such as by having sessions during daylight hours. Pakistani participants also reported the need for a community hall, whilst also suggesting that mosques would be the best place to disseminate health information to Muslim men in their own language.

Child care in the form of crèches was said to be needed to enable some parents of young children to seek health advice. Facilities that are suitable for women and that give access to female healthcare workers were also wanted. A Pakistani participant suggested that if such needs were met, it would encourage more women to access the services:

> *People, when they use these facilities such as crèche and transport, can spread the word to family and friends. Gestures like these make people more aware and prone to use these services. (P)*

Outreach health workers who would visit people at home were suggested by the Iranian and the Chinese participants as their communities are dispersed, making attendance at community-focused centres difficult. An Indian participant also suggested this:

> *. . . in my community they do need proper healthcare workers from the local communities who could actually go out and promote health awareness in their own communities. (I)*

The Pakistani group suggested a need for more health education in schools in their own languages, as they felt awareness about healthy living should start when children are young. Concern about drug taking among children was expressed by the minority ethnic women's group.

Information needed

Participants requested information on the diagnosis, treatment and prevention of disorders such as SARS, allergies, heart disease, hypertension, eczema, diabetes, sickle cell anaemia, tuberculosis, anaemia, migraine, and on the menopause, mental health problems, men's health and children's health. They identified a need for information on vaccinations, cancer screening, thalassaemia, dental health promotion, and information regarding self-medication with over-the-counter medication. Other information needs identified included how to access health promotion, when to seek professional medical advice, and how to live a healthy lifestyle.

They also suggested that people should be informed that NHS services are free at the point of delivery; that interpretation services are available if they need them, and that people can obtain information in their own languages.

Preferred formats for health promotion information

Many participants from several groups highlighted their preference for health promotion through personal interaction, such as consultations with health professionals and health promotion talks and events. The Iranian group particularly liked the immediacy and two-way nature of personal interaction when discussing health issues, especially those of an intimate or personal nature. Having verbal information from people who speak their own languages was preferred:

> *Many in the Pakistani community are not literate and cannot read their own language. So there has to be another way to communicate which I think is verbal method. There is a need to create an environment where they can go, talk, explain, discuss health issues which are very sensitive. I think there is a fundamental gap. . . . Not everyone can read Urdu. (P)*

Other groups also supported the preference for personal health advice in mother tongues. However, where this was not possible, then professional translation services were felt to be acceptable, as were properly translated good quality health promotion materials, such as leaflets that are written briefly and simply, preferably in their own language using illustrations. The benefits of health promotion leaflets were even noted by the Irish Travellers who have low levels of literacy:

> *. . . most of them [Gypsy Travellers] can read a bit and even passing out the leaflets because they can help the others if one can read, then the other can pass the message on to the others. . . . that rumour will carry on and on. (IT)*

Pictures in leaflets and other health promotion materials were thought to be particularly helpful to those who had difficulties reading.

Participants stressed, however, that it is important to ensure the pictorial representations are culturally sensitive and appropriate. The African Caribbean participants described stereotyping of black people in health promotion materials:

> . . . *speaking from a diabetic point of view any magazine with a black person is always a fat old black woman and my son is a young man. But it is changing.*

> *Our leaflets are very old and out of date and they still got the old afro and flares . . . (AC)*

Preferred information providers

Some groups, particularly the Gypsy Travellers, said they would prefer health advice and information to come from people within their own community. They explained that Gypsy Travellers are better at getting things across to other Gypsy Travellers and they are more likely to be listened to and trusted. Some participants also believed that health promotion activities or events would be better attended if they were run by people from their own communities.

> . . . *they had this short course sort of thing. They ran it in a mosque. The authorities, they took the skilled people to the mosque and asked the ladies to come there to get this. And if somebody is running it from their own community they do go. (EMW)*

Although professional interpretation services were highly valued, some participants felt it was important to be able to communicate directly with health professionals, emphasizing the issue of confidentiality.

> *Everyone has a problem, but they will not come and tell me because I might tell everyone in the city, but if there is a professional person then they can follow the secrecy code. That is what we need. (I)*

Pakistani participants preferred health promotion from professionals with high rank as they were thought to have more credibility.

Preferred modes of receiving health promotion information

A number of modes for receiving health promotion information were identified. Such variation is necessary because of the differences in language skills, literacy, education, acculturation, health and illness beliefs, and variations in access to services and technology.

Community radio and ethnic press

Chinese and Somali participants suggested that community radio should be used for health information. Others wanted health information to be conveyed through their community newspapers which use community languages.

Television and cinema

Some participants wanted discussions and chat programmes on health issues on Asian satellite and cable TV channels in community languages. Health promotion messages on TV were said to be given a lot of credence and the advice was thought to be more likely to be followed. The cinema, Pakistani participants mentioned, was also valued as a potential source of health promotion messages, but again if it was in community languages.

> When we go out to watch an Asian movie, any health promotion on the screen would be effective in raising awareness. (P)

Videos

The Gypsy Traveller and Chinese participants in particular were keen to get health information and advice via videos. The Chinese participants suggested videos were a good medium to promote exercise and suggested that the government should provide exercise videos free, or at low cost.

Text messaging

Pakistani participants suggested text messaging health promotion messages, such as 'drink clean water', 'exercise is good for you'. This was thought to be particularly good for targeting the younger generation.

Telephone advice lines

Many were unaware of the NHS Direct but reported that because it is difficult to get medical advice and treatment outside of office hours, and to avoid having to wait for a doctor's appointment, such a service would be useful, providing it is available in their own language. The few participants who had used this service were very complimentary about it.

Benefits of health promotion information and advice

The benefits of health advice and information were reported by the participants to include:

- positive changes in behaviour
- the uptake of screening
- prevention of illness
- quicker diagnosis and treatment
- increased confidence in dealing with health issues
- increased knowledge of where and how to access health services
- increased knowledge of self-care and less dependence on the NHS
- improved understanding of health issues
- more likely to talk about health problems
- better health.

THEME 5: ACTION FOR HEALTH IMPROVEMENT

The focus group participants recommended that the following actions were needed in order to improve the health of their communities.

Improve socio-economic circumstances

Participants felt strongly that reducing poverty would promote health, such as giving more financial support for single parents and enhancing the levels of social support particularly for the elderly.

Some wanted to see education schemes for Gypsy Traveller children enabling them to stay in their own community and the provision of literacy schemes for adult Gypsy Travellers with child care to enable education for mothers.

Improve the environment

More legal sites for Gypsy Travellers were wanted with clean and safe play areas for children and improved accident prevention measures, such as street lighting and good sanitation. A reduction in rubbish and dirt, and cleaner air were also suggested by a number of the other groups.

Facilitate positive lifestyles

Some wanted to see more action to encourage exercise and the following suggestions were made: government provision of exercise guide books and video tapes; raise awareness of physical exercises that can be undertaken in the home; group exercise sessions for the older generation; women-only sport and exercise facilities; the provision of transport to sports centres; concessionary rates at sport and exercise facilities; information about where to find exercise facilities in community languages; and the provision of exercise organizers.

Some suggestions were made relating to reduction of isolation including: more social mixing; separate social venues for men and women; places for children to play together; and encouraging Somali men to reduce use of khat and spend more time with their children. The Chinese participants said there was a need to help Chinese restaurant workers find ways of getting exercise as their hours of work make this difficult.

Address racism and discrimination

Suggestions for addressing racism and discrimination included ensuring the voice of the minority groups was heard, and getting more people from black and minority ethnic groups into positions of authority.

Public health policies on smoking and advertising

Banning smoking in public places and banning advertisements of unhealthy foods were suggested.

Provide culturally competent health promotion services

Participants described a need for services to be delivered using community languages, and for health promotion activities to be targeted more at their communities to ensure their specific health promotion needs are addressed. They also suggested a need to educate people about the benefits of complying with health promotion programmes.

DISCUSSION AND CONCLUSIONS

Although the participants in this study resided in Wales, we believe that minority ethnic groups (including Gypsy Travellers) resident in the UK hold similar views. Our study has indicated that minority ethnic groups have a holistic understanding of health promotion; they understand that health promotion requires action within many spectrums of life. For example, promoting access to clean air and a 'healthy' environment, access to adequate nutrition and shelter, appropriate and adequate social contact, access to good quality culturally competent health care, and fostering the ability to maintain a healthy lifestyle. They also illuminated how some groups who are marginalized in society, such as asylum seekers who do not have the protection of citizenship, and Gypsy Travellers who are particularly socially excluded, are especially liable to be exposed to deficiencies in the current health promotion system, and to the effects of socio-economic deprivation.

Novel ways of improving access to health promotion and health care generally have been developed or piloted over the years; for example, the single electronic patient record which could help continuity of care for highly mobile groups such as Travellers and asylum seekers, community health workers and health advocates, and community health initiatives. Our study highlighted a wish for more community-focused health promotion with workers from within local minority ethnic communities. Mainstream services need to be more flexible and creative in their approaches to enable a range of modes of service delivery to meet diverse needs and preferences. An example arising from our study is the use of a range of technologies, such as TV and the internet.

Efforts to reduce discrimination in British health-promoting institutions are also needed. For example, Gypsy Travellers need the help of local authorities to live on properly developed permanent and transit sites with modern facilities. This would help them access education, health and other services, as well as find employment and thereby improve their socio-economic status and their health. Training health workers to be culturally competent practitioners will contribute towards challenging discriminatory policy and practices. The policy of encouraging people from ethnic minorities and refugees into health professions including positions of authority would be supported by many of our participants. They want their opinions and needs reflected in health policies and services so they no longer feel 'invisible' within them.

The health promotion notions articulated by the participants in this study are not dissimilar to the notions advanced by Tannahill (1985) nor indeed to those expounded by the WHO (1998). This study has illustrated the need for the integration of health, economic, social and environmental policy, something that has been recognized by the Welsh Assembly Government as a way of improving health. This integrated approach is described in Wellbeing in Wales (Welsh Assembly Government 2002: 4) as a way in which 'different policies and programmes add value to each other'. It is also known as a 'cross cutting' approach as the issue of health cuts across all national policies in its aims to reduce social and health inequalities. The pan-agency strategies and inter-agency partnerships that have been recently fostered by the Welsh Assembly Government, as well as their approaches for enhancing user involvement and improving the collection and collation of population data, are examples that others can follow.

We have defined culturally competent health promotion as those policies and practices that have the capacity to provide effective health education, health protection and disease prevention taking into consideration people's cultural beliefs, behaviours and needs. To achieve this, it is crucial that health-promoting organizations embrace the findings of this study and staff must endeavour to become culturally competent practitioners. In summary, organizations must:

- work in partnership with other organizations
- involve user groups, fostering their empowerment
- have systems for harnessing appropriate data and ethnic monitoring
- ensure that staff have opportunities to develop knowledge and expertise in cultural issues
- have adequate resources to enable short and long term culturally competent health promotion
- be able to address the needs of non-English speaking and illiterate people
- deal with racism and discrimination appropriately
- provide information to aid clients' access to health promotion resources
- undertake health promotion needs assessment in order to customize health promotion
- target health promotion at identified need
- locate events and materials in appropriate places for the target groups.

REFLECTIVE QUESTION

1. The WHO Ottawa Charter for Health Promotion (1986) stated that health promotion action means:
   build healthy public policy
   create supportive environments
   strengthen community action
   develop personal skills
   reorient health services.

Reflect on the findings of the study described in this chapter and compare the above principles with those identified by the participants of our study.

Acknowledgements

We wish to thank all those who participated in the study. We also wish to acknowledge the contributions of Shelley Lees and Asanka Dayananda. We would also like to thank the Health Promotion Division, Office of Chief Medical Officer, Welsh Assembly Government for commissioning, funding and publishing the study. Finally our appreciation goes to Launa Harris and Kaori Onoda for their help and support.

REFERENCES

Acheson D (Chair) 1998 Independent inquiry into inequalities in health. The Stationery Office, London

Aspinall PJ 2005a Health ASERT Programme Wales: Enhancing the health promotion evidence base on Minority Ethnic Groups, Asylum Seekers/Refugees and Gypsy Travellers. Report 2. A Review of the Literature on the Health Beliefs, Health Status, and Use of Services in the Gypsy Traveller Population, and of Appropriate

Health Care Interventions. Cardiff: Welsh Assembly Government, Cardiff

Aspinall PJ 2005b Health ASERT Programme Wales: Enhancing the health promotion evidence base on Minority Ethnic Groups, Asylum Seekers/Refugees and Gypsy Travellers. Report 3. A Review of the Literature on the Health Beliefs, Health Status, and Use of Services in the Minority Ethnic Group, and of Appropriate Health Care Interventions. Cardiff: Welsh Assembly Government, Cardiff

Aspinall PJ 2005c Health ASERT Programme Wales: Enhancing the health promotion evidence base on Minority Ethnic Groups, Asylum Seekers/Refugees and Gypsy Travellers. Report 4. A Review of the Literature on the Health Beliefs, Health Status, and Use of Services in the Refugee and Asylum Seeker Populations, and of Appropriate Health Care Interventions. Cardiff: Welsh Assembly Government, Cardiff

Aspinall PJ 2005d Health ASERT Programme Wales: Enhancing the health promotion evidence base on Minority Ethnic Groups, Asylum Seekers/Refugees and Gypsy Travellers. Report 5. A Review of Databases and other Statistical Sources Reporting Ethnic Group and their Potential to Enhance the Evidence Base on Health Promotion. Cardiff: Welsh Assembly Government, Cardiff

Bahr R 2001 Sports medicine. BMJ 323:328–331

Barry J, Herity B, Solan J 1987 The Travellers' health status study: Vital statistics of Travelling people. Department of Health, Dublin

BBC 2004 Proposed Indian 'paan' ban panned. Online. Available: http://news.bbc.co.uk/1/hi/world/s/w_asia/82227.stm 15 Sept 2004

Cardiff Tourist Information 2005 Online. Available: http://www.aboutbritain.com/towns/Cardiff.asp 31 Mar 2005

Commission for Racial Equality 2004 Gypsies and Travellers: A strategy for the CRE, 2004–2007. Online. Available: http://www.cre.gov.uk/downloads/docs/g&t_strategy_final.doc 10 March 2005

Department of Health 2003 Department of Health Equality Framework: Priorities for Action. Online. Available: http://www.dh.gov.uk/assetRoot/04/07/89/10/04078910.pdf 16 Jan 2005

Department of Health 2004 Choosing health: Making healthier choices easier. Executive Summary. Online. Available: http://www.dh.gov.uk/PublicationsAndStatistics/Publications/PublicationsPolicyAndGuidance/PublicationsPolicyAndGuidanceArticle/fs/en?CONTENT_ID=4094550&chk=aN5Cor 16 Jan 2005

Doll R, Peto R, Boreham J, Sutherland I 2004 Mortality in relation to smoking: 50 years' observations on male British doctors. BMJ 328:1519

Downie R S, Tannahill C, Tannahill A 1996 Health promotion: models and values. Oxford University Press, Oxford

Drugscope 2004 Khat. Online. Available: http://www.drugscope.org.uk/druginfo/drugsearch/ds_results.asp?file=\wip\11\1\1\khat.html 15 Sept 2004

Henley A, Schott J 1999 Culture, religion and patient care in a multi-ethnic society. Age Concern, London

Immigration and Asylum Act 1999. The Stationery Office, London

Leininger M M 1995 Transcultural nursing. Concepts, theories, research and practices. 2nd edn. McGraw-Hill, New York

National Statistics 2004 2001 Census. Online. Available: http://www.statistics.gov.uk/census2001/default.asp 7 Sept 2004

Nazroo J Y 1997 The health of Britain's ethnic minorities: findings from a national survey. Policy Studies Institute, London

Nazroo J Y, Karlsen S 2001 Ethnic inequalities in health: social class, racism and identity Online. Available: http://www.lancs.ac.uk/fss/apsocsci/hvp/newsletters/10findings.htm 19 Dec 2003

Papadopoulos I 2005 Developing culturally competent researchers: a model for its development. In: Nazroo J (ed) Methods for health and social research in multicultural societies. Taylor and Francis, London

Papadopoulos I, Gebrehiwot A (eds) 2002 The EMBRACE UK Project. Middlesex University, London

Papadopoulos I, Lees S 2002 Developing culturally competent researchers. Journal of Advanced Nursing 37(3):258–264

Papadopoulos I, Tilki M, Taylor G 1998 Transcultural care: a guide for health care professionals. Quay Publications, Dinton

Papadopoulos I, Lay M and Lees S 2005a Health ASERT Programme Wales: Enhancing the health promotion evidence base on Minority Ethnic Groups, Asylum Seekers/Refugees and Gypsy Travellers. Report 7. Full Length Primary Research Report. Cardiff: Welsh Assembly Government, Cardiff

Papadopoulos I, Lay M and Aspinall PJ 2005b Health ASERT Programme Wales: Enhancing the health promotion evidence base on Minority Ethnic Groups, Asylum Seekers/Refugees and Gypsy Travellers. Report 1. Main Findings and Recommendations. Cardiff: Welsh Assembly Government, Cardiff

Papadopoulos I, Lay M and Lees S 2005c Health ASERT Programme Wales: Enhancing the health promotion evidence base on Minority Ethnic Groups, Asylum Seekers/Refugees and Gypsy Travellers. Report 6. Summary Primary Research Report. Cardiff: Welsh Assembly Government, Cardiff

Parry G, Van Cleemput P, Peters J et al 2004 The health status of Gypsies and Travellers in England. University of Sheffield. Online. Available: http://www.shef.ac.uk/content/1/c6/02/55/71/GT%20final%20report.pdf 5 Jan 2005

Race Relations (Amendment) Act 2000 The Stationery Office, London

Raphael D (ed) 2004 Social determinants of health. Canadian perspectives. CSPI, Toronto

Rawaf S, Bahl V (eds) 1998 Assessing health needs of people from minority ethnic groups. Royal College of Physicians, London

Refugee Council. Info centre statistics. Online. Available: http://www.refugeecouncil.org.uk/infocentre/stats/stats003.htm 31 Mar 2005

Silverman D 1993 Interpreting qualitative data: methods for analysing, talk, text and interaction. Sage, London

Tannahill A 1985 What is health promotion? Health Education Journal 44:147–148

Viner R, Booy R 2005 Epidemiology of health and illness. BMJ 330:411–414

Welsh Assembly Government 2002 Wellbeing in Wales: Consultation document. Welsh Assembly Government, Cardiff

WHO 1998 Health for all in the 21st century. World Health Organization, Geneva

PART 3

European perspectives on cultural competence

PART CONTENTS

Chapter **12**

Cultural healthcare issues in Finland

Marja Kaunonen and Meeri Koivula

LEARNING OBJECTIVES

After reading this chapter you should:
- achieve a higher level of awareness about cultural healthcare issues that relate to Finland in general
- become aware about some of the health and healthcare issues of minority ethnic groups in Finland
- increase your knowledge about cultural issues in Finland
- increase your level of sensitivity regarding the caring of people from different cultural backgrounds
- be able to apply this new awareness, knowledge and sensitivity to your practice, which should become more culturally competent.

INTRODUCTION

The chapter will begin by outlining the geographical and historical perspectives of Finland, which will help the reader to understand some cultural perspectives of our country. Some characteristics of Finnish culture as well as sociocultural aspects of Finland will be explained. We will also introduce some thoughts regarding the Finns' perception of migrant people living in Finland. Some examples of everyday life in Finland are discussed, as are examples of family life. The position of women has been unusually strong in Finnish culture; therefore some facts about it are offered in this chapter. Traditional health promotion methods are discussed as they represent illustrations of Finnish culture. The special emphasis given to cultural perspectives in Finnish nursing research is introduced through examples of research studies for both the majority culture and the Finnish minorities. Since coronary artery disease is a national disease in Finland nursing studies relating to the care of heart patients are included in this chapter. Death, dying and mourning processes and rituals offer an opportunity to understand life and culture from a Finnish viewpoint.

In this chapter culture is understood to be relevant to both the majority population of a country as well as being about the cultural richness and challenges that minority cultures bring to it. The word culture originates from the word *colere* in Latin, meaning to cultivate, to tend, to settle. In its original usage, the word referred particularly to agriculture, to taming the land for human needs. Later on, the concept expanded to include all human activities, including the way of life and traditions passed on to following generations (Reunala 2001).

Jokinen & Saaristo (2002) emphasized that cultures are multifaceted and changing all the time. There is not just one Finnish culture, but many different ones.

THE ETHNOHISTORY OF FINLAND

GEOGRAPHY

Finland belongs to the Nordic countries and stretches about 700 miles (1126 km) north and south from the Arctic Circle to the Gulf of Finland, with Sweden along its western and Russia along its eastern border. It is the second most northern country in the world but the climate is relatively mild because of the influence of the North Atlantic Current, the Baltic Sea, and more than 100 000 lakes. The landscape of southern Finland is characterized by its lakes and forests, and the northern part of Finland, called Lapland, by its fjelds and wilderness areas. Lapland is located north of the Arctic Circle and has unique summers when the sun does not set and winters when the sun does not rise (Kaunonen et al 2003).

HISTORY

To understand Finnish culture it is important to know the main points of the history of Finland. In the year 1323 AD Sweden and Novgorod (antecedent of Russia) signed the peace treaty of Pähkinäsaari which divided up the territory of Finland. Finland was a part of Sweden and could send representatives to vote in Sweden's royal elections. In 1397 the kingdoms of Denmark, Sweden and Norway united into the Kalmar Union. In 1493 Finland was mentioned for the first time on a printed map of Europe. Gustavus Vasa became king of Sweden and Finland in 1523. Bishop Mikael Agricola produced the first Finnish-language book, a volume of Finnish grammar in 1543. In 1640 Queen Christina of Sweden established Finland's first university, the Åbo Academi in Turku. The first complete Finnish translation of the Bible appeared in 1642. Under the treaty of Uusikaupunki (1721) Sweden ceded south-eastern Finland and the Baltic provinces of Livonia, Estonia and Ingria to Russia.

In 1808–1809 Sweden was defeated by Russia in the Finnish War and lost Finland, which became an autonomous Grand Duchy with the Czar as its ruler. Finland retained its own legislation and its old form of society, including the free status of the peasantry, the Lutheran religion and the old Swedish system of law and government. In 1860s sawmilling began to flourish and the paper industry started to develop. In 1882 the first Finnish women received a university degree. The period between 1850 and 1900 was a golden age of Finnish arts and nationalism. But in the early 1900s there was an economic depression and over 320 000 Finns immigrated to the USA and Canada.

Finland acquired its own national parliament in 1906. During the revolution in Russia, Finland declared itself independent in 1917 and Russia's government recognized Finnish independence. In 1918 there was civil or liberation war in Finland. The government forces, led by General C.G.E. Mannerheim battled against left-wing forces associated with the Bolshevik revolution.

In 1919 Finland adopted a new republican form of government and K.J. Ståhlberg became the first president. Finland and the Soviet Union signed a non-aggression pact in 1932 but in 1939 the Red Army attacked Finland. In the 'Miracle of the Winter War' the Finnish defence forces, commanded by Marshal C.G.E. Mannerheim, fought alone against the Soviet army for 105 days. Few at the time expected the tiny Finnish nation of 3.6 million to survive. But Finland reacted with desperate determination. Four months later, after the hardest fighting seen in Europe since the First World War and massive Soviet reinforcement, Finland's lines remained unbroken, while the Red Army lost up to 400 000 soldiers. In the peace of Moscow, Finland was forced to cede a large part of the Vyborg province to Russia. During 1941–1944 fighting resumed and defiant Finland aligned with Germany against the Soviet Union in order to regain the lost territory. In July 1944 the Finnish army halted a massive Soviet offensive. The Red Army's aim was to occupy southern Finland, but it could not do so because of the stubborn resistance of the Finnish army. Under the peace terms Finland lost the Karelian province and had to pay huge war reparations to the Soviet Union in the form of manufactured goods. The entire population of the lost Karelian territory, about 450 000 people, were resettled in Finland.

After the war Finland's industry, economy and the whole society developed expeditiously. In 1952 the Olympic Games were held in Helsinki. Urho Kekkonen's 25-year period as President of Finland came to an end in 1981. Finland became a member of the European Union in 1995 (Brady 2000).

FOUNDATIONS OF FINNISH CULTURE

The Finnish culture has been fashioned by Finland's history, and its geographical location both in terms of being the second most northern country in the world and in terms of being situated between the cultures of East and West. Finnish culture has its roots deeper in the forest than any other European culture. The oldest implication of the forest from the point of view of culture lies in the meaning of wild, untamed nature. Having the forest as one's source of life and livelihood has been considered in Western culture to be more primitive and less civilized than the practice of agriculture. In Finland, in the beginning of the 1900s the development of forest industries provided the necessary economic foundation for an independent state. In Finland wood is used in many ways; for heating, building material for houses, furniture and paper products. Furthermore, the forests had an important spiritual significance. Finnish artists who had studied abroad in the late nineteenth century discovered their national identity in the country's forests. The artists travelled in Finland's remote areas and collected the ballads for the Kalevala, which is the national epic of the Finns. In this way the artist Akseli Gallen-Kallela reinforced the Finns' belief in their own strong sense of identity with his paintings; Jean Sibelius did the same through his music (Reunala 2001).

The forest has had an impact on the social life of Finns. Long distances, large wilderness areas and poor roads have hampered people from meeting one other. The Finns are found to be shy and silent, which may have some connections to the social isolation imposed by nature. People in Finland appreciate their forest very much even today. In the forest they collect mushrooms and berries, they ski and hike during both the winter and summer. However, Finland's beautiful natural environment has also its dark side. The autumns and winters in Finland are very cold and dark. Many people feel depressed because of the long absence of sunlight. Nevertheless, many Europeans find the forests and lakeshores of Finland to be good places for calming down and relaxing.

SOCIOCULTURAL ASPECTS OF FINLAND

From the sociocultural viewpoint, Finland has been considered relatively homogeneous, even isolated. Altogether, 94% of its 5.1 million people are Finnish. There have been virtually no ethnic conflicts. Ethnic minorities, apart from the Sami and the Roma, have been almost non-existent and the small number of refugees and immigrants has not much altered the overall situation.

Finland has two official languages: Finnish and Swedish. About 6% of Finns have Swedish as their first language. In addition, there are two ethnic minorities, Sami (7000 people) and Roma (10 000 people). Finns study two to three foreign languages in school and their command of English and Swedish is good. There are about 107 000 foreigners living in Finland. The biggest groups originate from Russia (25 000 people), Estonia (13 500 people) and Sweden (8100 people). Each year only a few thousand people seek asylum in Finland; for example, in 2002 the number of asylum applications was 3443. Between years 1973 and 2003 a total of 22 250 persons immigrated as refugees to Finland (Statistics Finland 2004).

The Sami are one of the indigenous peoples of northern Europe. An ethnic group is considered indigenous if its ancestors inhabited the region before the establishment of present state boundaries. The Sami people live in the northern part of Finland, Sweden, Norway and Russia. In Norway, there are more than 40 000, in Sweden more than 20 000, in Finland 7000 and in Russia 2000 Sami people. In the Nordic countries, the definition of who is Sami is based on language criteria. There are nine Sami languages. North Sami is the most common language and it is spoken widely in the northern parts of the Sami region in Finland, Sweden and Norway. The reindeer are still fundamental to the Sami culture and society. Many Sami families and communities derive most of their income from reindeer, an economy that in most cases is combined with fishing, hunting and handicrafts. There are Sami political, cultural and youth organizations in all four countries and a Sami Parliament in each of the three Scandinavian countries. In 1992, a Language Act was passed in Finland to guarantee the official status and use of the Sami language. The Sami have the right to use their language when dealing with the authorities and Sami-speaking students have the right to study Sami at their comprehensive school (between the ages of 7 and 16). Most of the Sami in Finland also understand Finnish (Anon 2004a, 2004b).

The Roma people moved to Finland about 500 years ago from Sweden. In the 1600s there was a law in Sweden and Finland that all Roma people could be killed. Nowadays there are Roma people all over Finland, but most of them live in the cities in southern Finland. During the 1980s the legal and social position of Roma people was improved in Finland. In the basic law of Finland, discrimination is forbidden and Roma people have the right to maintain their own culture. The majority of the population have learned to appreciate the Roma culture. Despite these changes, Roma people in Finland remain poorer than the other Finns. They have higher unemployment and lower educational levels than other Finns. One of the reasons for this is that the Roma people have had negative attitudes towards education, which formerly was used as a tool of assimilation to the majority culture. Nowadays most young and middle-aged Roma people speak Finnish but also understand the Roma language. Important values in Roma culture are togetherness of families, social support for other Romas, respect for older people and their own culture. The Finnish government appointed the first Advisory Board on Roma Affairs in 1989. The Advisory Board functions in conjunction with the Ministry of Social Affairs and Health and half of the members represent the Roma population. The Advisory Board actively works to prevent work-related discrimination and to improve employment. The Advisory Board is paying close attention to the founding of the European Roma Forum, which is a result of an initiative made by Finland's President Tarja Halonen (STM 2004b).

In 2000, 89% of the Finnish population were members of the Evangelical Lutheran Church, 1% were members of the Greek Orthodox Church, and 0.1% were Catholics. In addition, 1165 people were Jewish and 962 were Muslim. Altogether, 2% of the entire population were not members of any religious group.

Finland enjoys one of the highest standards of living in the world (Kaunonen et al 2003). During the 1990s social problems such as unemployment, poor health and family problems increased and accumulated, because of the economic recession and its consequences which hit the country at that time (Forssen 1998, Jokinen & Saaristo 2002).

FINNS' PERCEPTION OF IMMIGRANTS

In an old proverb Finns explain their opinion of being a foreigner: 'In a country you must behave like the other citizens.' Or in Finnish: 'Maassa maan tavalla'. In a globalizing world and in a more international Finland this is not always possible, when immigrants have very different cultures to that of the indigenous people. The arrival of more refugees and migrants is posing a new challenge for Finnish society, which is beginning to realize that new cultures need to be understood and accommodated. For example, immigrant women from African countries have brought the practice of female circumcision to Finland (Haddi 2003).

Ethnic minorities and different cultures can often be used as a scapegoat by the majority community during times of economic crisis. This was the case in Finland during the 1990s, and migrants found themselves on the receiving end of racist actions. The European Commission carried out the Eurobarometer project in 1997, where the Finns assessed their own racist attitudes. Ten per cent of Finns assessed themselves to be very racist, 25% quite racist, 25% slightly racist and 22% not at all racist. The most unpopular immigrant groups in Finland are those who accentuate their culture and ethnic identity. In the Helsinki region about 5% of the population are immigrants. In the year 2000, the National Board in Finland accepted a plan of action against racism. Promoting positive opinions and attitudes among young people and the whole population towards migrants is a good way to minimize racism and to advance equality and respect for diversity (Makkonen 2000).

EVERYDAY LIFE OF A FINNISH FAMILY

The total number of families in Finland is 1.4 million. There are about 0.5 million married couples with children and also 0.5 million married couples without children. Cohabiting with children or without children is quite common (108 000 families versus 170 000 families). Almost 45% of all married couples divorce. The number of children (under 18) is two in 41.4% and one in 23.7% of families. Only 12% of families have four or more children (Statistics Finland 2004). Midwife-assisted hospital birth predominates. Finland has one of the lowest infant mortality rates in the world, at 3.0 per 1000 live births, whilst the rate of stillbirths is 3.3 per 1000 births (Statfin 2004, Vuori & Gissler 2004). Most fathers participate in the delivery and consider their presence at delivery important for their growth into fatherhood. After the delivery in hospital, rooming in is prevalent in Finland; in 2003, 79% of all mothers had returned home before the fourth day following the delivery (Vuori & Gissler 2004).

In the Nordic countries (Finland, Sweden, Norway, Denmark), the state has for a long time assisted families with the expenses of child care. Securing the welfare of families with children also contributes to the maintenance of a steady population growth. It can be argued that the Finnish family policy, including income transfers and social services, has been effective if studied with respect to child poverty reduction. However, Finland's family policy and social services did not survive the recession (1990–1993) without cutbacks. These affected single parent families especially (Forssen 1998). An important difference between Finland and many other industrialized countries is that high quality day care is available for every child under school age (Husu 2001).

Finland enjoys free education paid for by taxes. Most 6-year-old children go to pre-school to improve their capacity to learn. Comprehensive school starts at the age of 7. Comprehensive schooling is a 9-year system providing education for all children of compulsory school age (7–16 years). The upper secondary school offers a 3-year general education curriculum, at the end of which the student takes the national matriculation examination. Instead of the upper secondary school the student can choose to take the basic vocational qualification, which is a 3-year curriculum. The higher education system consists of two parallel sectors: universities and polytechnics. The polytechnic degree has a professional emphasis and takes 3.5 to 4 years to complete. The master's degree at university takes 3 to 5 years and a PhD takes 4–5 years. The purpose of universities is to perform scientific research and to provide higher education connected with it (Ministry of Education 2004). The cultural values and national identity of Finnish people are mostly formed by the school system. On the other hand, travel, the media, technology and globalization are causing schools to become more aware and open to other cultures (Tolonen 1999).

WOMEN'S SITUATION IN FINLAND

The Gender Equality Unit started its work on 1 May 2001. This unit is linked to the Ministry of Health and Social Affairs (STM 2004a). In a statement published in May 2004 the Ministry of Health and Social Affairs recognized equality between women and men as a central sociopolitical target in Finland. Equality between sexes means that the differences between women and men should not lead to unequal status or treatment within society. This is why the philosophy of equality in Finnish and Scandinavian societies emphasizes that providing the same opportunity is not enough; active work is also required to promote the status of women. Equality will be achieved when society places equal value and emphasis on the work, experience, knowledge and skills of women and men. The Government Act on equality between women and men is an important tool in the achievement of this target (STM 2004a).

The position of women in society started to change in the late nineteenth and early twentieth centuries, when new work possibilities opened up for women, such as teaching and nursing. Women's legal position also improved: for example, after 1864 an unmarried 25-year-old woman was able to apply for legal competency. This meant that she was able to decide independently upon her education, marriage or income. Married women were granted that status only in 1930, when the new Marriage Act brought an end of the husband's guardianship of his wife. After that married women were able to make their own agreements and have their own personal property (Table 12.1).

In Finland, the participation of women in the labour force has been high, and today it is almost identical with that of men. The reasons for this are the recognition of women's high level of education, women's wish for autonomy, and the necessity of a double income within a family. In some fields women still face problems at work when striving for the same status as men as well as the difficulties arising from their primary responsibility for the family and domestic duties (European Network 2004). In the Finnish Evangelical-Lutheran Church, women had to wait until 1988 to become professionally equal with men serving the Church. It was only then that the first women were inaugurated as church ministers (Ahola et al 2002). Throughout the 1990s women's average income from regular work was 81% of men's corresponding income, although the principle of equal pay had been recognized long before that. During the last quarter of 2003, monthly earnings for regular working time averaged 2322 euros, respectively 2581 euros for men and 2065 euros for women. The annual percentage changes in men's and women's salaries have remained the same over the last few years, indicating that the salary gap has not decreased (Statistics Finland 2004).

There is evidence that in Finland women with higher education degrees have their children slightly later than other women and have on average fewer children than women with less education. The average age of the primigravida is 27.6 years. Clearly, younger generations of academic women are combining motherhood with an academic career more often than previous generations (Husu 2001).

TRADITIONAL METHODS OF HEALTH PROMOTION IN FINLAND

Over the centuries, many nations have practised sweat bathing. The Finnish sauna is a sweat bath influenced by both Eastern and Western bathing cultures but has many national features (Valtakari 2004). In Finland the sauna is a national 'institution' which has been continuously cultivated through two thousand years of experience and practice. The

Table 12.1   Milestones in women's rights in Finland (source: STM 2004a)

1864	Unmarried women receive full rights (when 25 years old)
1878	Women and men receive equal rights with regard to inheritance
1890	The first public kindergarten is established in Helsinki
1901	Women receive the right to study at university, on equal terms with men
1906	Women receive voting rights for national elections (the first country to do so in Europe) and the right to be electoral candidates (the first country to do so in the world)
1907	The first women join the first Parliament (19/200)
1908	Brothels in Helsinki closed down
1917	Women receive general voting rights for local government elections
1919	Wives gain a right to work without their husband's permission
1926	The Act on women's eligibility in state posts is passed The first female minister for the Finnish government is instated
1930	The Marriage Act releases wives from the guardianship of their husbands and wives are given the right to their own property
1937	The Act on Maternity Allowance is passed
1943	Statutory school meals are introduced
1944	Acts passed instituting local government maternity and child healthcare clinics and also local government health visitors
1961	The contraceptive pill is accepted
1962	The principle of equal pay for work of equal value is established in both the public and private sectors
1970	The Abortion Act is passed Human relationships and sex education become part of the school curriculum
1972	First woman to be elected to be Minister of Finance
1975	First woman to be elected to be Minister of Justice Parents gain the right to share parental leave
1980	First Finnish government programme for promoting equality between sexes (1980–1985)
1985	The Act on Home Care Allowance is passed
1986	Finland ratified the UN Convention on the Elimination of All Forms of Discrimination against Women (Cedaw) Women are allowed to keep their family name even when married A child is entitled to have the mother's or father's family name
1987	The Act on Equality between Women and Men is passed
1990	Children up to the age of 3 are guaranteed a municipal child care place The first woman in the world to become Minister of Defence
1992	A woman becomes University Principal A woman becomes the Speaker of the Parliament Partial amendment of Equality Act Act on Women's Voluntary Military Service
1999	Act to prohibit unwanted approaching
2000	A women becomes President of the Republic of Finland

original, primitive sauna was a simple underground burrow or 'smoke sauna'. When one or more bathers crawled into the 'smoke sauna', they sweated their ailing bodies, chasing out devils and sicknesses. Previously when the doctor and the hospital were both miles away the sauna gave privacy and warmth for a woman during childbirth. An old traditional saying of Finns is that: 'If the sauna, tar, or alcohol doesn't cure a disease, it must be fatal' (Virtanen 1974). Sauna was known as the poor man's pharmacy and the folk healers practised their art in sauna (Valtakari 2004).

Sauna is still today a place for cleansing and revitalising the body, soul and mind for almost all Finns. The modern sauna is a building or room with wooden walls, floor and ceiling. There is a stove, called 'kiuas', which is heated with wood, electricity, oil or gas. The top of the stove is covered with natural stones, which radiate heat to the room. Humidity is regulated by small doses of water ladled repeatedly onto the 'kiuas' stones. The resulting vapour, rising from the stones, is called 'löyly'. The temperature varies between 70 and 100°C. Warming up is followed by washing and cooling off. Swimming in a lake after a sauna is especially relaxing. Sauna is nowadays a part of urban lifestyle in Finland too, and there are about 1.5 million saunas in Finland. Many families have sauna cottages by a lake or by the sea. Sauna is a standard element also in swimming baths and sport centres, hotels, holiday centres and camping sites (Finnish Sauna Society 2004).

Taken in moderation, sauna baths suit everyone who is aware of their own limitations. They alleviate both physical and mental stress, pain and tension. Saunas can also ensure good sleep and provide cosmetic care. Finns usually bathe in a sauna once or twice a week. Men and women bathe together only inside the family; in public saunas men and women have separate sections or different hours. Nakedness is natural in sauna and going to sauna is rarely connected to any kind of sexual behaviour. Haste and noise are out of place in the sauna (Viinikka 2004, Valtakari 2004).

One mode of sauna culture is winter swimming or 'ice hole swimming'. This means swimming in a frozen lake or sea where swimmers cut a large opening through the ice called 'avanto'. Swimmers take a quick plunge or swim for a few minutes at a time and most appreciate a hot sauna after the relatively cold swim. There has recently been a renewed interest in winter swimming, and swimming places are maintained throughout the winter by many local winter swimming societies. Winter swimming can be a risk for a heart patient. Most swimmers feel relaxation of muscles, body and mind, and pains, such as those resulting from rheumatic disease, can be decreased (Cankar 2004).

Medical care based on herbal drugs is quite popular in Finland and Finnish herbs are known to be very clear and flavoured because of the clean natural environment and bright summer nights. Certain forms of foreign alternative medicine, such as acupuncture, have become more commonplace and to some extent approved by the medical profession (Kaunonen et al 2003).

THE CULTURAL PERSPECTIVE IN FINNISH NURSING RESEARCH

In this part we are presenting examples of Finnish nursing studies from two perspectives: studies related to minority ethnic groups and the Finnish majority culture.

Tanttu's (1997) research aimed to describe the family dynamics of foreign families, their attitudes towards pregnancy and childbirth and their experiences and expectations concerning Finnish maternity care. Results indicate that life in exile, unemployment, a poor knowledge of the Finnish language were amongst variables having a weakening effect on family dynamics. The care provided during the pregnancy and delivery was reported to be different in Finland from that experienced in their own countries. The experiences of Finnish maternity care were positive, but the families expected to have interpreter services in the hospital. The lack of social support for the extended family in the hospital was seen as an isolating factor.

Vuorio (1997) studied the family dynamics and healthcare services of the Sami people in the north of Finland. The study was carried out in cooperation with health visitors, who distributed questionnaires to families. Family dynamics were assessed and the Sami families were found to have high mutuality and individuality. The family structure, functions and relations are flexible, but also stable. The family communication was clear and the family roles were reciprocal. The study found that Sami families were generally quite satisfied with their health care. But families had also experienced mistreatment and they found it hard to get care at weekends; there were often long distances between their homes and the health centre or hospital. Families also reported having to wait a long time for treatment.

Pursiainen (2001) studied the competence of public health nurses in providing culture-specific care for Muslim immigrant families. The study results indicated that participating public health nurses had not acquired their cultural care competence from their basic training, but rather they had gained their knowledge and skills relating to different cultures and the customs and values connected with them either on their own or during training arranged by their employer. Public health nurses perceived that difficulties encountered in meeting Muslim immigrant families were not caused by Islam, but rather by the problems created by refugeedom and their migrant status.

Haddi (2003) studied the health-related problems of Somali female circumcision and prospects for future changes. His study focused on the primary data of 60 Somali women residing in the Helsinki area. The study results indicated the existence of major health problems related to female circumcision, such as infection, pain, shock, trauma, gynaecological problems and difficulties in childbirth. This matter is relatively new for Finnish healthcare workers. Therefore the study recommended that healthcare workers in Finland should be given proper training in how to deal with the issues of female circumcision in Finland, which is prohibited by law.

CORONARY ARTERY DISEASE: A NATIONAL DISEASE IN FINLAND

In Finland the mortality from cardiovascular diseases (CVD) has been one of the highest in the world. In the early 1970s a large community-based programme (the North Karelian Programme) for prevention and control of CVD started in Finland. The results indicated that such prevention programmes have a high degree of generalizability, are cost-effective and can influence health policy (Nissinen et al 2001). Risk factors for CVD are smoking, unhealthy nutrition, physical inactivity, excessive use of alcohol and psychosocial stress. In Finland the programme largely addressed changes in lifestyle including smoking cessation and dietary changes. This resulted in a decrease in heart disease deaths by 75%. As a result of the programme doctors and nurses are providing advice to patients regarding smoking cessation (Puska 2002).

The nursing study by Koivula & Paunonen (1998) identified that 31% of 40-year-old Finnish men were smokers. The study used the Stages of Change scale (Leskinen et al 1995) and Men's Attitude scale (Koivula & Paunonen 1998) for smoking. Men were found to be at different stages of smoking cessation behaviour; 12% of men were found to be in the contemplation stage, and 11% in the preparation stage. One-quarter (25%) of men had recently given up smoking and were in the action stage. One-quarter (25%) of men regarded smoking as an integral part of their way of life (Koivula & Paunonen 1998).

According to a national health survey Finnish men's daily smoking has slightly decreased but women's daily smoking remains at the same level (Helakorpi 1999). In the same national survey food habits had improved: the use of full fat milk and butter has continued to decline. The consumption of alcohol has been increasing in Finland for many years. Overall, cardiac health has markedly improved according to this population survey (Helakorpi 1999). Because living habits and psychosocial factors are highly culture related, changes can be very slow. In Finland, the results of community-based cardiac health education programmes are good, because they are planned, run and evaluated according to clear principles and because they are closely linked to the national authorities (Nissinen et al 2001).

NURSING STUDIES RELATING TO THE CARE OF CVD PATIENTS IN FINLAND

Nursing studies in Finland have focused on the patients' perspective regarding heart disease. In Finland, 12 000 coronary arteriographies, 4500 coronary artery bypass operations and 2500 percutaneous transluminal coronary angioplasties (PTCA) are done every year. The number of bypass operations compared to the size of the population is the highest in Europe (Mustonen et al 2000). Patients have to wait for many months for heart examinations and then again for the operation. A study by Koivula et al (2002) reported that patients found waiting for care to be very difficult. Women were especially fearful, as were the young men. The spouse and the family were found to be very supportive to the family member waiting for heart surgery. The nursing care in the hospital was supportive and the information given by nurses and the care team decreased the fears of most patients (Koivula et al 2002). Caring for the family was found to be quite diverse in Finnish hospitals. Family members were not always given enough information which they need to support the patient. The study also found that patients sometimes rejected their own families during the acute stage of their illness (Koivula 2004). Finnish heart patients reported that information, inpatient treatment, and their own inner resources, such as faith and hope, helped them when feeling anxious and afraid. Nurses reported that after identifying the fear of the patient they were able to respond to the patient's emotions, thoughts and knowledge level. Finnish nurses reported that men often deny their fears whilst women behave in different ways and often speak about their fears. Talking about one's own possible death is difficult for Finnish men and women too (Koivula & Åstedt-Kurki 2004). Younger women with coronary heart disease have been shown to have a poor quality of life in Finland (Lukkarinen & Hentinen 1997, 1998). There is evidence from many countries that CVD is widely seen as a health problem of men, and that is why women and especially younger women have not been treated as actively as men. Other research with patients with coronary artery disease reports that women, the elderly, and patients with low levels of education had significantly more learning needs than men and young patients (Höltta et al 2002). Koivunen et al (2003) found that the rehabilitation processes of patients who had undergone coronary artery bypass surgery involved critical and difficult phases. Women's recovery involved loneliness, feeling unsafe, depression and physical sensations such as pain. Men attained a better balance in their recovery after 6 months, but even they had various problems such as depression.

DEATH, GRIEF AND MOURNING IN FINNISH CULTURE

For many Finnish people death is like a dark lingering shadow which reminds people of the ephemeral nature of life. Funeral songs were commonly improvised among Finns living in northern and eastern Europe. International comparisons (Achte et al 1987, Nenola 1994, 2002) indicate that Finland has an exceptionally large number of death- and grief-related songs. Laments were sung in eastern Finland, whilst in western Finland death psalms were common and in the village communities of Ostrobotnia people gathered to express their sympathy to the family and to pay their respect to the deceased person. Mourning rites served to facilitate death-related feelings and to show the community that the family was grieving by using black clothing (Pentikäinen 1990).

Most people in Finland die in a hospital setting. The first hospice in Scandinavia, Pirkanmaan Hoitokoti in Tampere, Finland, was opened in 1987. Currently there are three hospices in Finland. Sand (2003), a nursing researcher, has published an ethnography aimed at generating information on the substance and nature of Finnish hospice care. The study results indicate that Finnish hospices operate in keeping with the British hospice ideology and the care is based on meeting the dying patient's physical, psychological, social and spiritual needs. Finnish hospices have been characterized by charity, compassion and the traditional 'Niskavuori' ethos, meaning inner strength and hospitality towards visitors. As care environments, hospices send out strong messages and are marked by symbols of death. The cultural versatility and subtlety of hospice care stems also from collaboration with various groups, such as staff, volunteers as well as through cultural programmes and visits. Cultural programmes include visits by Finnish artists and also celebrations of Christmas and other traditional festivities. Visitors vary from local child groups who perform their own programmes to international professional groups.

Kaunonen's (2000) study on support for a family in grief found that while grief can be seen as a universal phenomenon, mourning has features that are culturally dictated. Nenola's (1994) study of Finnish mourning customs revealed that there are only a few collective mourning rituals, such as dressing in black or bringing flowers and candles to the graveyard. Väisänen's (1996) findings confirmed that after the death of a baby, rituals are few. The reason for this may be that death and grief is considered as private and almost as a taboo for the outsider. Kaunonen's study results revealed the importance of funeral and memorial services to a grieving Finnish family. In Finnish culture the funeral usually takes place 2–3 weeks after the death. The study found that survivors expressed their willingness to fulfil the deceased person's wishes concerning the funeral arrangements and were uncertain about their decisions when those wishes were left unexpressed. The funeral was seen as a turning point in the grieving process, after which the survivors were either starting to normalize their everyday life or had the most difficult time when being alone and having time to grieve (Kaunonen 2000).

Funeral rituals are important for grieving people as a way of expressing one's grief, especially since the old mourning customs, such as black clothing or black veils for widows have disappeared during the last decades. In Finland as late as in 1960s women wore a black dress and men a black grief button on their suit in order to express grief following the death of a close relative (Erjanti 1999). Funeral directors assist the family with after-death care. Burial is common practice but cremation is becoming more commonplace. A memorial service is usually held following the burial. The death is announced in newspapers either after the burial, but sometimes also prior to it, when the obituary serves as an invitation to the funeral. Family members often attend a church service the day after the funeral. Even though 58% of Evangelical Lutheran parishes offer bereavement support groups (Harmanen 1997), only 4–17% of bereaved family members participate in these groups. Family members and friends have been found to be the most important source of social support for grieving people (Kaunonen 2000).

The most recent features of the mourning culture include the collective expressions of grief such as that which occurred in Finland after the sinking of the ship Estonia in 1994; after the brutal murder of three policemen in October 1997; and after a bus accident where 23 youngsters were killed in the spring of 2004. Large numbers of people expressed their grief by bringing flowers and candles to places relating to these deaths.

Erjanti (1999) perceived the sociocultural connection among Finns to be linked with silent suffering and self-control, dominance of the culture of death, Lutheran mourning traditions and the relatively homogeneous structure of the population.

CONCLUSIONS

Finland is a large area in the northern part of Europe, but the population of Finland is small and the country is sparsely inhabited. Finland has had close connections to Sweden, Norway and Russia, which are also its neighbours. The original language, geographical situation, history and the Nordic nature have forged the homogeneous culture of Finland.

After the Second World War Finland rapidly developed economically, socially and culturally. Today Finland is part of the European Union. Previously there have been many emigrants from Finland and also during the Second World War Finnish refugees. Nowadays Finns are learning to accept immigrants from other European countries and undeveloped countries. Finnish society is becoming more and more a multicultural one. Health care and social conditions are rapidly responding to the standards of multicultural society. Finnish nursing research is building new knowledge about the needs of minority ethnic groups, without neglecting that of the majority culture.

REFLECTIVE QUESTIONS

1. Why is Finnish culture defined as homogeneous?
2. Is there a bathing culture in your country? Compare it with the Finnish sauna culture.
3. How has the country's history affected the current Finnish culture and habits?
4. Can you think of three ways in which nurses and other healthcare professionals can positively influence people's lifestyles?
5. Compare the status of women in your country with that in Finland.
6. Why is it important that healthcare workers know the grieving and mourning habits and rituals of the people they serve?

REFERENCES

Achte K, Lahti P, Rouhunkoski L (eds) 1987 Suomalainen kuolema (Finnish death, in Finnish). Yliopistopaino, Helsinki

Ahola M, Antikainen M R, Salmesvuori P (eds) 2002 Eevan tie alttarille (Eve's path to the altar, in Finnish). Edita, Helsinki

Anon 2004a Sami People. Online. Available: http://www.yle.fi/samiradio.saamelen.html 23 Aug 2004

Anon 2004b An introduction to the Sami people. Online. Available: http://www.its.se/boreale/samieng1.html 23 Aug 2004

Brady J 2000 A chronology of Finnish history. Virtual Finland. Online. Available: http://www.virtualfinland.fi/info/english/chrohist.html 10 Aug 2004

Cankar M 2004 Avantouinti. (Ice hole swimming). Online. Available: http://cankar.org/sauna/howto/avanto.html. 11 Aug 2004

Erjanti H 1999 From emotional turmoil to tranquillity. Doctoral thesis. Acta Universitatis Tamperensis 715, Tampere

European Network 2004 European network of the adult education organizations working on women's employment issues. A Socrates Programme. Women's specific situation in Finland. Online. Available: http://www.women-employment.lt/finland.htm 27 July 2004

Finnish Sauna Society 2004 Online. Available: http:// www.sauna.fi 11 Aug 2004

Forssen K 1998 Children, families and the welfare state. Studies on the outcome of the Finnish family policy. Research report 92. National Research and Development Centre for Welfare and Health, Helsinki

Haddi A–W 2003 The health related problems of Somali female circumcision and prospects for future. Master's thesis. University of Tampere, Department of Nursing Science, Tampere

Harmanen E 1997 Sielunhoito sururyhmässä – tutkimus ryhmän ohjaajan näkökulmasta Suomen evankelis-luterilaisessa kirkossa (Pastoral care in grief counselling groups – a study from the viewpoint of group leader in the Evangelical Lutheran Church of Finland). In Finnish, abstract in English. Academic dissertation, Suomen teologisen kirjallisuusseuran julkaisuja 207, Helsinki

Helakorpi S 1999 Health behavior and health among Finnish adult population: spring 1999. National Public Health Institute (Kansanterveyslaitos), Helsinki

Hölttä R, Hupli M, Salanterä S 2002 Patients' learning needs after coronary artery bypass surgery. In Finnish, abstract in English. Hoitotiede 14:11–18

Husu L 2001 Sexism, support and survival in academia. Academic women and hidden discrimination in Finland. Social Psychology Studies, University of Helsinki, Helsinki

Jokinen K, Saaristo K 2002 Suomalainen yhteiskunta (The Finnish Society). WSOY, Helsinki

Kaunonen M 2000 Support for a family in grief. Academic dissertation. Acta Universitatis Tamperensis 731, Tampere

Kaunonen M, Rask K, Sand H 2003 Finland (Republic of) In: D'Avanzo C E, Geissler E M (eds) Cultural health assessment. 3rd edn. Mosby, St Louis, p 275–281

Koivula M 2004 The importance of family and next of kin as experienced by CABG patients' and nurses. In Finnish, abstract in English. Tutkiva Hoitotyö 2:4–9

Koivula M, Åstedt-Kurki P 2004 How to reduce patients' fears of coronary artery bypass surgery in nursing care. In Finnish, abstract in English. Hoitotiede 16:50–60

Koivula M, Paunonen M 1998 Smoking habits among Finnish middle-aged men: experiences and attitudes. Journal of Advanced Nursing 27:327–334

Koivula M, Tarkka M-T, Tarkka M et al 2002 Fear and in-hospital social support for coronary artery bypass grafting patients on the day before surgery. International Journal of Nursing Studies 39:415–427

Koivunen K, Lukkarinen H, Isola A 2003 Rehabilitation of patients suffering from coronary artery disease following coronary artery bypass surgery and guidance as a part of rehabilitation process. In Finnish, abstract in English. Hoitotiede 15:62–73

Leskinen L, Pallonen U, Kääriäinen R et al 1995. Käyttäytymisen muutoksen vaihe ja prosessimallin soveltaminen tupakastavieroitukseen. (Stages of Change Scale applied to stopping smoking.) Kansanterveyden tutkimuslaitos, Kuopion yliopisto, Kuopio

Lukkarinen H, Hentinen M 1997 Assessment of quality of life with the Nottingham Health Profile among patients with coronary heart disease. Journal of Advanced Nursing 26:73–84

Lukkarinen H, Hentinen M 1998 Assessment of quality of life with the Nottingham health profile among women with coronary artery disease. Heart and Lung 27:189–199

Makkonen T 2000 Rasismi Suomessa (Racism in Finland). Ihmisoikeusliitto. Online. Available: http://www.ihmisoikeuslitto.fi (pdf) 11 Aug 2004

Ministry of Education 2004 Education. Online. Available: http://www.minedu.fi/education 11 Aug 2004

Mustonen J, Romo M, Airaksinen J et al 2000 Sepelvaltimotaudin invasiivisen tutkimuksen ja hoidon toteutuminen Suomessa ja muualla Euroopassa. (How invasive examinations and the care of the coronary artery disease patients fulfil in Finland and other European countries). Suomen Lääkärilehti 55:2883–2886

Nenola A 1994 Suremisen perinteistä (Mourning traditions, in Finnish). In Suominen T, Hupli M, Iire L et al (eds). Hoitotiede 1994. Pro Nursing ry:n vuosikirja. Pro Nursing ry, Turku, p 98–106

Nenola A 2002 Inkerin Itkuvirret. Ingrian Laments. Suomalaisen Kirjallisuuden Seura/Finnish Literature Society, Helsinki

Nissinen A, Berrios X, Puska P 2001 Community based non-communicable disease interventions: lessons from developed countries for developing ones. Bulletin of the World Health Organization 79(10):963–970

Pentikäinen J 1990 Suomalainen lähtö. Kirjoituksia pohjoisesta kuolemankulttuurista (Finnish death. Writings on the northern death culture). Sisälähetysseura, Pieksämäki

Pursiainen P 2001 Terveydenhoitajan valmius hoitaa kulttuurin mukaisesti islamilaista maahanmuuttajaperhettä (Public health nurse competence in cultural care of Muslim immigrant families). In Finnish, abstract in English. Master's thesis. University of Tampere, Department of Nursing Science, Tampere

Puska P 2002 European medical newsletter on smoking cessation. Interview with Prof. Pekka Puska. Online. Available: http://www.hon.ch/emash/news 12 Aug 2004

Reunala A 2001 Forests and Finnish culture: 'There behind yonder woodland . . .' Virtual Finland. Online. Available: http://virtual.finland.fi/finfo/english/forest.html 10 Aug 2004

Sand H 2003 Sateenkaaren päästä löytyy kultaa (There is gold in the end of the rainbow). In Finnish, abstract in English. Academic dissertation. University of Tampere, Tampere

StatFin 2004. Statistics Finland's StatFin – Online Service. Online. Available: http://statfin.stat.fi 12 Oct 2004

Statistics Finland 2004. Finland in Figures. Online. Available: http://www.stat.fi/tup/suoluk/ taskue_vaesto.html 5 Aug 2004

STM 2004a Ministry of Social and Health Affairs. Equality between women and men in Finland. Online. Available: http://www.stm.fi/Resource.phx/tasa-arvo/english/ milestones/index.htx 5 Aug 2004

STM 2004b Ministry of Social Affairs and Health. Suomen romanit. (Roma people in Finland). Online. Available: http://pre20031103.stm.fi/suomi/pao/julkaisut/ romanit.htm 7 Sep 2004

Tanttu K 1997 Vierasmaalainen perhe äitiyshuollon asiakkaana – monikulttuurinen näkökulma perheen toimivuudesta ja lapsen syntymään liittyvistä käsityksistä ja kokemuksista (Foreign family as a client in maternity care – multicultural aspects of family dynamics, beliefs and expectations concerning childbirth). In Finnish, abstract in English. Master's thesis. University of Tampere, Department of Nursing Science, Tampere

Tolonen T 1999 Suomalainen koulu ja kulttuuri (The Finnish School and Culture). Vastapaino, Tampere

Väisänen L 1996 Family grief and recovery process when a baby dies. A qualitative study of family grief and healing processes after fetal or baby loss. Academic dissertation. Acta Universitatis Ouluensis, Medica D series, 398, Oulu

Valtakari P 2004 Finnish sauna culture – not just a cliche. The Finnish Sauna Society 2004. Online. Available: http:// www.sauna.fi 11 Aug 2004

Viinikka L 2004 Sauna and health. The Finnish Sauna Society 2004. Online. Available: http://www.sauna.fi 11 Aug 2004

Virtanen J 1974 The Finnish sauna. Peace of mind, body, and soul. Continental Publishing House, Portland

Vuorio B 1997 Saamelaisten perhedynamiikka (Family dynamics of the Sami people, English abstract). Master's thesis. University of Tampere, Department of Nursing Science, Tampere

Vuori E, Gissler M 2004 Parturients, births and newborn infants – preliminary data for 2003. STAKES, Statistical Summary 15/2004. Online. Available: http://www. stakes.fi 13 Oct 2004

Chapter **13**

Dealing with cultural plurality in health and social care settings: the case of Germany

Monika Habermann

LEARNING OBJECTIVES

By reading this chapter you will:
- learn about some facts and figures regarding health and migration in Germany and be able to compare them with other countries in Europe, which are outlined in this volume
- be able to consider migration policies and the impact on health and social care, as perceivable in Germany
- be able to analyse theoretical discourses in health and migration and compare them with those of the other European countries in this volume
- be able to identify cornerstones of communal and organizational developments in Germany in improving the health of migrants
- get to know some 'best practice' examples, which you could consider transferring to your own work settings.

INTRODUCTION

Compared to some of its European neighbours, Germany has been somewhat late in dealing coherently with migration and its impact on society. A substantial political and public discussion about Germany as a country of immigration started only a few years ago. The incentive for this was not only the recognition of decades of immigration into Germany but also the alarming demographic trends. These indicate that an active immigration policy is necessary to balance persistent low birth rates and prevent low economic productivity in the future (Ulrich 1998). In addition, the mediocre position of Germany in comparative outcome studies, such as those dealing with the educational system, led to public discussions. It was realized that one reason for this unfavourable development is a failed integration policy. It became clear that some Germans but especially migrants could not benefit from an education system that seems to favour the privileged.

Reflecting the recent general debates, deficits in health and social support for the migrant population have also been focused on. In addition to the minority of scientists and health practitioners who have been concerned about these issues for decades, welfare organizations, community health planners and professional bodies have now also become involved. It seems that in the context of globalization German people are finally ready to discover and accept plurality, not only when enjoying exotic travel but also within their own country.

This chapter outlines health and social issues with regard to cultural plurality in three sections. First, some facts and figures about health and social care for migrants are given. Secondly, theoretical debates and their impact on the practice field are discussed. The last section provides some examples of practice developments in Germany.

MIGRATION TRENDS AND POLICIES IN GERMANY: SOME FACTS AND FIGURES

MIGRANTS IN GERMANY

The International Organization for Migration (2003: 8) defines migration 'as movement of a person or a group of persons from one geographical unit to another across an administrative or political border, wishing to settle definitely or temporarily in a place other than their place of origin'. Migration is not a new phenomenon of the industrial and post-industrial era. It has been a constituent of nation-building processes. For instance, Germans left the country in large numbers in search of a better life during the last three centuries, North America being the main target. Numerous Polish workers were brought to the country in the first decades of the last century to strengthen the workforce of the coal mines in north-western Germany (Projekt Ruhr 2002: 7) The Nazi regime enforced another exodus of threatened people, mainly of Jewish origin. The aftermath of the Second World War caused the flight and exodus of an estimated 12–14 million people from eastern parts of Europe, who were resettled within the boundaries of the current Federal Republic of Germany (Faulenbach 2002).

However, it was only in the 1950s and 1960s that there was a growing awareness within the population of Germany of being a plural society. In the wake of the Cold War, Germany was divided into two states, with a closed frontier, the so-called Iron Curtain. The booming economy, known as the 'Wirtschaftswunder', lacked the workforce of the eastern parts of Germany. This was balanced by recruiting workers first from southern countries of Europe like Italy (especially south Italy and Sicily), Spain and Portugal, followed by the recruitment of workers from Turkey. The recruitment procedure was simple: agencies focused on young and healthy people, checking this in some areas in a rather rude manner: teeth, a quick health check and some questions concerning mental orientation. Upon a positive result, a ticket to one of the industrial centres was handed out. Over 3 million workers came to Germany by 1970 (Münz et al 1997: 38). They were called 'Gastarbeiter' (guest workers) because of the perception that they would return to their home countries after some years of work. However, the majority did not return. Because of the ongoing demand for workers and the realization that this workforce needed a better social embedding within the country, the government allowed family members to follow their breadwinners to Germany. Since 1973, in the context of an economic crisis, this recruitment has been stopped and immigration of family members has been handled more restrictively since then. Only selected work fields, which have a shortage of applicants, such as nursing or information technology, have since been allowed entry permits.

The recruited workers and their families constitute the highest number of foreigners. Since they cannot apply for dual citizenship, many are still living with a foreign passport in Germany, being statistically counted as foreigners, even though they might be third-generation migrants and were born in Germany. It is evident, that the presence of the guest workers and their families in Germany has had a lasting impact on city lives, habits, attitudes and cultural self-perception of the German population; even so, reservation and even hostility towards the strangers were widespread in the beginning.

Apart from these workers, the so-called 'Aussiedler' (referred to also as 'remigrants' in this chapter) are the largest group of migrants. These are the descendants of former German settlers in the eastern part of Europe and former Russia who used to live in German-speaking communities until the Second World War. After the war they were allowed to return to Germany as citizens, if they had proof of their origin. This is based on German law, which follows the 'ius sanguinis' in acknowledging citizenship: the origin of the family counts, not the actual place where a person is born.

During the last four decades an estimated 3.7 million 'Aussiedlers' re-immigrated to Germany (Europäisches Forum Migration 2003). This caused repeated controversial public debates challenging the basis for German citizenship and finally led to successful attempts to limit the number of those being allowed to return to Germany, to roughly 100 000 people per year.

In many regards, these remigrants have to be considered as immigrants, even though they have German origins and a German passport. Like other migrants, they constitute a potentially vulnerable group, due to lack of or mediocre German language abilities, low average income, and living in regional fringe groups. Like other foreigners they often experience reserve and sometimes even hostility. It is also evident from the health statistics that adaptation to life in post-industrial Germany seems to involve specific stress for these families, especially amongst young people and the elderly (see section on health and social care issues below).

In addition to the groups already mentioned, immigration is also determined by asylum seekers and war refugees for whom German law has several different categories including 'asylum seekers', 'person and their families who are entitled to asylum', 'Convention refugees' and 'quota refugees', 'homeless refugees' or 'Jewish emigrants from former UDSSR' (see, for example, the Federal Government's Commissioner for Foreigners' Issues 2000: 27).

SOME HEALTH AND SOCIAL CARE ISSUES

As indicated earlier, detailed integration policies for migrants have been missing in many fields, including the health and social care sector. Migrants are regarded worldwide as a high-risk group with regard to health problems (International Organization for Migration 2003: 87f). Their health often depends on the reasons and motives for migration, their citizenship status, and their socio-economic position in the host country. To put it simply: being abroad for several years as a manager, scientist or student will not necessarily create specific risks. If they occur, for instance due to psychological and mental stress, these migrants usually have the social skills and networks as well as the financial resources to seek sufficient support. In contrast, migrants who are illegally in the country or have an unsettled legal status, as for instance asylum seekers, may experience severe health risks, often without having the means to deal with them appropriately. Migrants such as the above-mentioned guest workers or the remigrant 'Aussiedler' are somewhere in between on this continuum. This has to be taken into account when reading the available data, as necessary distinctions with regard to legal and socio-economic status are often not made when 'migrant' issues are addressed. Also population surveys and health-related research did not produce extensive data on migrants in the past. Ten years ago Flatten (1994: 41) stated that 'available data on the health status of foreigners are insufficient with regard to morbidity and mortality as well as data concerning the volume and structure of utilization of medical and social services in the communities' (translated by M.H.). According to the annual report of the government this has not basically changed with recent developments (Federal Government's Commissioner for Foreigners' Issues 2000: 159; see also Razum 2000).

The following list of specific health risks for migrants must therefore be seen as tentative. Most data need further clarification especially in evaluating frequencies.

- Psychiatric and psychosomatic diseases are obviously important issues due to migration experiences and strenuous social adaptation. In the remigrant population, juveniles show a higher incidence of psychiatric illness than the comparable population in Germany and the comparable population in the countries of origin. This is also evident with regard to drug addiction of all kinds (Marschalck 2000, Weber 2000, Zenker 2000, Collatz 1998, Ramazan 1998).
- Higher rates of mother and infant mortality have been reported constantly during the last decades amongst migrants who have the legal status of foreigners. (The Federal Government's Commissioner for foreigners' issues 2000:160).
- Frequently, anxiety reactions in migrant children are mentioned (Marschalck 2000),
- There is evidence that a stronger somatization of psychosomatic disorders leads to higher rates of prolonged diagnostic procedures, such as radiological examinations and invasive investigations, establishing additional risks which seem to cause a higher number of iatrogenic diseases (Flatten 1994, Collatz 2000).
- First-generation migrants show work-related diseases earlier than in the average German population due to 'dirty work effects' (Collatz 2000, Flatten 1994).
- Rehabilitative measures are less frequently granted to migrants than to Germans (Flatten 1994).
- Traumatized persons often receive no adequate therapy due to a lack of resources and failures in diagnosing post-traumatic stress disorders (Zenker 2000).
- Illegal migrants have no access to healthcare services unless they risk deportation (Federal Government's Commissioner for Foreigners' Issues 2000: 163). Unlike other countries in Europe, there are no healthcare institutions available for this group on a legal basis, creating enormous health risks for this group.

In addition, it is necessary to consider the problems that may face the ageing population amongst migrants. Guest workers in particular form a growing part of the migrant population in need of services such as home care, day care, meals on wheels or nursing homes. However, as in the medical field, available support is often not made use of by migrants (Brucks & Wahl 2003). Sociocultural barriers and the resulting lack of adequate information are discussed as factors preventing migrants from accessing the health and social care services they need. Again, representative data are missing. The following factors have been identified as barriers in some regional, community-commissioned studies (Geiger 1998, Habermann 2004a):

- Verbal communication problems. Many migrants do not have such a good command of German that they feel able to verbalize needs and expectations when confronted with professionals.

- Communication problems based on a non-verbal sign system.
- Unsatisfactory experiences with the medical and social care system seem to get generalized with regard to nursing care. There seem to be low expectations that the services will accept and support cultural norms and habits.
- Ethnically constructed communities which do not share the information channels, such as television/newspapers, which forward health-related information to the broader German population.
- Lack of experience from the countries of origin with social care and nursing care services. For instance, the concept of nursing homes or home-based nursing care and other services is unknown to many migrants. Even though the corrosion of family network traditions is also perceivable in the migrant population, an approach to the concept of care for the elderly outside families has yet to be achieved.

Adding to sociocultural barriers, general deficits in the German health-care system might have a major impact on delivering adequate care for migrants. Social care, hospital care, consultations with the general practitioner and specific nursing care have to be integrated services, if they are to succeed in supporting the population. The lack of such integrated services creates communication problems, additional health risks and economical loss (Advisory Council for the Concerted Action in Health Care 2003). Migrants are especially likely to get lost in the maze of fractured care delivery services; no studies have so far been undertaken in this specific field.

A growing awareness of the above listed shortcomings has caused an ongoing debate within the health and social disciplines and the practice fields. How can these deficits be met? What does it mean to develop sensitivity to the needs of migrants in terms of organizational changes? How should the caring professions be educating their members to become culturally competent? Some of the answers will be outlined in the next two sections, first in the form of theoretical considerations and secondly as practice examples.

THEORETICAL DEBATES – CULTURE IN HEALTH AND SOCIAL CARE SETTINGS

The reception of the work of medical anthropologists from Anglo-Saxon countries, such as Arthur Kleinman or Cecil Helman, did not have a decisive impact on developing the theoretical discourse. To date there is no chair in a German university representing this discipline. The bits and pieces of research that had been done (Verwey 2003), followed by recommendations for the practice field, had been wrecked by the medically oriented routines in the hospitals and community-based care. This can only be understood when taking the powerful position of the medical profession into consideration. Priority-setting and the definition of quality had been almost wholly in the hands of medical practitioners with a strong therapeutic, cure orientation. Even though the move from complete medical domination has been slow, the nursing profession, with its focus on the client, has played an important role in bringing about this change.

The nursing profession in Germany is powerful in terms of numbers – there are nearly one million nurses and midwives in Germany. Nursing gained access to university education in the 1990s. Even though this university education is still limited to certain areas such as education of teachers, managers and experts (basic nursing education is still linked to hospital-based schools) and research is continually underfunded, theoretical debates focusing on the care for migrants have developed rapidly. The nursing discourse borrows from other disciplines and builds on developments in Anglo-Saxon countries. However, one may also discern a specific German dimension, related to the concept of nursing.

CULTURE AND CARING

In contrast to the medical symptom orientation and the dominance of cure in the medical profession, nursing concepts are based on human caring affirming the person as a bio-social-mental and spiritual being. Nursing concepts in Germany are derived from Henderson's (1969) principles of nursing, based on elementary needs and their conversion into activities of living, as described by Roper et al (1993), or variations of these (e.g. Krohwinkel 1992 or Orem 1996). A biographical orientation is recommended as the most appropriate method of addressing the bio-social-mental oneness of patients. The culture of patients, their individual history, beliefs and value orientations, constitute the centre of care. Taking this as the point of departure in professional nursing, cultural issues in German patients as well as in the care of migrants should be routinely addressed and responded to. However, qualitative research studies at Master's level, focusing on the care of migrants in different nursing settings (Giesen 1992, Hunstein et al 1997, Kutschke 1999, Schilder 1998), have produced alarming findings. Migrants who had been interviewed claimed to receive less favourable care. Communication problems dominated the care settings and the steps involved in the nursing process. Due to the lack of financial resources, quantitative approaches including a comparison with German patients of similar socio-economic status have so far not been carried out. However, the findings seem to indicate that in Germany, as in most other European countries, 'culture' is not yet a well-integrated part of nursing actions in the practice field. It might be taken into consideration in some special areas of nursing, but more often it is neglected. Nursing theories based on the above-mentioned patient-centred approaches are not guiding daily work. As in other disciplines, e.g. social and cultural anthropology (Berg & Fuchs 1993) or pedagogy (Auernheimer 2002), analysis of the encounter with foreigners exposes the gap between theory and practice within the nursing profession.

This has led to debate about the theory and practice of 'intercultural nursing' in Germany. Due to theoretical considerations and in line with the terminology used in other disciplines, this term is usually used to address issues that are known in the USA and UK as 'transcultural nursing'.

INTERCULTURAL NURSING – GERMAN DISCOURSES

As in many other countries the debate about cultural dimensions in nursing started with Leininger's transcultural nursing theory and her Sunrise model (Leininger 1998). Following criticisms of Leininger's transcultural model (Culley 1996) as one which focuses primarily on foreigners, her theoretical concepts were disregarded in Germany and instead an approach that stresses the integration of cultural competencies in all nursing actions, focusing on German as well as foreign patients, has been favoured (Habermann 2002, 2003a, 2004b, Kollak 2003, Uzarewicz 1999). In this conception intercultural settings are regarded as special cases, insofar as they might demand more concerted efforts to put a general professional standard of nursing into action: an individualized care. As a consequence, a 'specific theory' for intercultural settings is not favoured but rather a learning process that incorporates cultural issues in all care planning. In teaching and counselling, models of intercultural or transcultural care which avoid 'prescription knowledge' about ethnic orientations and provide a general view on cultural dimensions in nursing care are regarded as helpful, as outlined also by Papadopoulos in this volume.

Ten years of theorizing, teaching and some research in Germany brought another recognition: that enhancement of good nursing care within a plural society cannot be achieved only by teaching nurses who are responsible for direct care. These nurses need social support by an interculturally open organization and a similarly devoted management. Structural dimensions and new actors therefore came into focus. With this development, healthcare and nursing institutions encounter challenges, which are also met by social care organizations. The last section of this chapter will outline some best practice examples from the social and healthcare settings in general and from special nursing institutions such as nursing homes.

PRACTICE DEVELOPMENTS: EXPERIENCING PLURALITY AS RESOURCE

Some welfare organizations and some well-funded projects have managed to focus on intercultural organization development in the last few years in order to motivate personnel to develop individual, intercultural competencies and improve services (Arbeiterwohlfahrt 2004, Friebe & Zalucki 2003, Sozialreferat Landeshauptstadt München 2003, Haus Neuland 2004). The focus of these projects has been support for intercultural teams, intercultural management, and the development of a quality policy, integrating intercultural aspects. For each item an example will be given in the following sections.

INTERCULTURAL WORK TEAMS

Intercultural teams are helpful for delivering services for a plural population. Additional cultural competencies in form of language abilities and knowledge of cultural backgrounds are provided for the clients. The integration of migrants in the workforce can also signal intercultural openness of the organization to potential clients, though they may not be represented by a member of their own country of origin. The common experience of migration often seems sufficient to establish special confidence in the intercultural team (lacking research findings, this statement is based on narratives during seminars and training with cultural heterogeneous staff of health care and social care settings). Learning is also affected when working in teams with different educational backgrounds and this can provide another positive aspect. Creative solutions for practical problems can be found more easily in intercultural settings as research findings in international companies indicate (Apfelthaler 1998).

However, there are also potential problems with intercultural teams, as research in internationally operating companies has discovered (Apfelthaler 1998: 168).

- taking into account other people's viewpoints in formulating problems.
- the preferred procedures to be followed in conducting work.
- differentiating the tasks they believed could be best achieved through individual effort from those that could best be achieved through combined efforts.
- setting task priorities and time guidelines for their accomplishment.
- the acceptance of the work roles to which they were assigned in the group.
- the definition of quality work in the group.
- the way they thought resources should be allocated to group members.

When such problems dominate a group, special support by an interculturally informed leadership may be necessary. The objective for interventions in the social and healthcare sector is to profit from the plurality as outlined above and minimize deficits due to interculturally defined problems.

However, interventions can only take place when an awareness of the development potential of intercultural groups exists. In Germany, intercultural teams in the field of health and social care have long been regarded primarily as deficient by managers and clinical staff. Employers disregard the positive contribution that professionals from other countries can make to an intercultural healthcare team functioning within a pluralistic society. There remains a strong preference for employing German nurses (and other health and social care professionals) whilst the employment of health professionals from other ethnic groups is reluctantly taking place, primarily as a response to the shortage of German health professionals. The negative orientation in the organization creates problems for the intercultural team and its members by denying special support to the many workgroups.

Group development was the focus on the agenda of a practice development project which was scientifically evaluated (Haus Neuland 2004).

Supervised by a psychologist, members of intercultural group settings in social and healthcare institutions worked together over a period of about one and a half years to identify typical problems and discuss possible strategies to deal with them. Some of the strategies that were brought forward were the creation of space and time to develop and cherish a narrative culture in the team, rules about work language, which is supposed to be German, and the creation of zones of private language speaking which might be in other languages than German. The acceptance of the need to address cultural backgrounds in the team and the creation of certain basic rules about how to do this was also seen as important. Getting support from the management was seen as essential in moving towards a productive team culture by the team members.

LEADERSHIP AND MANAGEMENT IN THE INTERCULTURAL SETTING

Communication, motivation and control are central tasks of leadership. They are also of importance in the intercultural setting. Several projects and workgroups in Germany have tried to outline specific intercultural competencies for managers in social and healthcare settings in recent years (Friebe & Zalucki 2003). An in-depth analysis of literature in this field of management, however, led to the conclusion that there are only a few additional competencies required. These focus mainly on the development of attitudes such as the willingness to reflect plurality and one's own reactions, for openness and tolerance, as well as a genuine interest in personal traits and actions of staff members which are perceived as culturally tainted. Another interesting competence that was convincingly outlined was the readiness to accept that one might not understand; or, to put it another way, managers who believe in their quick and comprehensive understanding of what they consider to be cultural issues frequently produce major misunderstandings (Habermann 2003b, Hinz-Rommel 1994). Based on the results of exploring necessary competencies, workshops for nurses, social workers, teachers and managers, aimed at raising cultural awareness, have been conducted by experts and evaluated after their initial introduction in several areas in Germany (Friebe & Zalucki 2003).

Some of the considerations brought up in these workshops are outlined in the following examples.

Creating open communication, seeking participation possibilities for staff members, and identifying and communicating the mission and objectives of the organization are held to be central aspects of good leadership. But not all staff members might be willing to fulfil the expectations of a leadership that intends to be participatory. Due to cultural and biographically based experiences some members might feel overburdened. When participation has not been expected in previous work and learning experiences, leaders who ask for it might be readily identified as weak and indecisive leaders. Clear and more authoritarian instructions are then preferred. This was experienced by the managers with staff members from diverse cultural backgrounds. In Germany, this is especially true for remigrant nurses who were trained in eastern Europe or the former UDSSR and need time to adapt to participatory leadership styles. The lack of readiness and of specific competencies to act out a flexible leadership style was therefore seen as a major ongoing challenge for managers.

Forms of motivation are further items that were considered as important in the above-mentioned projects. What motivates people to deliver good work results? How can the work of staff members be approved? For instance, do they appreciate public praise or do they need a more private pat on the shoulder? The answer to that must be culturally informed to meet the different demands. There are books available which outline specific cultural regions with regard to advice for management actions. However, the recommendations often seem to be 'cook-book' in style. An orientation focusing on the individual was therefore held to be most promising for the healthcare and social settings in the projects mentioned above. Awareness and attention to raising the right questions, flexibility in leadership styles and a tolerant view towards the differing demands of staff members – whether they fit in easily with management concepts or are rather contradictory to it – are found to be sound recommendations for health and social care settings.

Staff development targeting cultural plurality was another issue that was frequently addressed by members of the workshops on intercultural management competencies. Leaving behind the view that cultural plurality in an organization is a problem, one outcome of the workshops was the recommendation of an active policy for healthcare and social organizations to recruit staff from diverse ethnic backgrounds, and the outlining of the steps needed to set this into action. In addition, the members elaborated management strategies that would actively involve cultural experiences of staff members by addressing them in their personal development plans.

QUALITY DEVELOPMENT: TOWARDS AN INTERCULTURAL ORGANIZATION

Leadership orientation and intercultural orientation are two important foundations for an intercultural organization. One recently finished project in the city of Munich showed how to proceed (Sozialreferat Landeshauptstadt München 2003). To support an intercultural orientation for all sub-organizations the social services department initiated a process to ameliorate structures and processes for a plural clientele. Besides considering leadership, team and staff development, they took time to elaborate a mission statement with staff members. Structural and process standards were checked and reworked to fit coherently into the mission and objectives of the organization. For instance, the question of whether counselling processes are interculturally adequate and how to improve them were part of the analysis. The department involved staff members extensively, thus creating a process that needed more financial support, but might be more sustainable.

SUMMARY

This chapter has looked at German policies regarding immigration. It has been highlighted that late and inadequate responses to the challenge of migration are also reflected in the lack of intercultural orientations in institutions of health and social care, as some of the health-related data of migrants show. Theoretical approaches and their impact in the practice field, drawing on the developments in the medical and nursing professions, have also been considered. Catching up with the decades of theoretical development in the Anglo-Saxon countries, nursing theory in Germany found the intercultural focus to be futile in exemplifying general problems in achieving individualized care. A consensus has developed that the theoretical basis of general nursing should include intercultural nursing and focus on plurality in society instead of working with specific theories focusing mainly on foreigners. Finally, the chapter dealt with some practice developments that are centred on organizational changes. The improvement of the dual relationship between professionals and clients requires the commitment both of political/ administrative institutions and the health and social care organizations; as discussed, some major projects are currently aiming to investigate this further.

REFLECTIVE QUESTIONS

1. A high incidence of psychiatric and psychosomatic diseases have been reported among young 'Aussiedler'. Consider the reasons for this and suggest three ways in which healthcare professionals could help to reduce this morbidity.
2. Elderly migrants do not use home care services as frequently as the German population does. Consider the reasons for this and suggest ways in which this could be influenced.
3. Migrants in Germany have significantly higher health risks as outlined in this chapter. How is it in your country? Choose three of the mentioned risks and analyse them with respect to data in your country.
4. Have you ever experienced an intercultural team? Were there 'cultural issues'? What did they mean for you?
5. Due to a shortage of nurses in Germany (as indeed is the case for many other countries), nurses are being recruited from many developing countries. Identify problems that relate to this practice and suggest ways to address them.

REFERENCES

Advisory Council for the Concerted Action in Health Care 2003 Health care finance user orientation and quality, Vol 1 and 2. Online. Available: http://www.svr-gesundheit.de/gutacht/gutalt/gutaltle.htm 15 Feb 2005

Apfelthaler G 1998 Interkulturelles Management als soziales Handeln, Servicefachverlag, Vienna

Arbeiterwohlfahrt Bundesverband 2004 Sozialbericht 2003/2004. AWO-Bundesverband eV, Bonn

Auernheimer G 2002 Interkulturelle Kompetenz und pädagogische Professionalität, Leske & Budrich, Opladen

Berg E, Fuchs M 1993 Kultur, soziale Praxis, Text. Suhrkamp, Frankfurt aM

Brucks U, Wahl W–B 2003 Über- Unter-, Fehlversorgung? Bedarfslücken und Strukturpobleme in der ambulanten Gesundheitsversorgung für Migrantinnen und Migranten. In: Borde T, David M (eds) Gut versorgt? Migrantinnen und Migranten im Gesundheits- und Sozialwesen. Mabuseverlag, Frankfurt, p 15–34

Collatz J 1998 Kernprobleme des Krankseins in der Migration – Versorgungsstruktur und ethnozentristische Fixiertheit im Gesundheitswesen. In: David M, Borde T,

Kentenich H (eds) Migration und Gesundheit. Mabuse, Frankfurt, p 33–58

Culley L 1996 A critique of multiculturalism in health care: the challenge of nurse education. Journal of Advanced Nursing 23:564–570

Europäisches Forum für Migrationsstudien. Online. Available: http://www.uni-bamberg.de/~ba6ef3/impressumd.htm 13 Aug 2004

Faulenbach B 2002 Die Vertreibung der Deutschen aus den Gebieten jenseits von Oder und Neiße. Zur wissenschaftlichen und öffentlichen Diskussion in Deutschland. Online. Available: http://www.bpb.de/publikationen/ 13 Aug 2004

Federal Government's Commissioner for Foreigners' Issues 2000 Facts and figures on the situation of foreigners in the Federal Republic of Germany. Berlin

Flatten W 1994 Gesundheitsprobleme der ausländischen Bevölkerung, ihre ambulante medizinische Versorgung und dringliche Forschungsmaßnahmen. In: Illhardt F J, Effelsberg W (eds) Medizin in multikultureller Herausforderung. Gustav Fischer, Mainz, p 41–58

Friebe J, Zalucki M 2003 Einleitung. In: Friebe J, Zalucki M (eds) Interkulturelle Bildung in der Pflege. Bertelsmann, Bielefeld, p 7–12

Geiger I 1998 Altern in der Fremde – zukunftsweisende Herausforderungen für Forschung und Versorgung. In: David M, Borde T (eds) Migration und Gesundheit. Mabuse, Frankfurt, p 167–184

Giesen D 1992 Die Pflege von Patienten mit unterschiedlichen kulturellen Hintergründen. Eine ethnographische Studie. Fachhochschule, Osnabrück

Habermann M 2002 Interkulturelle Pflege und Therapie. Qualitätssicherung auch für Migranten? Dr med Mabuse (27)136:22–26

Habermann M 2003a Pflege und Kultur. Eine medizinethnologische Exploration der Pflegewissenschaft und -praxis. In: Lux Thomas (ed) Kulturelle Dimensionen der Medizin. Reimerverlag, Berlin, p 192–210

Habermann M 2003b 'Interkulturelle Kompetenz' – Schlagwort oder handlungsleitende Zielvorstellung in der Altenpflege? Pflege und Gesellschaft 8(1):11–15

Habermann M 2004a Interkulturelle Aspekte in der Pflege. In: Arbeiterwohlfahrt Bundesverband Sozialbericht 2003–2004. Arbeiterwohlfahrtsbundesverband eV, Bonn, p 121–127

Habermann M 2004b Denken Sie sozialglobal. Interkulturelles Management in sozialen Einrichtungen. In: Handbuch Sozialmanagement. Raabe, Berlin, p 1–17

Haus Neuland 2004 Qualitätsentwicklung im multikulturellen Arbeitszusammenhang Altenpflege. Haus Neuland, Bielefeld

Henderson V 1969 The basic principles of nursing care. International Council of Nursing, Genf

Hinz-Rommel W 1994 Interkulturelle Kompetenz. Waxmann, Münster

Hunstein D, Dreut M, Eckert S et al 1997 Kopf draußen – Füße drin. Wie erleben Patienten aus anderen Kulturen das deutsche Gesundheitswesen? Teil I. Pflege 10(4):193–198

International Organization for Migration World Migration 2003 Managing migration. Challenges and responses for people on the move. IOM World Migration Report Series, Vol 2. Geneva

Kollak I 2003 Pflegepädagogik und Kultur: Anforderung und Wirklichkeit. In: Friebe J, Zalucki M (eds) Interkulturelle Bildung in der Pflege. Bertelsmann, Bielefeld, p 47–60

Krohwinkel M 1992 Rahmenbedingungen zur Einführung und Sicherung ganzheitlich-fördernder Prozesspflege. In: Krohwinkel M (ed) Der pflegerische Beitrag zur Gesundheit in Forschung und Praxis. Nomos, Baden Baden, p 48–58

Kutschke M 1999 Untersuchung von Pflegeerfahrungen bei Migranten vor dem Hintergrund eines dynamischen Kulturbegriffs. Unveröffentlichte Diplomarbeit an der Katholischen Fachhochschule Nordrhein-Westfalen

Leininger M 1998 Die Theorie der kulturspezifischen Fürsorge zur Weiterentwicklung von Wissen und Praxis der professionellen transkulturellen Pflege. In: Osterbrink J (ed) Erster internationaler Pflegetheorienkongress Nürnberg. Huber, Basel, p 73–90

Marschalck P 2000 Öffentliche Gesundheitspflege und die Einwanderung: 'Gastarbeiter', Aussiedler und Flüchtlinge in Deutschland. In: Gardemann J, Müller W, Remmers A (eds) Migration und Gesundheit: Perspektiven für Gesundheitssysteme und öffentliches Gesundheitswesen. Dokumentation der Tagung. Akademie für öffentliches Gesundheitswesen, Düsseldorf, p 31–42

Münz R Seifert W, Ulrich R 1998 Zuwanderung nach Deutschland. Suhrkamp, Frankfurt aM

Orem D 1996 Strukturkonzepte der Pflegepraxis. Huber, Basel

Projekt Ruhr Demographischer Wandel im Ruhrgebiet 2002 Ethnisches Mosaik des Ruhrgebietes. Typisierung der Stadtteile und Potenziale der Migranten. Zentrum für Türkeistudien, Essen

Ramazan S 1998 Spezifische gesundheitliche Lage und Belastungen der Migranten. In: Czycholl D (ed) Sucht und Migration. Verlag für Wissenschaft und Bildung, Berlin, p 31–38

Razum O 2000 Gesundheitsberichterstattung für Migranten in Deutschland. Abschlussbericht, Robert-Koch-Institut, Hamburg

Roper N, Logan W W, Tierney A J 1993 Die Elemente der Krankenpflege: ein Pflegemodell, das auf einem Lebensmodell beruht. 4th revised edn. Recom, Basel

Schilder M 1998 Türkische Patienten pflegen: Erfahrungen Pflegender mit Pflegebedürftigen und ihren Familien im ambulanten Bereich. Kohlhammer, Stuttgart

Sozialreferat Landeshauptstadt München 2003 Offen für Qualität. Interkulturell orientiertes Qualitätsmanagement in Einrichtungen der Migrationssozialarbeit. Sozialreferat, München

Ulrich R 1998 Grau oder bunt? Zuwanderungen und Deutschlands Bevölkerung im Jahre 2030. In: Borde T, David M, Kentenich H (eds) Migration und Gesundheit. Mabuseverlag, Frankfurt, p 17–32

Uzarewicz C 1999 The concept of culture and transculturality. In: Kim HS, Kollak I (eds) Basic concepts of nursing. Springer, New York, p 71–86

Verwey M 2003 Hat die Odysee Odysseus krank gemacht? Migration, Integration und Gesundheit. In: Lux T (ed) Kulturelle Domensionen der Medizin. Reimerverlag, Berlin, p 277–307

Weber K 2000 Ambulante nervenärztliche Versorgung von Migrantinnen und Migranten. In: Gardemann J, Müller W, Remmers A (eds) Migration und Gesundheit: Perspektiven für Gesundheitssysteme und öffentliches Gesundheitswesen. Dokumentation der Tagung. Akademie für öffentliches Gesundheitswesen, Düsseldorf, p 49–56

Zenker H-J 2000 Betrachtung der psychiatrischen/ psychotherapeutischen Versorgung in Bremen. In: Gardemann J, Müller W, Remmers A (eds) Migration und Gesundheit: Perspektiven für Gesundheitssysteme und öffentliches Gesundheitswesen. Dokumentation der Tagung. Akademie für öffentliches Gesundheitswesen, Düsseldorf, p 171–179

Chapter **14**

Cultural healthcare issues in Greece

Athena Kalokerinou–Anagnostopoulou

LEARNING OBJECTIVES

After reading this chapter you should be able to:
- understand the ethnohistory of Greece, the Greek political system and its membership of the European Union
- consider traditions, customs and practices which comprise Greek culture/s
- appreciate the changing demography of Greece, the differing ethnic groups which make up Greek society and the shift from net migration to immigration
- examine the health and social care system in Greece with particular reference to the care and support of minority ethnic communities
- explore the contribution of nursing to health care in multicultural Greece.

A BRIEF ETHNOHISTORY OF GREECE

HISTORY, GEOGRAPHY AND THE ORIGINS OF MEDICINE

Increasingly nursing and other health professionals recognize the international context within which health care is practised. Mass movement of populations throughout the world creates demographic, cultural, socio-economic effects in Europe. Nursing science is concerned with promoting health, preventing illness and providing care, treatment and rehabilitation to people who are ill. Nursing is a demanding profession which requires personal involvement and commitment. The fundamental values of life that spring from Classical Greece relate to responsibility, respect for human dignity and heroism. Values of sacrifice, faith and love are also found in many religious writings. They are all consistent with the values of nursing and are fundamental to the process of transcultural nursing, which is an essential component of nursing within an international community.

The origins of modern medicine and health care can be traced back to Ancient Greece. Donahue (1985) writes that Apollo, the Greek god of sun, was also the god of health and medicine. His son Asklepios, who had a human mother, was the chief healer of Greek mythology. Two of his sons were physicians in the Trojan War. His six daughters included 'Hygeia' the goddess of health, 'Panacea' the restorer of health, 'Meditrina' the preserver of health (supposedly the ancient forerunner of the public health nurse) and 'Iaso', who personified the recovery from illness. As Greek civilization progressed the healing arts did too, particularly during the birth of the 'age of reason' which culminated in the classical philosophy of Socrates, Plato, Aristotle and others. Thales (640–546 BC) was the first Greek scientist-philosopher. But it was Aristotle (384–322 BC) who had a profound influence on medicine and he is credited with laying the foundation of biology and comparative anatomy. Hippocrates (460–370 BC) is credited with the establishment of rational and scientific medicine. He is known as the 'Father of Medicine'. He taught that disease was not the work of spirits, demons or deities but the result of the breaking of natural laws. According to Hippocrates, hygiene, good diet, exercise and avoidance of sexual excesses should be our way of life. His emphasis on the role of environment in the spread of disease as presented in 'Airs, Waters and Places' provided a basic epidemiological text. The Hippocratic method rested on four principles: observe all, study the patient rather than the disease, evaluate honestly, and assist nature.

The Greek literature also contains many references to nurses, primarily in their role as children's nurses, wet nurses and midwives. Greek tragedies describe traditions around birth, marriage and death, the family structure, religious and cultural traditions, health and illness theories and practices and other areas of science, philosophy and politics. Much later in Greek history, during the Byzantine period, the social profile of nursing was raised and was transmitted to the Western world (Dolan 1963).

Just as history influences a people's culture, so does geography. O'Hagan (2001) wrote that the relationship between individuals and the land is the most continuous and enduring aspect of culture. Patterns of thoughts, feelings, spirituality and values evolve from this relationship and over time they become features of the individual's personality. Differing physical environments produce different diet choices, dress codes, customs, and so on.

Greece, also known as Hellas, is located in the south-eastern part of Europe. It is the eighth largest country and one of the least densely populated in the European Union (EU) with an area of 132 000 km^2 and a density of 78 people per km^2. The coastline of the mainland is around 4000 km, while 9841 islands (114 of them inhabited) add another 11 000 km of coastline (Hellenic Ministry of Internal Affairs 2003). Even though the country is mountainous it is blessed with the Mediterranean climate and it enjoys over 250 days of sunshine annually. It also has beautiful beaches; the sea (*thalassa*) has always influenced Greek people and remains central to their way of life in terms of employment, food production, customs, leisure and transportation. Even the name of their main inheritable medical condition, thalassaemia, is associated with the sea, literally being translated as sea in the blood (*aima*).

Greece in its modern history went through political turbulences, and its political system changed many times from kingdom to dictatorship to democracy. Greece became a constitutional democracy in 1974 with an elected president and a parliament. The population of Greece is in the region of just over 11 million people (2001 census). Life expectancy at birth is high at 75.8 years for males and 81.1 years for females, while 17% of the population is over 65 years of age.

There is a tendency to view Greece as a culturally homogeneous society and when asked, more than 95% of people identify themselves as ethnically Greek or Hellenes. Dascalopoulos (2004) argues that half of the population of Greece are second- or third-generation descendants of Greek people who were expelled, exchanged or otherwise ethnically segregated. They come from all parts of Anatolia, Turkey (following the Greek–Turkish War of 1921–1922 when a huge population exchange took place between Greece and Turkey, as Greeks left Turkey and Turks left Greece), Romania, Egypt, the Caucasus, Russia, Ukraine, as well as from eastern Thrace and the neighbouring Balkan states of Bulgaria, Yugoslavia and Albania. Dascalopoulos also highlights several Greek subcultures originating in the different groups of Greek islands, as well as Cyprus, communities of Turkish origin, and nomadic Roma, some of whom have different languages and dialects.

In contemporary Greece, Dascalopoulos (2004) estimates that up to 30% of new births registered in Athens have a parent either born abroad or of non-Greek origin and that about 25% of families in the urban centres of Greece have a multicultural composition.

Greece was an exporter of migrants, especially following the Second World War and the Civil War (1945–1949). Between 1950 and 1970 emigrants went mainly to North America, Australia, Canada, Germany and other western European countries (Kassimis & Kassimi 2004). Greek migration to the industrialized nations of northern Europe functioned as a reserve army of labour in industry and other low-pay employment sectors. Since 1974, after the collapse of a seven-year military regime, Greece has known a period of political stability, with a socialist government for most of that time. With a mixed economy and a fairly large public sector, Greece has recently entered a period of restructuring with a privatization plan mostly in the areas of telecommunications, energy, industry and tourism. Greece entered the European Economic Community in 1981 and having met the Maastricht criteria joined the economic and monetary union in 2000, converting its currency from the drachma to the euro with other EU countries in January 2002.

RELIGION AND ITS IMPACT ON CULTURE

The majority of Greeks belong to the Greek Orthodox Church. The following paragraphs draw on an article about Greek Christian Orthodoxy by Papadopoulos (2002).

Religion is a central plank to the Greek culture. However, unlike Islam which is seen as both a religion and a way of life, the Greek Christian Orthodoxy occasionally conflicts with the Greek culture, way of life and sometimes the official legislation. Those who identify themselves as Greek Orthodox do not always strictly adhere to the teachings of the Greek Orthodox Church. Home and family life is central to the Greek Orthodox lifestyle. Marriage is one of the seven sacraments of this religion, the others being baptism, confession, holy communion, holy ordination and the anointment of the sick. Marriage is regarded the only appropriate and morally fitting place for a sexual relationship. Premarital and extra-marital sex as well as homosexuality are considered immoral and are viewed as attacks on the institution of marriage. Despite the legal position in Greece which accords homosexuals equal rights (with a few exceptions such as marriage) the attitudes of many Greeks are closer to the Church than the State.

According to the Greek Orthodox religion, all persons are entitled to be treated with dignity and respect because they have been created in the image of God. This dignity affords them fundamental human rights whilst at the same time they are also expected to respect the rights and dignity of others.

The Greek Orthodox Church condemns the control of the conception of a child by any means. In practice, most Greek people plan their families very carefully by using the whole range of birth control methods despite the position of the Church.

Greek Orthodox babies are baptised soon after birth. Unless a person is baptised they cannot marry in the Greek Orthodox Church. Many parents often name their children after their own parents' names out of respect. Most Greek Orthodox names come from the Bible or are names of saints. However, this is not a requirement, and many parents choose names from Greek mythology or from lists of more modern, often universal names.

Abortion is absolutely condemned as an act of murder except in certain very special circumstances such as when the life of the mother is in grave danger, or the pregnancy of a young girl as a result of rape. In practice, a number of women, particularly those who are unmarried, have legal abortions, as the negative consequences of having a baby out of wedlock are felt to be more severe than the consequences of an abortion.

The Greek Orthodox Church is strongly pro-life. It sees death as evil and the opposite to life-giving God, and Christ's victory over death through his resurrection. It therefore strongly opposes euthanasia, which is seen as suicide on the part of the individual and murder on the part of others.

Despite the views of the Church about euthanasia, the Church does not support an excessive or extraordinary use of technology to prolong life. The Greek Orthodox religion teaches that individuals have a responsibility to take care of their lives given to them by God but at the same time it does accept the inevitability of death.

Greek Orthodox people have no dietary restrictions except during the fasting periods when they abstain from animal and dairy products. Fasting is also seen as a spiritual catharsis. The Church requires healthy adults to fast at least three days before taking communion, on Wednesdays and Fridays, and during the holy periods of Easter (50 days before Easter), the Assumption of the Virgin Mary (1 to 14 August), and Christmas (40 days before Christmas). However, in practice very few – usually older people – observe the fasting rules. Most commonly, people who wish to take holy communion fast for three days during ordinary periods and for one week before Easter and Christmas.

The selected glimpse of Greek culture through its history, geography and religion illustrates the evolving nature of culture. Today, this evolution is very evident within the Greek family structure and values. Customs around marriage, choice of partner, family size, residence, familial obligations and norms around inheritance are continuously changing. Each family adopts aspects of culture that suits it, adopting practices and customs, maintaining them for the next generations, modifying or rejecting them according to their circumstances and needs. The increased multiculturalism is also impacting on the Greek culture and way of life.

THE CHARACTERISTICS OF IMMIGRANTS

Greece has undergone major changes in the last decade, shifting from being a major provider of migrant labour to one with increasing numbers of immigrants arriving at its borders. The age-related composition of immigrants shows that the overwhelming majority are of working age and while not always made welcome, they are needed to fill gaps in the labour market. There is a need particularly for unskilled labour due to a combination of demographic factors, increased prosperity and better levels of education. Over the years remittances from former emigrants and more recently membership of the EU have contributed to an improved Greek economy. Higher levels of education and material advantage have created the need for an unskilled workforce as locals are unwilling to do many of the jobs they did previously (Danopoulos 2004).

Table 14.1   Profile of ethnic groups living in Greece (Census 2000–2001: total population 11 006 377)

Ethnic group	No.
Albanians	438 036
Bulgarians	35 104
Romanians	21 994
Georgians	22 875
Americans (USA)	18 140
Cypriots	17 426
Others	208 616
Total immigrants	762 191

Source: http:/www.statistics.gr.

Table 14.2   Social profile of immigrants living in Greece (Census 2000–2001: total population 11 006 377)

	No.
Legal immigrants	413 214
Repatriates	51 694
Joining the family	99 168
Foreign students	20 787
Seeking asylum	9 880
Refugees	2 368
Others	165 080
Total immigrant	762 191

Source: http:/www.statistics.gr.

Today, immigrants living and working permanently or temporarily in Greece can be divided into different categories. Table 14.1 details the ethnic distribution of immigrants and Table 14.2 their social profile, according to the 2001 census. The first category are legal immigrants, who have permits to work and stay. The second category of immigrants includes political refugees and those seeking asylum, who are the smallest number. As in other countries in Europe, they work in the informal economy, with poor and unsafe working conditions often exploited by employers (Patiraki 2002). The third category are students. There are also a large number of illegal immigrants, mainly from the Balkans, and their number is estimated at around 300 000.

In Greece, political refugees claim asylum through a series of official processes and provided their claims are accepted they are allowed permission to stay. In special humanitarian circumstances a refugee can remain in the country even if political asylum has not been granted. However, the legal process of claiming asylum in Greece is very time-consuming. The Greek state has a Centre of Reception of Political Refugees in Lavrion Attica and in other areas of the country (Patiraki et al 2002).

Refugees in Greece have the right to use the services of healthcare centres and hospitals, provided they have evidence of their identity and their authorized asylum or permit to stay for humanitarian reasons. Illegal immigrants who have not been granted asylum or leave to stay are either reluctant to or believe they are not allowed to use the services provided by the National Health Service (NHS). They are entitled, however, to use the NHS in an emergency. If they are not registered for certain social services they can seek healthcare services in the polyclinics of Doctors of the World and Doctors Without Frontiers and other non-governmental organizations, where volunteer doctors and nurses provide health care. However excellent these facilities are, some cases will inevitably require acute hospital care.

THE INFLUENCE OF IMMIGRATION ON THE DEMOGRAPHY OF GREECE

According to the 2001 census, of the declared total population of around 11 006 377, 10 244 186 are Greeks and 762 191 are non-Greeks, representing 6% of the population. However, it is probable that this percentage actually underestimates the real size of the non-national population in Greece considering that the illegal immigrants are not declared. It is argued that the real percentage of non-nationals in Greece is around 10% of the overall population (OECD 2002). However, this overall figure does not represent the concentration patterns of immigrants in cities, major industrial towns and the poorest parts of those areas. Over half (51%) of non-nationals live in the cities of Athens and Thessalonika.

The demographic profile of Greece has changed with the entry of immigrants, reversing some of the trends shared with other parts of Europe. The increasing numbers of older people and the reduction in birth rate has created a problem for the future. The total fertility rate is 1.3 compared with 1.5 in other parts of Europe. This is considerably lower than the 2.1 needed to replace the productive population in order to address some of the concerns about the cost of an ageing population (http:/www.statistics.gr). Population trends have begun to change due to the entry of immigrants and the repatriation of others such as Pontic Greeks (Kaitelidou et al 2004). Data from the National Observatory of Employment (1998) show that 51% of immigrants are married and two out of three have up to five children. This demographic shift is most evident in urban areas where there is a larger concentration of non-nationals.

CONTEMPORARY GREECE: HEALTH AND SOCIAL CARE SYSTEM AND POLICY

The Greek NHS was established in 1983 and aimed to provide universal coverage and equity in the distribution of health services. The guiding principle was the decommercialization of health, implying greater equity, state responsibility for financing and delivery of services, and a reduction of the private sector's role. In some respects the 1983 health reforms lagged behind other European countries, as many of the principles and policy objectives prevailing in Europe were ignored until then (Berman 1995). It is argued that many of the proposed reforms have not materialized and there is still a fragmentation of primary healthcare services in urban areas and no organized referral system (Tountas et al 2002). Contrary to expectations, the private healthcare sector is growing and there is increasing private health expenditure resulting in considerable inequality in access to health care. However, despite evidence of some socio-economic and geographic inequalities, health indicators for the Greek population are generally positive.

A national network of health centres serves as the focus of public health activities and includes public health campaigns, health education activities and health screening. A mixture of taxation and compulsory health insurance contributions by employers and employees finances the public health system. Tax revenues are derived by both direct (mainly income taxation) and indirect taxes on goods and services. The increase in total health expenditure during the 1980s and early 1990s from 6.6% to about 8.5% of GDP (gross domestic product) was a move in the opposite direction compared with other EU countries (OECD 1990) where cost-containment policies were put into effect (Abel-Smith & Mossialos 1994). The increase was in part due to efforts to establish a national health system and to compensate for under-financing of the public sector in previous decades, but it was also due to the growth in private health expenditure (Liaropoulos 1995).

Policing the right to health services by refugees and asylum seekers is a contentious issue and many nurses and other practitioners are uncomfortable in asking patients about their legal status. Unfortunately, there are fears that the Greek NHS is being exploited by the so-called 'smugglers of health' who 'import' people who are not entitled to use the NHS services for free. Thus, routine incidents and chronic diseases are labelled urgent and are illegally hospitalized, overloading the Greek NHS. It is argued by the Ministry of Health that 80% of the beds of certain NHS obstetric clinics are occupied by non-EU women hospitalized as urgent incidents having arrived in Greece sometimes only 24 hours prior to requiring health care.

To tackle this major problem the Ministry of Health has published guidelines around medical, pharmaceutical and hospital care for people from outside the countries of the EU. This states that the approval of the Greek Minister of Health is required before medical-pharmaceutical or hospital care is given to people from outside the EU. There are some exceptions to this regulation. Tourists will receive care providing they are able to demonstrate appropriate travel documents.

THE COST OF IMMIGRANT HEALTH CARE

Data on the origin of immigrants admitted to hospital show that Albanians represent 60% of those hospitalized, followed by Bulgarians (7.57%)

Table 14.3   The mental health problems of immigrants

Disturbances of dispersal	14%
Schizophrenia	7%
Psychosomatic problems	45%
Stress	29%
Alcoholism	2%
Family problems	3%

Source: Polyclinics of Doctors Without Frontiers (Mpoufidis 2000).

Russians (6.11%) and others representing smaller percentages (Gaitanidou 2001a).

According to the Centre for Control of Communicable Diseases, 10–15% of immigrants – mainly from African countries – are HIV positive (Chimonas et al 1985).

Refugees often experience considerable difficulties prior to arriving in Greece. Many have been suffering from a variety of problems such as open wounds, infections and symptoms of malnutrition. Research conducted by the Social Service of Refugees and the Greek Council for the Refugees showed that 13% present with certain serious or chronic health problems (Chimonas et al 1985). Refugees have also been found to suffer from health problems related to the liver, kidneys, stomach, as well as deafness, blindness, hepatitis, diabetes and cardiovascular problems (Chimonas et al 1985). There is evidence in other parts of the world that migrants experience an excess of mental health problems and Greece is no exception. Data from a study of polyclinics run by Doctors Without Frontiers show a high level of mental distress for which help is sought (Mpoufidis 2000). Table 14.3 shows the mental health problems suffered by immigrants.

THE HEALTH OF IMMIGRANT CHILDREN

A recent study by Siafas et al (2000) showed that 25% of the children visiting the outpatients department of Agia Sofia children's hospital are children of immigrants. Given the size of the Albanian immigrant population it is not surprising that 20% of the children are of Albanian origin while only 5% are of other nationalities. This mirrors the profile of the catchment area for the Agia Sofia children's hospital in Athens (Bakoula 2002), where 25% of 850 children attending 40 kindergarten schools were of non-Greek origin, with 16% being of Albanian origin. The composition of non-Greek populations differs from one geographical area to another (Davros et al 2002). For example, data from the outpatients departments of regional hospitals in Peloponnese showed that between 1998 and 1999, 17% of the children examined were of Roma origin and 7% were of other non-Greek background.

Spiridis et al (2000) demonstrated an increase in the level of tuberculosis among children and this reflected demographic changes associated with immigration to Greece. The percentage of non-Greek foreign children treated for tuberculosis was 7% up until the year 1995. Following a recent wave of immigration largely from areas without access to immunization, the percentage of non-Greek children treated for tuberculosis reached 29%. Since the publication of this evidence the children's hospitals of Athens have developed a special programme consisting of a check-up and follow-up for tuberculosis of non-Greek children and Roma children. The programme takes account of the special needs of children and parents and pays particular attention to communication. Additional time is allowed to compensate for language difficulties. Appointments are prioritized and open visiting is encouraged. Medicines are free and special efforts are made to ensure the parents understand and comply with medical advice, using interpreters and advocates as necessary. Instructions are given in written form in the language appropriate for the family, such as Albanian, Russian, Arabic, Filipino, and so on. In view of the relationship between poverty, poor housing and tuberculosis, every help and support is given to facilitate the issuing of a 'green card', which will allow for a temporary stay.

In a study by Arvanitidou et al (1989) it was reported that the children of immigrants presented more often and with more serious psychological problems in comparison to other children. The study demonstrated psychological problems related to the configuration of the children's personalities, their sociability, school performance, food and sleep behaviours, memory/recall, tics, difficulties in making social relationships, and expression of feelings of inferiority. These disturbances were found in 24% of the children of immigrants, while in the children of Greek working mothers these were found in 15.5%, and in the children of Greek non-working mothers in 13.7%.

THE COST BENEFITS OF IMMIGRATION

Greece has changed from a country of emigration to being a recipient of immigration. Many of the problems in the health sector appear to coincide with the increasing numbers of immigrants entering Greece. However, this issue has not been adequately explored and while the health of immigrants clearly incurs a cost, this has to be balanced against the potential benefit to the economy as a whole. It is commonly understood that the use of the health system by non-Greek nationals who are not insured is an economic burden. The hospital costs of non-insured immigrants have risen and are expected to continue to rise. The costs of dealing with public health problems and individuals with HIV are high. Because of this a specialized department in the Ministry of Health and Social Welfare was recently formed, to ensure health insurance for immigrants. This department functions as a centre for the follow-up and coordination of health care of immigrants in the NHS hospitals. The centre will contribute to the creation of a database where all the hospitalized immigrant data will be recorded. It will facilitate the retrieval of information about hospital inpatients and outpatients and enable collaborative working between organizations concerned with the different facets of immigrants' health.

However, while there are real costs associated with the health needs of immigrants, refugees and asylum seekers, there is also a need to acknowledge their contribution to the economy as a whole. Despite a general misconception that immigrants are a source of evils, from criminality to disease, there is evidence that this is not the case (Tsaoussis 1997). On the contrary, it is recognized that migrant communities positively influence business and public services, scholarship, politics and social justice. They also impact on and enrich sport, music and fashion, media, faith and conventional health practice. Demographic change and the expansion of the Greek economy have created the need for immigration as is the case in all EU countries. Migrants of differing legal status not only fill a range of unskilled jobs in the labour market but they are also willing to work for lower wages. They will work in any job even in the dirty and dangerous sectors of the workforce and are invariably more flexible in reacting to market needs. The increasing participation of Greek women in paid employment outside the home has created a market for domestic work, childcare and other services. Notwithstanding the costs of health and social care, the host community gains from the productive work of non-nationals without being burdened with the cost of their upbringing and education (Emke-Poulopoulou 1990).

The process of the European enlargement means there could be now freedom of movement between 25 different European countries. This expansion has created questions and potential problems about the right to access the healthcare services in another country. A policy for the social insurance systems of all EU countries is required. This could be accomplished by the creation of a pan-European insurance fund for immigrant workers, which would operate in parallel to the national insurance systems (Sakellaropoulos 2001). In order to reduce the bureaucratic burden associated with accessing health care in another country, a proposal aimed at introducing the 'European Health Insurance Card' (Commission of the European Communities 2003) was made in 2003. This aims to rationalize the paperwork used for medical and pharmaceutical care in different member states and to simplify processes whilst maintaining all the existing rights and obligations of European citizens (Hermans & Berman 1998).

NURSING IN MULTICULTURAL GREECE

The above evidence makes it imperative that nurses in Greece make an effort to take account of the child and family's cultural background and religious beliefs. This can be difficult for nurses who are predominantly Greek and of Greek Orthodox Christian background. It is easy to blame parents who are not familiar with the Greek healthcare system or who do not understand the importance of complying with medication and health advice. However, if nurses had greater understanding of the clients' culture, religion and their health beliefs and behaviour they would be in a better position to advise and support parents.

Nurses must be able to care in culturally competent ways, and in a clinical practice discipline such as nursing there are limitless opportunities for exploring viable options to enrich the practice. Immigrants to Greece contribute to economic growth directly and indirectly and have rights to quality, culturally competent health care. Being new to Greek society they face considerable problems in the healthcare system and it is a nurse's responsibility to be informed so that people are not excluded. There is a growing body of transcultural nursing knowledge from the USA, UK, and elsewhere to draw upon and there are also some early developments in Greece. A study in the University of Athens Faculty of Nursing demonstrated that only 23.5% of students had had some information on transcultural health care (Kalokerinou-Anagnostopoulou et al 2001); 41.2% reported having some social contact with immigrants and 26.5% had had contact with refugees. However, both the undergraduate (Guide of ND/UOA 2003) and postgraduate (Ministerial Decision 2002) curricula of the Faculty of Nursing, University of Athens have included courses in transcultural nursing since 2002/3. Although theoretical knowledge learned from a textbook or in the classroom is important, nurses can learn a lot from each other and from their clients and families. Patients and families are the richest possible source of information about culture but nurses must recognize their own ethnocentricity and know which questions to ask. Nurses must value the skills, experiences and practices that colleagues from other cultures bring and reflect on how this could be incorporated to improve the care of clients from other cultures.

REFLECTIVE QUESTIONS

1. Policing the right to health services by refugees and asylum seekers is a contentious issue in many countries. Reflect on how this issue is dealt with in your country and how you may have been involved in this.
2. 'Patients and families are the richest possible source of information about culture but nurses must recognize their own ethnocentricity and know which questions to ask'. Do you agree with this statement and if so how will you know which questions to ask?

REFERENCES

Abel-Smith B, Mossialos E 1994 Cost containment and health care reform: a study of the European Union. Health Policy 28:89–132

Arvanitidou V et al 1989 Problems of immigrant children who live in their home. Pediatric of North Greece 1(2):106–116

Bakoula C et al 2002 Risk factors of premature birth in Greece. A population study. 40th Hellenic Pediatric Congress, Thessaloniki 21–23 June 2002, p 45 (EA082 Abs)

Berman P 1995 Health sector reform: making health development sustainable. Health Policy 32:13–285

Chimonas C, Alexakis A, Charalambidis S 1985 The frequency of infections of foreign students in Aristoteles Thessaloniki University from intestinal vermin. Greek Medicine 48(5):335–346

Commission of the European Communities 2003 Communication from the Commission concerning the introduction of a European health insurance card. Brussels 17 02 2003 COM(2003), 73 final

Danopoulos A 2004 Albanian migration into Greece: the political, sociological and political implications. Online. Available: http://www.newbalkabpolitics.org.mk/napis.asp?id=9&lang-English 18 Dec 2004

Dascalopoulos S 2004 Linguistic and ethnic diversity. Online. Available: http://www.Aegean.gr/culturaltec/dasc/Dasc_pap2_lediv.htm 23 Dec 2004

Davros I et al 2002 Otitis: Frequent reason for attending the Children's Outpatients Department. 40th Hellenic Pediatric Congress, Thessaloniki 21–23 June 2002, p 238 (AA335 Abs)

Dolan J A Goodnow's History of Nursing. Philadelphia: W. B. Saunders Company, 1963

Donahue M P 1985 Nursing. The finest art. An illustrated history. Mosby, St Louis

Emke-Poulopoulou H 1990 Immigrants and refugees in Greece 1970–90. Selection of subjects in social care. Panteion University 85/86, Athens

Gaitanidou E 2001a The immigrants and their care in our country. Online. Available: www.istoselides.gr

Guide of ND/UOA 2003 National and Kapodistrian University of Athens Faculty of Nursing 2004 Students guide. EKPA, Athens Online. Available: www.ek-ekpa@elke.uoa.gr 16 Jan 2005

Hermans H, Berman C 1998 Access to health care and health services in the European Union: Regulation 1408/71 and the E111 process. In: Leidl R (ed) Health care and its financing in the single European market. IOS Press, Amsterdam, p 324–343

Kaitelidou D, Siskou O, Liaropoulos L 2004 The use of health care services of immigrants and refugees in Greece. In: Kalokerinou A (ed) Transcultural nursing. University lectures, Athens, 47–61

Kalokerinou-Anagnostopoulou A et al 2004 The social profile of refugees and immigrants in Greece. 12th Biennial Conference of WENR, Lisbon

Kassimis C, Kassimi C 2004 Greece: A history of migration. Online. Available: http://www.migrationinformation.org

Leininger M M 1978 Transcultural nursing: Concepts, theories and practice. Wiley, New York

Leininger M M 2001 Culture care diversity and universality: A theory of nursing. National League for Nursing, New York

Liaropoulos L 1995 Health services financing in Greece: a role for private health insurance. Health Policy 34:53–62

Liaropoulos L, Kaitelidou D 1998 Changing the public-private mix: an assessment of the health reforms in Greece. Health Care Analysis 6:277–285

Liaropoulos L, Kaitelidou D 2000 Assessment in health care. International Journal of Technology 16(2):433

Ministerial Decision 2002 B7/93913 1136/23/12/2002 Governmental Gazette

Mpoufidis S 2000 Cancelled dreams, psychopathetic conditions and immigrants. Online. Available: www.msf.gr/library/health3.html 19 Sep 2000

OECD 1990 Health care systems in transition: The search for efficiency. OECD, Paris

OECD 2002 Trends in international migration. Annual report, OECD, Paris

O'Hagan K 2001 Cultural competence in the caring professions. Jessica Kingsley, London

Papadopoulos I 2002 Nursing with dignity. Part 4: Christianity II. Nursing Times 98(12):36–37

Patiraki E, Kalokerinou A, Sourtzi P 2002 The positive contribution to health of host community by immigrants and refugees. In: Papadopoulos I Changing context of European nursing: Promoting cultural competence. Reader for Intensive European programme. Middlesex University, London, p 39–43

Sakellaropoulos T 2001 Hyperethnic social politic in the season of globalization. Critique, Athens, p 118–120

Siafas K et al 2000 Why children with non-severe illnesses attend Outpatients Departments at working hours. 38th Hellenic Pediatric Congress, Kos, 16–18 June 2000, p 148 (286 Abs)

Spiridis P, Tsolia M, Gelesme A et al 2000 Demographic and epidemiologic study about tuberculosis alterations in children (1988–1999). 38th Hellenic Pediatric Congress, Kos, 16–18 June 2000, p 285 (560 Abs)

Tountas Y, Karnaki P, Pavi E 2002 Reforming the reform: the Greek national health system in transition. Health Policy vol 62 p 15–29

Tsaoussis D 1997 Social demography. Gutenberg, Athens

Chapter 15

Transcultural healthcare issues in Spain

Silvia Garcia Barrios

LEARNING OBJECTIVES

After reading this chapter you should be able to:
- understand how national policies on immigration, the economy and health care in contemporary Spain impact on the health of its non-European Union immigrant population and on other minority ethnic groups, such as Gypsies
- understand the mechanisms through which immigration status in Spain can determine health and access to health care
- gain an insight into how countries who do not have a long history of immigration respond to increased pressures to settle immigrants from non-EU countries.

INTRODUCTION

In this chapter I take a sociocultural perspective in aiming to describe the health needs of the new immigrants to Spain and of the Gypsy population who are a long-standing minority ethnic group. I also explore the impact of Spanish immigration law and health policy on the health of these groups. I begin this account with a brief ethnohistory of Spain.

BRIEF ETHNOHISTORY OF SPAIN

Spain is situated on the Iberian Peninsula in the far south-western corner of Europe. It is bordered by the Bay of Biscay to the north, the Mediterranean and Balearic seas to the east, and the North Atlantic Ocean to the south-west and north-west, and Portugal to the west. It is also bordered by the Pyrenees Mountains and the south-west of France to the north-east. The terrain is very varied with mountain ranges, fertile valleys and vast arid plains. The weather is temperate, with hot summers and cold winters inland but more moderate and cloudy weather in coastal regions. Spain is divided into 17 autonomous communities including the Balearic Islands, the Canary Islands, and three small Spanish provinces off the coast of Morocco. The capital city is Madrid (CIA 2004).

Spain has a history chequered with invasion, colonisation and domination by a number of nations. Significantly Spain has also been a coloniser. By 1200 BC Celtic tribes from the north entered the peninsula and mixing with Iberians created the Celt-Iberians. By 1100 BC Phoenicians arrived in the peninsula and founded colonies, the most important of which was Gadir (today's Cadiz). Greeks also founded colonies in southern Spain and along the Mediterranean coast early in the first millennium BC but were expelled between the sixth and third centuries BC by the Carthaginians (http://www.red2000.com/spain/primer/hist.html).

The Romans conquered the whole peninsula from 217 BC to 19 BC. The Roman Empire started to fall in 409 AD, during the invasion by Gothic (Germanic) tribes who established their kingdom in 419 AD. They dominated Spain until 711, when Muslim armies crossed the Strait of Gibraltar and defeated Roderic, the last Visigoth (German) king. The Moors (African Muslims with a mixed Berber and Arab descent) conquered major parts of the country until they were defeated for the first time by the Visigoth king Pelayo at Covadonga in northern Spain in 722. Although small Christian kingdoms in the north formed a nucleus of resistance, the Arabian culture thrived in the rest of the country and Muslim Spain gained independence from the Arabian Empire. However, in the eleventh century conflict between various Arabian noble families became increasingly common. It was then that the Christian kingdoms in the north started the re-conquest of Spain, which was facilitated by the marriage of the Catholic monarchs Isabella of Castilia and Ferdinand of Aragon in 1469, whose combined forces were able to drive the Moors from their remaining stronghold in Granada. Isabella and Ferdinand succeeded in uniting the whole country under their crown, and their effort to 're-christianize' Spain resulted in the Spanish Inquisition, when thousands of Jews and Moors who did not want to convert to Christianity were expelled or killed (http://www.floatingfree.co.uk/History_en.html).

After the discovery of America by Christopher Columbus in 1492, tons of gold and silver were brought in from the new continent, and Spain became one of the most powerful nations of this epoch called the Golden Age. Areas in the Americas under Spanish control included most of South and Central America, Mexico, parts of the Caribbean and much of the United States. In Africa, Spain's empire included the Spanish Guinea, the Spanish Sahara, Ifni and Spanish Morocco. In 1898, the United States won the Spanish–American War and occupied Cuba and Puerto Rico, finally ending the Spanish occupation in the Americas.

The twentieth century saw many changes in Spain. An economic crisis in the early 1920s led the country to the brink of civil war. Increasing conflicts between the Republican government and the Nationalist opposition led to the Spanish Civil War (1936–1939). The Nationalists, led by General Franco, received extensive support from Nazi Germany and fascist Italy and succeeded against the Republicans. Although Franco kept Spain neutral during the Second World War, his military dictatorship led to political and economical isolation. During the 1950s and 1960s every effort was taken to improve international relations, and the country's economy recovered. In 1969 Franco proclaimed Juan Carlos de Borbón, the grandson of Alphonse XIII, his successor with the title of king. Franco died in 1975, and a constitutional monarchy was established. Spain entered the European Community in 1986. In 1992 Barcelona hosted the Olympic Games, and Madrid was declared European Cultural Capital.

CONTEMPORARY SPAIN – KEY DEMOGRAPHICS

Spain has one of the largest populations in Europe with just over forty million people living there in 2004 (40 280 780). In 2004 it had 10.11 births per 1000 population, a birth rate of 1.27 children per woman (amongst the lowest in the European Union), and 9.55 deaths per 1000 population. The estimated net immigration rate in 2004 was 0.99 migrant per 1000 of the population. Demographic trends indicate an ageing population. Unemployment for the whole population is high at 11.3% (CIA 2004).

The Basques are a distinct cultural group numbering around 2 million. They occupy a region straddling France and Spain. Basques are seeking political independence from Spain.

There are several Spanish languages: Castilian Spanish 74%, Catalan 17%, Galician 7% and Basque 2%. Castilian is the official language nationwide; the other languages are official regionally. Most (94%) of the Spanish people are Roman Catholic.

THE SPANISH HEALTHCARE SYSTEM AND HEALTH POLICY

The Spanish National Health Service is publicly financed through taxes raised by central government and provision is mostly publicly owned and managed; approximately 15–20% of public hospital provision has been contracted out to private non-profit providers. The Spanish healthcare system has undergone major changes since the devolution of power to regional governments in the early 1980s and early 1990s. However, for 10 out of 17 regions some powers are retained by central government through the INSALUD (the national health institute). Autonomous regions hold health planning powers as well as the capacity to organize their own health services. Coordination between regions is hampered by this divided system.

Insurance companies have a minor but increasing role and private voluntary schemes cover one-tenth of the population. There are also three publicly funded mutual funds exclusively for civil servants, who are free to choose between public or private provision. There are also other providers including the military. Public health and health services are coordinated by the Ministry of Health. The Ministry is also responsible for health policy and any basic enabling legislation, for coordination of health and social services with the Ministry of Labour and Social Affairs, and for the INSALUD.

People who are economically disadvantaged are covered by a special means-tested non-contributory scheme. Healthcare rights have recently been extended to the adult immigrant population.

The healthcare system is still centred on hospitals rather than primary health care. The functions of primary care in Spain are principally health promotion, disease prevention, curative care and rehabilitation follow-up. Primary health care is completely publicly owned and staffed by salaried personnel. The general practitioner is the patient's first point of contact, acting as 'gate keeper' to other health services (European Observatory on Health Care Systems. Spain 2002).

MIGRANTS' ACCESS TO HEALTH SERVICES

Generally, immigrants do not have difficulties accessing the Spanish health centres and services (Informe España 2003). However, despite all the health facilities offered to immigrants in Spain, an unspecified number of them do not use them; these are generally those without identity papers ('illegal immigrants').

The collaboration of non-health professionals who can promote social integration and provide translation services is imperative; without such assistance, patients who are not Spanish speaking may receive suboptimal levels of care and treatment and will have difficulties in accessing the services. However, Comelles et al (2000) report that to date little importance has been placed on the need of health services to provide interpretation services.

LAW AND POLICY RELATING TO HEALTH CARE FOR IMMIGRANTS IN SPAIN

The Spanish Constitution (article no. 43) guarantees the right to health of all Spanish people; in contemporary Spain health is a universal right by law (WHO 2000). In 2000, a law on foreigners' rights in Spain (Ley Orgánica 8/2000) came into effect. This law facilitated social integration and the recognition of the right to health care for those immigrants in Spain who are on the municipal register, or who are aged under 18 years. These foreign nationals receive a health card giving them the right to access health care on condition that they do not have sufficient economic resources.

The same law gives pregnant foreigners the right to antenatal, birth and postnatal care. Health care of those having a health card is provided on the same terms as for Spanish nationals (Ministerio de Trabajo y Asuntos Sociales 2004). However, there are many delays in obtaining a health card. This issue was highlighted in 2002 by the legal coordinator of Doctors without Frontiers in 2002 (Médicos Sin Fronteras), who declared that one in five immigrants registered in Madrid had not received their health cards (Confederación Estatal de Sindicatos Médicos 2004).

SPANISH CITIZENSHIP AND IMMIGRATION LAW

Eligibility for Spanish citizenship depends upon parentage, current nationality and duration of residence in Spain. People automatically acquire citizenship if they have a Spanish parent, if they were born in Spain, or if a parent was born in Spain, whatever their nationality. People who have held a resident permit for 10 years or more can apply for Spanish citizenship, except those who have been granted political refugee or asylum status, who can apply after 5 years. Nationals of Latin America, Portugal, the Philippines, and Jews of Spanish origin may apply after just 2 years. In all cases the period of residence in Spain must have been immediately prior to the application. Foreign children (aged under 18) who are adopted by Spanish parents automatically become Spanish citizens. Applications for Spanish citizenship are made to the Minister of Justice, who can refuse it on grounds of public order or national interest. In addition to producing the required evidence of identity, applicants must produce a supporting statement from two Spanish citizens to show that the applicant is a good citizen and one who has integrated into Spanish society (Quintero 2005).

WHY IMMIGRANTS CHOOSE SPAIN

Spain is a country with weather conditions and a lifestyle that have attracted migrants from wealthy developed countries for several decades, for example those who come to live off their income from investments and retired people who enjoy a lower cost of living and weather more conducive to health than in northern Europe. Opportunities for people to improve their quality of life and their chances for future enhancement are an important attraction. It is foreseeable that relatively high levels of migration to Spain will continue in the future (Informe sobre la inmigración y el Trabajo en España 2004). Like most developed countries, there is economic migration between regions within the country. However, there are currently very few refugees (Balance de Extranjería 2004). At the end of 2003, Spain hosted about 230 refugees in need of protection. During 2003, 5900 asylum seekers filed applications in Spain, an 8% decrease from 2002. The largest numbers came from Nigeria (1700), Colombia (520), Algeria (350), Congo-Kinshasa (270), Côte d'Ivoire (240) and Liberia (190) (US Committee for Refugees 2004).

THE RECENT HISTORY OF SPANISH IMMIGRATION

Immigration has only posed a challenge to Spain in the past 10 or 15 years to the extent that it has now become a priority on the political and social agenda (OECD 2003). Increased immigration occurred after Spain was admitted to the European Union (EU) in 1986, prior to which emigration was more common. The only significant migrant group coming to Spain prior to the late twentieth century were Gypsies. These formed one of the largest minority ethnic groups in Spain and one of the oldest, having first settled there in the fifteenth century. In recent years, however, there has been a large influx of people from Africa, Central and South America, and Asia as well as from eastern Europe. Although Spain has lower levels of immigration than many other EU countries, the sudden influx has necessitated urgent reviews of immigration legislation and policy. The Migration Policy Group (2003) reported that legal immigrants made up 2.7% of the Spanish population and that the percentage with legal resident status had particularly increased in 1998 by 18.01% and in 2001 by 23.82%.

On 31 December 2003 the number of foreigners with residence permits in Spain was 1.6 million, a quarter (406 199) of whom were from EU countries; 154 001 were Europeans from non-EU countries, 432 662 were Africans, 541 485 Latin Americans, 16 183 North Americans, 121 455 Asians, 1018 from Oceania and 1028 whose nationality was not stated. In Spain most immigrants have settled in Catalonia, Madrid and Andalusia (Instituto Nacional de Estadística Decenio 1994/2003).

Reasons for the increase in non-EU immigrants include increasing inequity in the distribution of economic activity and disparities in income between the most and the least developed areas of the world. Economic, political or military crises have also led to increases in migration to southern Europe. It is likely that the globalization of the media has influenced people's decisions on migration by increasing their awareness of the attractiveness of other countries. Demands in the labour markets in the destination countries have also attracted migration either due to expansion in certain areas of the economy, or due to demographic imbalances causing a decrease in potentially economically active people, and the relatively high salaries available in western and southern Europe. Spain's proximity to Morocco in North Africa means that Morocco is a common point of departure for illegal immigrants to Spain. The Spanish language adds to its attraction as a destination for Latin Americans, whose home countries have been colonized by Spain.

In 2001, of the six main countries of origin of non-EU immigrants (Morocco, Ecuador, Colombia, China, Peru, Dominican Republic), only China has no historical ties with Spain (http://www.migpolgroup.com/uploadstore/Spain.pdf).

In 2002, after the regularization and the noticeable increase in people coming from North Africa, it was forecast that the number of migrants from developing countries would increase to be in line with other European neighbours, outstripping perhaps those coming from Latin America and Asia (Informe sobre la inmigración y el asilo en España 2003).

ILLEGAL IMMIGRANTS IN SPAIN

Moroccans and Bulgarians make up the major contingent of illegal immigrants reaching Spanish territory by sea. As regards immigrants from Latin America, there are reported to be more without authorized documentation than there are those who have become nationals with a valid residence permit (Migration Policy Group 2003).

There has been much concern about the growing number of persons illegally present in the country, many of whom are vulnerable to being exploited in the Spanish black economy as a result of the high demand for unskilled workers particularly in agriculture, construction and domestic work (Comisión de Derechos Humanos 2003). Many steps are being taken to control the influx by improving the administrative management of immigration, strengthening social policies, and promoting policies to help the influx of legal immigrants. Two of the government's main objectives regarding immigration are the integration of legal immigrants and the pursuit of human traffickers. The government claims that Spanish legislation and the system of guarantees protects the human rights of any person, Spanish or not, including immigrants and asylum seekers. Spain has also implemented the 'Schengen Agreement', which is the agreement for free movement of people between EU member countries, on condition that there are effective controls on external (non-EU) borders. Spain signed the agreement in 1991.

Immigrants in Spain have the right to free legal assistance and interpretation, which are under the control of the judicial authority. A 'Forum for the Social Integration of Immigrants' facilitates the contribution of non-government officers to take an active part in achieving these goals. The government is also running campaigns to promote positive attitudes toward immigration and against racism and xenophobia known as the 'Permanent Campaign for the Intercultural Coexistence and against Racism and Xenophobia' (Informe SOS Racisme 2004). Additionally, an improvement in the speed of processing foreigner's applications has been targeted.

Increasing numbers of family reunification permits have been given and the number of foreigners with valid resident permits has also seen an increase, as has the number of those being repatriated. Those who were repatriated in 2003 were predominantly Romanians, Moroccans, Bulgarians and Ecuadorians. Delays in the processing of immigrants are believed by the government not to be the cause of illegal immigrants, but the consequence. The Spanish government, at the request of Spanish businessmen, has revised immigration law to regularize all immigrants who are in employment (Ministerio de Trabajo y Asuntos Sociales 2005).

SOCIO-ECONOMIC DETERMINANTS OF THE HEALTH OF IMMIGRANTS IN SPAIN

The problems of access to regular employment, illegal residence, living in areas of high social risk (including risk of drug addiction, which is a major problem in Spain), communication problems associated with language, and cultural differences are the main health determinants of immigrants. These are compounded by high levels of geographic mobility with frequent changes of address, which causes problems associated with lack of continuity of care, including health promotion; children may suffer most from this lack of continuity. Immigrants are also exposed to all the diseases associated with life in advanced and complex societies, developing new illnesses, such as asthma, coronary heart disease, strokes and certain types of cancer.

THE GYPSY MINORITY IN SPAIN

The first documentary evidence of Gypsies in Spain dates back to 1425. Today there are more than 600 000 Gypsies in Spain (Unión Romaní 2004). Andalusia has the largest number (300 000), constituting about 5% of the population of that area.

Gypsies in Spain were subject to laws and prejudice designed to eliminate them from Spain during three hundred years of oppression. Settlements were broken up, they were required to marry non-Gypsies, and were denied their language and rituals. They were also excluded from public office and from craft workers' guilds (e.g. of jewellers, clock makers. etc.). In 1560 Spanish law forbade Gypsies (gitanos) from travelling in groups of more than two and Gypsy dress and language were also forbidden. This meant that Gypsies could no longer be nomad people (http://www.flamencoshop.com/gypsy/historicalnotes.htm).

In contemporary Spain Gypsies are a heterogeneous, albeit disadvantaged group consisting of unemployed families living in state-subsidized houses and others living in extreme poverty. Some Gypsy families are well established and socially integrated but many more are marginalized and impoverished. Gypsies have always been people with an oral tradition; consequently their rates of illiteracy are very high. Traditionally they worked as blacksmiths, horse traders, musicians, dancers and fortune tellers. The majority of Gypsies in Spain today try to make a living as traders; however, local authorities are reported to be reluctant to give them trading licences (Unión Romaní 2004). Problems finding more regular and consistent work are compounded by their lack of professional qualifications and the racial discrimination and prejudice of many would-be employers. Few businessmen dare to employ them and, even less, give them jobs of responsibility. Consequently the unemployment rate among Gypsies is reported to be quite high (although there are no robust data on this).

Although there is diversity in terms of the reception of Gypsy children in schools and Gypsy attitudes to schooling, with some still not recognizing its importance for success in the workplace, there has been a rise in school attendance over the last two decades. Now almost all Gypsy children have a school education. Some of them are also studying at university (Unión Romaní 2004).

In summary, lack of academic education and employment, and the poor recognition and acceptance of their cultural idiosyncrasies has led to many living in poor socio-economic conditions (often living in caves), being marginalized and excluded from the majority population. Some are driven to crime as a way to survive, which reinforces discrimination against them (Oliván 2002). There is an almost automatic association of the word 'Gypsy' with criminal activities, although violent racism suffered by the Gypsies is not frequently reported (Vega Cortés 1998).

Today the state provides aid to Gypsy people through the central, regional or local administration in different ways, but often through Gypsy Associations.

HEALTH PROBLEMS OF THE GYPSY COMMUNITY IN SPAIN

References to Gypsies' health are rarely found in health science journals. Neither are they taken into account when developing health programmes. It is important to distinguish between Gypsies who are settled (the minority), who often maintain steady employment and good compliance with preventive and health promotion programmes, and the majority Gypsy population, who are marginalized and whose access to health care is extremely limited. Here we concentrate on this more underprivileged group.

According to a study carried out in Catalonia, the degree of marginalization experienced by Gypsies in Spain depends on their place of residence (Cabedo García 2000). In recent years they have tended to live on the outskirts of big cities alongside immigrant groups who also live in poverty and share the same poverty-related diseases. Their paediatric health problems are similar to those acquired in Spain by immigrant children. These Gypsy families have the highest birth rates, but also the highest rates of child mortality. Gypsy children are at greater risk of having tuberculosis, malnutrition, accidents, tooth decay, and of taking drugs, and they are less likely to be immunized. They are a group recognized as being at risk of anaemia due to iron deficiency and at risk of lead poisoning. Their hospitalization and emergency visits rates are high (Corretger 2000).

High levels of hospitalization among this disadvantaged group of Gypsy children are due in part to the unhealthy conditions in which they live, making them prone to transmissible and environmental diseases. They also have poor access to primary healthcare disease prevention services and planned secondary treatment and care. They are prone to chronic diseases consequent to a lack of treatment in the early stages of disease. Some health professionals may contribute to this in their desire to avoid confrontation with families who are potentially difficult. Gypsies often have no choice but to resort to using emergency services (Sánchez Serrano 2002).

THE HEALTH PROBLEMS OF NON-EU IMMIGRANTS IN SPAIN

A review of the literature relating to surveys carried out in the European Union regarding health and immigration shows that the perspective taken is almost invariably that of health and disease and the supposed health risks they may bring to the country of destination. This may contribute to a negative perception of immigrants in Spain. Though immigrants may carry a wide variety of diseases, the infection risk to the native population is minimal, since the circumstances for transmission (such as the vectors) necessary for that infection may not be present and the standards of hygiene may not be conducive to transmission. Intestinal parasitism and tuberculosis are the most studied diseases in the field of immigration and health (Jansà Joseph & García de Olalla 2004).

Contrary to the common misconception of immigrants as diseased, many people arriving in Spain are young and healthy, and seeking employment. For the 'healthy immigrant', the impact of low socio-economic status and mental health problems are the main health risks (Vall Combelles & García-Algar 2004). This risk tends to grow with time if their economic circumstances do not improve and if they remain socially marginalized. Immigrants also have a higher number of industrial accidents and psychiatric and psychosomatic disorders. The often poor living and work conditions suffered by many also impact negatively on their health.

AIDS AND TUBERCULOSIS IN IMMIGRANTS

AIDS/HIV and tuberculosis are the two transmissible diseases which mainly concern the Spanish health authorities. The majority of immigrants who have arrived in Spain since the beginning of the AIDS epidemic come from countries where the prevalence of HIV infection is low. Spain has more cases of HIV infection than any other EU country (except

Portugal), higher also than South America and North Africa. Infection rates, however, are lower than in sub-Saharan Africa and some Caribbean and Asian countries. The HIV/AIDS epidemic in Spain is native and immigration has not meant a significant increase in the number of cases. From the beginning of the epidemic the number of AIDS cases in immigrants has been 1076 people, 1% of the total of the 58 092 cases notified in Spain in 2000 (Plan Nacional sobre el SIDA 2004).

Studies of prostitutes corroborate the low proportions of infection in immigrant women, including those coming from countries where it is endemic. There are no differences regarding the number of HIV infections between Spanish women and immigrants who are equal in terms of risk behaviours. However, immigrant males who practise prostitution are at higher risk due to their social vulnerability (Del Amo 2001). As a consequence of the illegal trafficking of people, a growing proportion of immigrants are appearing within the groups that practise prostitution; this situation of marginalization makes them more vulnerable to risky sexual behaviours.

Tuberculosis (TB) in Spain is also native, although it has increased in the last six years in some areas and among the immigrant population. Tuberculosis in people of origin other than Spanish is especially associated with situations of social exclusion and in people from countries with a high prevalence; these cases are diagnosed in more advanced stages of the disease. This is believed to be due to the under-use of health services and not to delays in treatment (Díaz de Quijano et al 2001). The abandonment of the policies of prevention and control has led to an increase in TB incidence and resistance to the usual medicines. There has been an increase in the number of studies in Spain on TB among immigrant and native at-risk populations (Anuario Medico Internacional 2003).

CONCLUSIONS

The phenomenon of immigration in Spain does not have the same characteristics as that of Germany, France or the United Kingdom, which have a longer and more consistent history of immigration. It is foreseeable that the need for workers in some sectors will increase in the following years. Without adequate systems for legal migration of such workers, people trafficking will increase. More resources are needed to enable legal migration to help fill jobs in Spain and to bolster the contribution of workers to pensions for future generations. Many of the migrant workers will be from developing countries such as North Africa, some Latin American countries, some others from sub-Saharan Africa and China.

Improved knowledge of immigrants' health needs and of effective preventive measures is needed as a priority for the health services. The main health needs that require addressing are those of immigrant children, particularly the need to improve the proportion of those receiving vaccines; mental health needs; oral and dental health needs; and managing the increase of tuberculosis in immigrants (Salazar et al 2003). Furthermore, due to the increasing numbers of immigrant women and the higher birth rate in mothers of foreign origin, many of them teenagers, some of the health services most needed by immigrants in Spain are those for women and children (Perez Cuadrado 2004).

Not having immigration papers, work permits and so on makes migrants vulnerable to economic exploitation leading to poverty-related diseases, but also makes them reluctant to use health services despite health care being a universal right by law.

A large number of scientific studies in the European Union have centred on immigrants' diseases and on the risks they pose for the health of the resident population. This may offer a negative impression of immigrants. But generally the immigrant is a young and healthy person who is seeking work. He or she should not be perceived as a health risk to the general population; although there has been a small increase in HIV cases, the impact of immigration on this has not proved to be very significant. On the other hand, there has been a considerable increase in cases of tuberculosis, but this is being studied and controlled.

Gypsies appear to have health problems and needs different in some respects to the newer non-EU immigrants. The Spanish Gypsy community's health is at risk not only because of socio-economic and cultural factors, suffering from health inequalities leading to higher morbidity and mortality as a consequence of their poor living conditions, but also because of the limited use they make of the health services. More work is needed to ensure the Spanish health service can respond in a culturally sensitive way to the needs of Gypsies.

Immigrants from non-European countries are at increased risk of suffering ill health consequent to their socio-economic status, especially as they frequently are brought in to fill low-paid positions in the economy. More can be done to reduce health inequalities among them, such as by increasing the coordination between all public bodies that impact on the health of minority ethnic groups. An increase in the number of health professionals who are trained to provide a culturally competent service (appropriate and sensitive to cultural difference) would also help. Much can be learned from those countries that have a longer history of immigration, such as the UK. Comelles et al (2000) advocate that in multicultural Spain it is essential that health professionals be prepared in culturally competent ways in order to ensure equality of rights of immigrants and to provide culturally competent care to all of Spain's peoples.

REFLECTIVE QUESTIONS

1. How has Spain's ethnohistory impacted on the nature of its migration trends?
2. In your view how should the European Union be addressing the health issues of migrants at policy level?

Acknowledgements

I would like to thank Margaret Lay for her contribution to this chapter.

REFERENCES

All about Spain. Online. Available: http://www.red2000. com/spain/primer/hist.html Dec 2004

Anuario Medico Internacional 2003 Epidemiological and clinical study of patients diagnosed with tuberculosis in the northeastern area of Madrid 2003. Anuario Medico Internacional 20(1):10–15

Balance de Extranjería. Balance que realiza anualmente el Gobierno Español sobre Extranjería e Inmigración 2004. Online. Available: http://www.acoge.org/ Jul 2004

Cabedo García V R 2000 Cómo son y de qué padecen los gitanos. Atencion Primaria 26:21–25

Central Intelligence Agency (CIA) 2004 The world fact book. Online. Available: http://www.odci.gov/cia/ publications/factbook/geos/sp.html#Geo Dec 2004

Comelles J M, Mascarella L, Bardaji F, Allue X 2000 Some health care experiences of foreign migrants in Spain. In: Vulpiani P, Comelles J M, van Dongen E (eds) Health for all, all in health. European experiences on health care for migrants. EU Commission. Cidis/ALISEI, Perugia, p 144–167

Comisión de Derechos Humanos 2003 Andalucia Acoge. Informe presentado por la Relatora Especial, Sra. Gabriela Rodríguez Pizarro, de conformidad con la resolución 2003/46 de la Comisión de Derechos Humanos. Online. Available: http://www.acoge.org/ Jul 2004

Confederación Estatal de Sindicatos Médicos (CESM). Online. Available: http://www.cesm.org/Jul 2004

Corretger J M 2000 Marginalidad, grupos étnicos y salud. Anuario Especialidad Pediatrica 36(suppl 48):115–117

Del Amo J, Belza M J, Castillo S, Llácer A 2001 Prevención del VIH/SIDA en inmigrantes y minorías étnicas. Ministerio de Sanidad y Consumo, Madrid

Díaz de Quijano E, Brugal MT, Pasaria MI et al 2001 Influencia de las desigualdades sociales, la conflictividad social y la pobreza extrema sobre la morbilidad por tuberculosis en la ciudad de Barcelona. Salud Pública, Barcelona 75:517–528

European Observatory on Health Care Systems. Spain 2002 Online. Available: http://www.euro.who.int/document/ Obs/SPAsum112002.pdf Jan 2005

Informe España 2003. Fundación Encuentro. Online. Available: http://www.fund-encuentro.org/informes/ notapr03/00–2pIIinmi.pdf Jul 2004

Informe sobre la inmigración y el asilo en España 2003. Ministerio de Trabajo y Asuntos Sociales. Online. Available: http://www.imsersomigracion.upco.es/ Jul 2004

Informe sobre la inmigración y el Mercado de Trabajo en España 2004. Online. Available: http://www.extranjeria. info/publico/revista/016/16–11.pdf

Informe SOS Racisme 2004 Informe anual 2004 sobre el racismo en el Estado Español. Catalunya. Online. Available: http://www.sosracisme.org/ Jul 2004

Instituto Nacional de Estadística Decenio 1994–2003 Inmigraciones procedentes del extranjero, por país de residencia. Resumen de datos. Online. Available: http:// www.ine.es/inebase/cgi/ Jul 2004

Jansà Joseph M, García de Olalla P 2004 Salud e Inmigración: nuevas realidades y nuevos retos. Gaceta Sanitaria 18(suppl):207–213

Migration Policy Group (2003) EU and US approaches to the management of immigration. Online. Available: http://www.migpolgroup.com/uploadstore/Spain.pdf Jan 2005

Ministerio de Trabajo y Asuntos Sociales 2004 Secretaría de Estado de Inmigración y Emigración. Modelos de solicitud. Online. Available: http:/www.dgei.mir.es/es/ general/Procedimientos_Solicitudes_index.html 21 Jul 2004

Ministerio de Trabajo y Asuntos Sociales 2005 El Consejo de Ministros, en su reunión del día 30 de diciembre de 2004 ha aprobado el nuevo Reglamento de la Ley Orgánica 4/2000, de 11 de enero, sobre derechos y libertades de los extranjeros en España y su integración social.
Online. Available: http://www.seg-social.es/inicio/

OECD 2003 Comparative analysis of the legislation and the procedures governing the immigration of family members in certain OECD countries 2003. Online. Available: http://www.oecd.org/document/ Jul 2004

Oliván G 2002 The health status of delinquent gypsy youths in Spain. Public Health 12:308

Perez Cuadrado S, Munoz Avalos N, Robledo Sanchez A et al 2004 Characteristics of immigrant women and their neonates. Anuario Pediatrico, Barcelona 60(1):3–8 (in Spanish)

Plan Nacional sobre el SIDA 2004 V Reunión Nacional sobre la vulnerabilidad de las personas inmigrantes a la infección por el VIH/sida. Resumen y conclusiones. 29 y 30 de abril, Madrid Online. Available: http://www.msc. es/profesional/preProSalud/sida/prevencion/ inmigrantesMinorias/pdfs/InformeReunion.pdf Jul 2004

Quintero J Spanish Citizenship: A guide to the Law in Spain. Online. Available: http://www.andalucia.com/ law/citizenship/home.htm Jan 2005

Salazar A, Navarro-Calderon E, Abad I et al 2003 Diagnostics upon hospital release of immigrants in the city of Valencia, Spain (2001–2002). Revista Espanola de Salud Publica 77(6):713–723 (in Spanish)

Sánchez Serrano F J 2002 Diferencia étnica en la actividad asistencial de urgencias. Aproximación a la realidad gitana. Anuario Especialidad Pediatrica. 56: 17–22

Unión Romaní 2005 Unión del pueblo gitano. Organism acknowledged by the United Nations. On line. Available: http://www.unionromani.org/ April 2005

US Committee for Refugees and Immigrants 2004 Refugee conditions by country. Report, Spain. Online. Available: http://www.refugees.org/ April 2005

Vall Combelles O, Garcia-Algar O 2004 Immigration and health. Anuario Pediatrico 60(1):1–2 (in Spanish)

Vega Cortés A 1998 Los Gitanos en España. Unión Romaní. Pueblo Gitano. Online. Available: http://www.unionromani.org/news.htm Jul 2004

World Health Organization (WHO) 2000 Health care financing and expenditure. Spanish immigration 2000. Online. Available: http://www.euro.who.int/observatory/Hits/Updates/20031031_7 Jul 2004

PART 4

Global perspectives and cultural competence

PART CONTENTS

Chapter 16

A trisomial concept of sociocultural and religious factors in healthcare decision-making and service provision in the Muslim Arab world

Zbys Fedorowicz and Thomas D. Walczyk

LEARNING OBJECTIVES

After reading this chapter you should have:
- an understanding of the historical context of medicine in Islam
- a recognition of the three main components contributing to healthcare decision-making in an Islamic society

- a greater awareness of the distinction between medicine in secular and non-secular societies
- an insight into the factors differentiating healthcare decision-making in Islamic society from that in 'Western society'
- an understanding of the critical differences between 'scientific medicine' and the holistic approach of Islamic medicine.

INTRODUCTION

This chapter, which explores the knowledge, attitudes and practices of healthcare providers and users in the Middle East, does so within the framework of a trisomial concept of sociocultural and religious factors. It draws on the combined knowledge of the authors who have over two decades of healthcare experience in the Middle East.

The trisomial concept we advance is a tripartite distribution of factors that have the potential to influence both healthcare decision-making and the provision of health care. It brings together social and cultural perspectives that are dominant in secular societies with religious factors that predominate in non-secular societies such as those of the Arab world.

As there is a readily accessible wealth of information on Islam, this chapter will not dwell on the doctrinal minutiae of the Islamic religion other than where they can help to better illustrate the historical development, and the integration of medicine, healthcare beliefs and practices within Islam.

The fundamental impact of sociocultural and environmental factors on health has been widely acknowledged (Davey Smith 2003) but significant gaps remain in our understanding of their individual, proportional and joint contributions. More recently, ethnicity and sociocultural determinants of health have been thoroughly explored by Papadopolous et al (1998), and Mares et al (1985) who reviewed the necessity for an increased awareness and understanding of the needs of specific cultural groups. However, while emphasis in transcultural healthcare research continues to focus on the sociocultural sensitivities of ethnic groups, the cultural competence of providers and the effects of culturally inappropriate care, there is clearly a lack of information on the impact of religion on health care. The extensive text by Koening et al (2000) comprehensively covers the interaction between religion and health but fails to explore the significant and intricate relationships that exist between these two issues in Islam.

In their groundbreaking book, Henley & Schott (2003) describe some of these issues and discuss ways of meeting the healthcare needs not only of people of minority cultures but also of minority religious groups. Although the Islamic community may currently represent a minority religious group in the United Kingdom and other European countries, there are parts of the world where Islam is the 'state' religion and those religion-influenced healthcare needs may already be met. Conversely in some counties, e.g. Saudi Arabia, where religions other than Islam are proscribed the religion-specific healthcare needs of other religious groups may not be met. Regular attendance for Islamic religious services is approaching the figures of other mainstream religions in the UK and thus the necessity of meeting the spiritually influenced healthcare needs of Muslims may be a matter of increasing urgency.

A comprehensive description of some of the intriguing religion-influenced health beliefs and practices to be found in Egypt was presented by Fedorowicz in Kemp & Rasbridge (2004). Until recently there has been very limited debate on the influence of religion or the proportionality of its impact on healthcare provision and decision-making. This omission may perhaps reflect the general lack of awareness of the significant effect that religion has on the health and lives of certain communities.

We will illustrate how knowledge, acquired through religious scripture, combined with the traditions and sayings of the Prophet Muhammad has guided the development of healthcare beliefs and practices in Islamic society. In addition, we aim to demonstrate to what extent these healthcare beliefs may play a role in healthcare provision and decision-making in the Muslim Arab world.

SOCIOCULTURAL FACTORS AND SECULAR AND NON-SECULAR SOCIETY

As long ago as the early 1950s a study conducted in the UK by Mogey (1956) confirmed the prevailing attitude of indifference to religion, and in particular churchgoing. Consequently, over the last few decades most Western societies have witnessed an expansion of secularism, accompanied by an increased emphasis on materialism and a concurrent de-emphasis of religion. However, it is acknowledged that part of the void left by this sharp decline in religion has been filled by a rekindling of spirituality and the emergence of new 'communities' and societal groupings that uphold profound religious beliefs but which may only be loosely affiliated to mainstream traditional religions.

Secularism, as defined, implies an indifference to, or the exclusion of religion, and in this context secularism and Islam are conceptually irreconcilable. Secularization in the 'revolutionary West' was described by Van Leeuwen (1964) in a historical perspective, which he related to the advent of the scientific and technological age. In his comprehensive work he refers to the term 'secularization' in a number of ways, but primarily in a positive sense, as a process of emancipation or freedom from religious constraints. However, there is a discernible lack of agreement on what is secularization. This disagreement in part stems from the absence of an accurate definition of religion, with the differing concepts of religion leading to widely varying views of secularization. An attempt was made by Haralambos & Holborn (2000) to clarify the issue of secularization by classifying it in terms of concept and measurement, specifically of attendance at religious services, with a decline in attendance seen as evidence of secularization. Yet the word 'secular' continues to be inaccurately applied to Western societies, most of which may never achieve the total exclusion of religion but are in a transitional state of partial secularism and even religious pluralism with its multiplicity of denominations and sects. Conversely, in Muslim society, religion is fundamental to, an integral part of, and axiomatically indivisible from the sociocultural aspects of daily life in which attendance for worship is mandatory. This difference has significant importance with respect to healthcare perceptions, knowledge and practices in Islamic society.

Muslims are acutely aware of the minor role that religion plays in secular society, and it is this reduced role of religion and the increased penetration of materialism and secularism into their society that are sources of increasing concern (Moracco 1983). Some researchers have implied that truly religious societies have one faith and one place of worship or church, key characteristics which although not unique are integral to Islamic society. Thus, central to the Islamic 'way of life' are powerful religious beliefs, perceptions, traditions and healthcare practices that operate within the ordered and comparatively confined sociocultural boundaries of Muslim society, thereby fulfilling Durkheim's (1961) composite view of religion, as society, community and place of worship.

Social, cultural and religious beliefs are capable of influencing individual behaviour patterns. Thus in secular societies there may be a notional acceptance of health-damaging behaviour and lifestyle choices that are freely made by individuals, whereas in Islamic society these types of unrestricted lifestyle choices are proscribed. Moreover, in secular societies these lifestyle patterns are often associated with low indices of socio-economic status, decreased access to care, reduced health aspirations, and poor health choices (Scambler 2003). The resultant inequalities in health have been extensively investigated by Davey Smith et al (1998), who compared gender and socio-economic and ethnic groups across a wide range of measures of health and determinants of health. However, studies correlating social stratification, health and healthcare beliefs and practices are virtually unknown in Muslim society, which in general discourages this form of 'intrusion'.

A recognition of the significance of this *trisomial concept* will help open some of the 'closed doors' and assist in the development of an understanding of how aspects of healthcare decision-making and provision of healthcare services can be explored by considering religious, in addition to, social and cultural dimensions.

ISLAM A RELIGION NOT A CULTURE

Henley & Schott (2003: 2) defined culture as 'how we do and view things in our group'. Macpherson (1999) portrayed it as a collective resource for the management of everyday behaviour, challenges and difficulties. It is widely accepted that culture constitutes a core set of values, assumptions, perceptions and conventions, chiefly derived from a common history and language, and which permit individual members of a community to function collectively. Quite significantly, these definitions and attributes of culture do not include any direct reference to religion, and although there are frequent references to 'Islamic culture', evidently it is no more appropriate to refer to Christian or Buddhist culture than it is to Islamic culture.

As a religion, Islam is one of the three great faiths, with the Arabic word *Islam* meaning to surrender, specifically to God, and its religious principles are based on what Muslims believe to be the word of God (Mortimer 1982). It is the predominant religion in a number of countries, each with its own distinctive culture, yet quite clearly there is no readily recognizable universal or international 'Islamic culture'. Nevertheless, Islam does have an influence on culture, and it is reasonable to expect that some of these cultural values, which have been influenced by Islam, may be a common thread in some of these countries. In keeping with other religions, Islam has been exposed to a wide range of cultural influences characterized by the cultural diversity seen throughout the Islamic world. However, even when taking sectarian diversity into account, the more prescriptive and orthodox characteristics of Islamic doctrine are unlikely to be influenced by cultural factors.

It is universally accepted that culture is not inherited but is a segment of a single layer of human mental programming conducted throughout childhood and part of a process through which we may acquire the values and norms of the society that we live in (Hofstede 1991). Thus, cultural mental programming is recognized as part of human development whereas the not dissimilar cultural and religious 'mental conditioning' occurring in Muslim society is often considered, by ill-informed non-Muslims, as a form of 'brainwashing'. This is an approach that is expressly forbidden and totally inappropriate to Islam yet there has been an unbalanced focus on Islam, more so than on a number of non-mainstream religious cults that have employed this form of 'brainwashing'.

Regrettably, recent global events have led to a stereotyping of all Muslims as Arabs, yet somewhat surprisingly only 20–25% of Muslims are Arabs (Luna 1989). In the predominantly Islamic Arab world, each Arab society has its own distinctive culture. Thus the religiously orthodox Saudis take pride in the Bedouin origins of their cultural traditions, whereas the more secular Lebanese have integrated elements of European culture with their own unique Arab culture and disavow any Bedouin ancestry. Consequently in the more secular parts of the Arab world where there is more likely to be a wider divergence between religion and culture, there is also a more distinctive boundary between religion, culture and health. However, in the more traditional Islamic societies, sociocultural factors subtly influenced by Islam are interwoven with a complex mosaic of compelling religious beliefs and customs, and as will be seen, may play a significant role in healthcare decision-making by both provider and user.

MEDICINE AND SECULAR AND NON-SECULAR SOCIETIES

Haralambos & Holborn (2000) recognized that in the West the practice of medicine, even though it is based on Christian societal values that dictate community responsibility for the individual, is no longer surrounded by religious ritual. Thus in the increasingly secular societies of the West the influence of religious beliefs and social values on health is changing, and nowadays, unlike in the past, hospitals are more frequently seen as secular institutions.

Secular and non-secular societies were examined by Jansen (2000), who noted that the 'religion and medicine mix' can have one of two scenarios, ranging from the acceptance of a possibly unbridgeable gap as in a secular society, to that of a close relationship which is presented as 'religious medicine' in some non-Western societies. Secularization within Western society appears to have begun in the aftermath of the First World War with the crumbling of the old patterns of European culture.

Five key conditions were identified by Shiner (1967) as having contributed to the phenomenon of secularization:

- decline of religion
- de-sacralization of the world (i.e. conscious removal or reduction of sacred symbols from religious life and worship)
- disengagement of society from religion
- achievement of global conformity
- transposition of beliefs and patterns of behaviour from the 'religious' to the 'secular' sphere.

It is clear that the religious and sociocultural patterns and trends that are an inherent feature of close-knit Islamic societies are diametrically opposed to those seen in the increasingly secularized Western society. Thus there is a readily visible impact of religious and sociocultural factors on traditional Islamic society, more so than in 'Western' secular societies, resulting in marked differences in perception, knowledge, attitudes and practice in health and health care.

HEALTH IN PRE-ISLAMIC ARABIA

A graphic illustration of life and health in pre-Islamic Arabia was provided by Khan (1986). In pre-Islamic times the Arabian Peninsula was inhabited by nomadic tribes of camel- or sheep-herding pastoralists who wandered between sporadic settlements and pockets of habitation. The society was polytheistic and numerous deities were recognized and worshipped. A harsh climate in conjunction with a rudimentary awareness of medicine resulted in a poor level of general health among these inhabitants of the Arabian Peninsula. Health care was primitive and combined folk medicine with magic; the little surgery that was performed was limited to cauterization, branding and cupping (Tabbara 1989). As in other traditional societies, past and present, the pre-Islamic Arabs believed in mythical treatment that included sorcery, witchcraft, talismans, spells, incantations, amulets, folk medicine, potions and magic charms. A detailed and fascinating description of these practices and this system of medicine can be found in Shiloh (1961).

Khan also informs us that promiscuity was widespread, women had a low social status and infanticide was common. Intriguingly, alcohol was widely available and as is seen these days, its use in the alleviation of the stresses of daily life encouraged widespread abuse (Badri 1978).

'ISLAMIC MEDICINE' AND MEDICINE IN ISLAM

Whilst the concept of 'Islamic medicine' dates back to the earliest times in Islamic history, the terminology arose in the late 1960s as a response to the encroachment of the 'Western' biomedical model within Arab and Muslim nations (Adib 2004). In reality it was a product of the integration of the universally held tenets of Islam with the art of medicine. Although it is enjoying somewhat of a renaissance in some parts of the world there are currently no Islamic medicine training programmes in any Arab country. Quite significantly, Islamic medicine does not appear to have been universally accepted as a comprehensive health alternative comparable to other non-Western health models.

The term 'Islamic medicine' (*tibb islamiya*) is semantically more acceptable than 'Islamic culture' and refers more specifically to those healthcare prescriptions and practices based on Islamic teaching that have been handed down through traditional healers and still find ready acceptance today. 'Medicine in Islam', however, refers more specifically to the practice of contemporary medicine that has been tempered with the societal and cultural norms that are characteristic of present-day Muslim society.

'ISLAMIC MEDICINE', THE PROPHET, QUR'AN, HADITH AND PROPHETIC MEDICINE

Islamic medicine arose in the early part of the Islamic era as a body of medical knowledge that was assimilated by Muslims in the earliest phase of Islamic history (661–861 AD). This knowledge came mostly from Greek sources but subsequently incorporated medical practices from, Persia, Syria and India. It embodied physiological concepts based on Hippocratic and Galenic thinking and included a recognition and understanding of 'humors' and 'natures' that had to remain in balance to prevent disease. These concepts and prescriptions of Galen, Hippocrates and others were eventually translated into Arabic, the literary and scientific lingua franca of the time, and were exhaustively added to and subsequently 'Islamicized'.

Early progress in medicine and health in the Arabian Peninsula may be linked to the arrival of Islam, which was preceded by the birth of the Prophet Muhammad in 570 AD. It is acknowledged that his 'doings and sayings', the Hadith, had a significant impact on improving the lives and health of the inhabitants of the Arabian Peninsula. The Hadith, as the second source of authority in Islam, complements the Qur'an and assists with its ultimate understanding in the context of the Prophet Muhammad's life and the ways in which he demonstrated and applied the Qur'anic message. Several historical sources recount that the Prophet gave advice about health and hygiene, yet most of these pieces of advice are not mentioned in the Qur'an. It is widely accepted that the Qur'an is not intended as a book of medicine or of health sciences, but in it there are hints and guidelines to health and the prevention of disease, with specific mention made of the healing properties of honey. Sura an-nahl (the Bee: Qur'an 16: 68–69), 'there comes from their bellies a drink of many colours in which there is healing for mankind'.

The requirement of all Muslims to fast in the month of Ramadan and the prohibition on alcohol and the consumption of pork, which are all documented in the Qur'an, are well known to most non-Muslims.

The Hadith consist of the 'doings, sayings and traditions' of the Prophet that were originally circulated orally and were assembled between the tenth and fifteenth centuries by clerics rather than physicians. These traditions were grouped according to subjects, with each subject constituting a book or *kitab* and each tradition a chapter or *bab*. The Sahih al-bukhari, which is the most renowned of these books, covers a wide range of subjects in medicine and includes a section on nursing the sick, two books dealing with patients (70) and with medicine (71). This collection of Hadith is considered to be the most reliable, a result of their compliance with the most stringent of criteria.

Inevitably portions of these Hadith were shaped into a genre of medical writing called *at-tibb an-nabawi, or* Prophetic medicine, and became a guide to medical therapy that was acceptable to the religiously orthodox. The treatise by the religious scholar Jalal u'Din As-suyuti (1994) is the most celebrated and was based almost exclusively on what was known of medical practices during the time of the Prophet. It was derived from the Qur'an and the Hadith, and included some of the practices of the early Muslim community and provides a striking insight into their perceptions of the causes of disease and the theory and practice of medicine. Quite remarkably for its time, it emphasized a holistic approach to health and health care, concepts that would find a ready acceptance by adherents of currently fashionable trends in homeopathic and alternative medicine.

These 'doings and sayings' advocated the traditional medical practices of the Prophet Muhammad and those mentioned in the Qur'an, rather than the practices assimilated from Greek medical tradition. Primarily, these edicts expounded on the virtues of diet 'eat and drink but not excessively' (Qur'an 7: 31), the use of natural remedies, the management of simple ailments such as headache, fever 'if any of you has a fever then pour cold water over him' (Hadith Aisha: Volume 7, Book 71, Number 621), sore throat, conjunctivitis, and included injunctions against contact with persons having contagious diseases, 'if you hear that plague is in a place then do not go there but if the plague has already arrived then do not try to run away from it' (Hadith Abdullah bin Abbas *Volume 7, Book 71, Number 625*).

In addition to these 'pieces of advice', a large number of traditions and sayings were assembled and are known as 'spiritual medicine' or *Ruqyah*. These are a collection of verses from the Qur'an or prayers to the Almighty, which invoke blessings and may be used in healing. There are numerous examples of this form of healing in the Hadith and it is said that the

Prophet would recite the last two *surahs* (verses) of the Qur'an whenever any member of his household was ill.

Although he was not a physician, the Prophet Muhammad made medical care a sacred duty and asked his followers to not avoid any necessary medical treatment. The Hadith highlights the significant interest of the Prophet in health and is replete with his quotations and recommendations. He said, 'there is no illness without a cure as God had created a cure for all disease, except the cure for old age' (Hadith: usamah). Prophet Muhammad is quoted as saying, 'there are two gifts of which many men are cheated – good health and leisure' (Hadith: al-bukhari). A further quotation of the Prophet Muhammad states that, 'whoever wakes in the morning with a healthy body, and a self that is sound, and whose provision is assured, he is like the one who possesses the whole world' (Hadith: at-tirmidhi).

Prophetic medicine (*at-tibb an-nabawi*), as it was based exclusively on the Hadith, proved to be extremely popular amongst the multitude of Muslims, chiefly because of its doctrinal and theological content. It contrasted with the scientific and analytical approach of Islamic medicine that had already been accepted by a majority of Muslim historians and physicians. Gradually, Islamic and Prophetic medicine have become more integrated and the dividing line between them is less distinct such that the terms are often used freely and interchangeably. The reader will find an interesting and extensive collection of the Hadith on many of the excellent Islamic websites listed in the References.

A number of traditional Islamic medicine healthcare practices are still in common use, but they have no doctrinal support from the Hadith, and are therefore not acceptable as 'orthodox' Prophetic medicine. Some of these practices and remedies include vestiges of witchcraft, sorcery and casting of spells, and although most of these date from the earliest period of Islam they continue to enjoy varied support.

ISLAMIC MEDICINE AND 'WESTERN' SCIENTIFIC MEDICINE

El Kadi (2003), in attempting to draw a distinction between Islamic and modern medicine, suggested that Islamic medicine includes all the significant qualities of modern medicine, but differs from it by fulfilling the following criteria:

- it excels above all other genres of the healing arts
- it is a healing art that takes cognizance of faith and divine ethics
- it is guided (divinely)
- it comprehensively includes the body and spirit, the individual and society
- it is universal in offering its services to all humankind
- it is scientific.

He contends that Islamic medicine is comprehensive, spiritual, holistic, divinely inspired and guided, all of which may be considered fine attributes but perhaps to some observers may seem more of a 'wish list' than a reality. In contrast, few healthcare providers would dispute the increasing application and major contribution of the rigorously scientific and evidence-based approach of modern medicine (Sackett et al 1996). Yet there has been a more recent and quite remarkable acceptance and integration of alternative and holistic practices into mainstream modern medicine. However, in secular society the belief in divine guidance of medical care has diminished somewhat since the time of Hippocrates, 'may the physician be given strength from God almighty'.

Nevertheless it would be difficult to argue for or against the criteria listed by El Kadi referring to divine guidance as these constitute some of the fundamental tenets of Islamic belief which command absolute faith in God.

'Western' scientific medicine has to a large extent replaced the core of the healthcare systems in most Islamic countries, but Islamic medicine retains its popularity and having undergone a 'renaissance' continues to be practised ever more widely. It enjoys official status in some of the countries in the Indian subcontinent, where a number of medical schools have been established that teach 'Tibb or Unani' medicine (which is translated as a knowledge of the state of the human body in health and disease).

DEVELOPMENT OF KNOWLEDGE, ATTITUDES AND PRACTICES BY THE HEALTHCARE PROVIDER AND THE TRISOMIAL CONCEPT

ISLAMIC MEDICAL EDUCATION PAST AND PRESENT

The early history of Islamic medical education can be traced back to the School of Medicine at Jundishapur or 'Gondeshapur', a city in Khuzestan in western Iran (Browne 2001). The town was conquered by Muslims in 738 AD and at that time it already had a well-established hospital and medical school which would serve as the model for future medical schools throughout the region. Lectures and clinical sessions incorporated the major concepts of Islamic medicine by placing a greater emphasis on treatment that augmented the body's natural defence and healing mechanisms through the use of herbal medicines.

Much has changed; currently almost all medical schools in the Arab world follow the Western medical curriculum with its emphasis on technology and scientific medicine. This curriculum focuses on the learning of skills that are test and procedure oriented and which ultimately equip the graduate with the knowledge and skills required for the disciplines of medicine, surgery and the other specialties. As in the Western milieu, a significant majority of these graduates will become highly skilled technicians, scientists and experts in curative medicine but with a limited awareness of disease as a manifestation of poor lifestyle choices and socio-environmental factors. Many of these clinicians may, with further training, become specialists in the disease of 'one organ or system' or may simply cross into the 'business' of medical practice and lose sight of their primary role as a healer.

Conversely, an education in Islamic medicine is said to teach and emphasize the recognition of the links between disease and the spirit (soul), and that physical disease is not merely a manifestation of poor lifestyle choices and environment.

RELIGIOUS BELIEFS AND CLINICAL PRACTICE

Uniquely Muslim healthcare providers, unlike their secular counterparts, may be confronted daily with clinical decisions that question the religious legitimacy of their clinical activities and decisions. It is in this decision-making that they will be expected to use their combined knowledge of Islam and medicine. Some of these patient encounters will include potentially controversial issues on which instant decisions may be required: e.g. birth control, abortion, extrauterine conception, end of life issues and euthanasia. Thus the clinician may have to make decisions on matters that are not covered by the laws of the land but are subject to Islamic law (Rispler-Chaim 1989). Accordingly the practice of medicine in Islam requires a combined knowledge of the sharia, the Islamic legal system, as well as contemporary Islamic teachings, for which a solid background knowledge of Islam is essential. This background must include a profound understanding of the moral, ethical, spiritual and philosophical issues that reflect current precepts in Islam (Ajlouni 2003). The ordinary physician cannot be expected to have a full working knowledge of the sharia and thus at times the interpretation of aspects of Qur'anic law and their relevance to health care may require the expertise and advice of a Muslim cleric.

Therefore a healthcare provider to Muslim patients must not only be aware of the contemporary views on the causes of disease, but also of the other influences on health which are supported by Islamic beliefs. To that extent their care should attempt to integrate the traditional medicine of the past with the best medicine of the present.

There is a wide range of reference books offering guidance to the non-Muslim healthcare provider to ensure the provision of care appropriate to social, cultural and religious beliefs (Mares et al 1985, Papadopoulos et al 1998, Henley & Schott 2003, Aziz 2000).

Increasingly, we are seeing calls for Muslim physicians to revitalize the concepts of Islamic medicine and work towards applying some of its principles to contemporary health care, scientific research and education. In this respect the Hadith obligates physicians to not only find cures for diseases, but also to be conversant with the preventive aspects of all illnesses whether they are physical, mental or spiritual.

And He makes for them good things lawful, and bad things forbidden. (Qur'an 7: 157)

In many aspects the recommendations in the Hadith closely parallel the fundamentals of the Hippocratic oath by endorsing standards of care expected from the healthcare provider. Physicians must offer appropriate care and advice after careful consideration of both physical and spiritual aspects. They must not recommend or administer anything harmful, refuse needed help regardless of financial ability or ethnic origin of the patient, compromise a patient's confidentiality, examine a patient of the opposite sex in the absence of a third person, or criticize another physician in the presence of patients or health personnel. Moreover they should strive to use wisdom in all their decisions and must refuse payment for treatment of another physician or the physician's immediate family. Additional responsibility is placed on the healthcare provider to proffer Islamic perspectives in health and ethical issues and to be able to give scientific explanations for Islamic principles and prohibitions.

Much has been written about how non-Muslim healthcare providers can best care for Muslim patients but it is apparent that there are deeper issues than just the physical aspect of providing care. To be able to satisfy the recommendations of the Hadith in caring for a Muslim patient requires religious 'competency' beyond that of the average non-Muslim physician and signifies that cultural competency may well include a significant religious dimension.

Scant mention is made of the nursing profession in the Islamic medical literature and regrettably there has been a historical perception of nurses as helpers, not healthcare professionals, and whose suggestions and advice are not taken seriously. The culturally linked hierarchical stratification within the medical profession and its not uncommon paternalistic attitude towards other healthcare professionals often means that nursing professionals may not be directly involved in the care or decision-making process but may merely 'receive orders' from doctors. The establishment of nursing colleges and professional training programmes in the Arab world is driving much needed changes to this outmoded approach.

In summary, the Hadith expects that the Muslim physician believes in God and in Islamic teachings and puts these into practice in both private and public life. The Hadith places emphasis on the realization that God is the maker and owner of the patient's body and mind and that this patient must be treated within the framework of God's teachings. These teachings stress that life was given to man by God, that human life starts at the time of conception and that it cannot be taken away except by God. Moreover, the Hadith informs the medical practitioner that God is watching and monitoring his every thought and deed. It exhorts him to stay abreast of current medical knowledge, continuously improve his skills, seek help whenever needed, and comply with legal requirements governing his profession. However, in order to achieve this the healthcare practitioner needs not only to excel in contemporary knowledge and skill but also to comprehend the philosophy of Islam and Islamic medicine.

KNOWLEDGE, ATTITUDES AND PRACTICES, THE HEALTHCARE USER AND THE TRISOMIAL CONCEPT

Arab culture and the Islamic religion emphasize the importance of maintaining good health, especially through personal hygiene practices and a healthy diet. It is these concepts of health and illness that are shaped by the strong religious belief in *predestination* which may influence healthcare decision-making.

Although Arabs place a high value on Western medicine and have confidence in the medical profession, some will resort to traditional healthcare practices when other treatment fails.

PREDESTINATION

Muslims in general are fatalistic about ill health and disease and accept that these are preordained and to a certain extent beyond individual control. Predestination (*al-qadar*) is a pillar of Islamic belief, 'every small and great thing that men do is recorded in God's books' (Qur'an 54: 53), demanding acceptance that all that happens, good and bad, occurs according to God's divine preordainment and decree. Furthermore, that every human will is subordinated to and controlled by God's will, 'while the very will to walk straight does not exist in man's heart unless it be that Allah willeth, the Lord of creation' (Qur'an 81: 29). And that whatever man does and whatever happens to him is directly willed by God. 'If God touches thee with affliction, none can remove it but He' (Hadith: Jabir). Such a deterministic view of human existence arose from the ancient Judeo-Christian heritage but has through time undergone 'progressive' modification to permit a more decisive and individualistic role in Judaism and Christianity. Conversely, in Islam neither an individual nor any external factors can change a person's God-given character, which remains with him throughout his life and which destines him to a prescribed lifecourse. He has no choice but to go through the course of events which have been preordained for him right down to the smallest detail. Thus a Muslim patient views his life with all its vicissitudes and deprivations from a long-range perspective which extends into the afterlife. However, this spiritual outlook, in which predestination is an indispensable element, has a positive spin-off in that it provides composure and peace of mind which is maintained even in the face of great adversity, illness and disease.

It is this total submission to the will and orders of God, the ultimate provider of health, that guides the conduct of life in this world, while the role of disease is to test patience and faith and will erase sins in preparation for the next world. When a Muslim is afflicted with any disease it is his belief in the mercy of God, his faith in destiny and the requirement for forbearance and patience which give him strength to stand fast and endure his ordeal. Accordingly, most Muslims are remarkably stoic and enduring towards disease, even those diseases that are relentless or incurable. They are instructed to accept it as the will of God and pray for its removal or its cure.

TRADITIONAL HEALTHCARE BELIEFS AND PRACTICES IN THE ARAB WORLD

Science and medicine have been linked to Arab culture since the tenth century AD and certain folk remedies and practices that may provide psychological comfort and some physical improvement still persist. Some of these traditional beliefs incorporate *djinn* (or *jinn* meaning devil) and aspects of animism that are not accepted by mainstream Islam. They are often characterized by harsh treatment modalities: branding, cutting and use of purgatives, emetics and other powerful potions. They have been used primarily to avoid illness and harm to a healthy person. They may include the wearing of amulets for protection against the 'evil eye' or the burning of incense to keep the evil eye away from the sick. The evil eye is said to be invoked when an individual or family receives something positive which evokes jealousy in others, prompting the eyes of others to inflict harm on that person or family. In its simplest form it was understood to be the deliberate projection of a ray of occult energy with the malicious intention to cause harm, ill health or death. The effect was believed to be fatal if the person 'overlooked' by the evil eye actually met the malicious gaze directly. There are references in the Hadith to the evil eye and the treatment of those who have been affected by it, 'the evil eye is true, and if there is anything that precedes predestination it would be the evil eye' (Hadith: Ibn Abbas). 'The Prophet ordered me or somebody else to do Ruqyah (if there was danger) from an evil eye' (Hadith: Aisha).

It would be difficult to accept that there is no such thing as the evil eye, when the belief is so widespread across both time and cultural boundaries. Al-Jauziyah (2003) covers the topic extensively and states that the effect of the evil eye on health is less physical and more spiritual or psychological in nature and is invoked by the soul on the victim.

Just as the evil eye finds its influence and ultimate destructive effects on some susceptible individuals, an equally pervasive and universal force, the 'Hand of Fatima', exists to remedy the eye and any 'evil spirits'. Fatima was the Prophet Muhammad's daughter and was often called upon for protection and compassion. The hand is considered to be a healing symbol (the laying on of hands) and thus the 'Hand of Fatima' is a representative name for any article or object that is capable of healing and repelling the evil eye. It may adorn the body or be conspicuously placed at the entrance to a dwelling where the distinctive blue object (the colour of healing) is said to protect vulnerable inhabitants and visitors. Silver amulets worn around the neck or wrist are also alleged to help ward off sickness and a variety of diseases. There is some degree of uncertainty about the orthodoxy of wearing these amulets but prophetic traditions appear to prohibit them even though they may contain Qur'anic verses.

CULTURAL ATTITUDES TO MEDICAL CARE AND HEALTHCARE DECISION-MAKING

The Prophet Muhammad encouraged Muslims to seek early medical attention: 'servants of God seek treatment; God has not set a disease without setting a cure to it, known to whoever knows it and unknown to whoever does not know it' (Hadith: Abu Huraira).

In general, a patient and family will not wait long to seek professional help. One or more family members may accompany a patient to a medical appointment and it is common for the family members to stay with the patient and to help answer questions about the patient's health. The extended family occupies a position of great importance in Arab society; and older male members (grandfather, father, eldest son and eldest uncle) play significant roles in the process of decision-making in the health care of individual family members. Even though their knowledge may be rudimentary and supported by no more than personal experiences, their opinions are sought and often inordinate weight is attached to their perceived medical wisdom.

At clinical examination some Arabs are reluctant to disclose detailed information about themselves and their families to strangers. They tend to give as little information as possible and may not give enough for a proper diagnosis and may be embarrassed by questions about their sexual relationships and other personal questions.

Culture dictates that patients are only told the good news about their disease whereas severe illness and its possible sequelae are generally reported to a selected family member. An overriding theme found in Arabic culture is the family's need for hope, optimism and belief in the positive advantages of treatment. They will answer questions, will listen carefully to the healthcare provider's advice, explanations and warnings, and will follow the provider's directions carefully. Some patients may question the necessity of laboratory testing, X-rays and medication but in the end will accept the provider's advice.

Patients are usually anxious to receive medication as soon as possible and pain relief is expected to be immediate and pleas for relief may be persistent although displays of pain are expressed privately and only among close relatives or family friends. However, once symptoms have improved, many patients will stop taking the prescribed medication or may not return for a scheduled follow-up appointment.

In summary, healthcare decision-making by Muslim patients may be governed by a complex mix of religious, social, cultural and traditional beliefs. Religious perspectives pervade and subtly influence all of these domains, emphasizing how significant it is for the healthcare provider to have an understanding of social, cultural and religious aspects in healthcare provision for Muslim patients.

CONCLUSION

This chapter has described the early development of Islamic medicine with its visionary holistic approach to health, in a model that is now finding wider acceptance in Western medicine (Ewles & Simnett 1999). This model consists of three concentric rings: societal, environmental and an inner ring with six discrete dimensions one of which is spiritual (Fig. 16.1) (Naidoo & Willis 2003). The similarity in the concept of Islamic medicine to Ewles & Simnett's holistic model is not coincidental but is an illustration of how medicine has turned full circle. Western medicine with its philosophical roots in the Cartesian revolution, which separated mind and body, now increasingly recognizes these wider socio-environmental determinants of health, and that healthcare needs are best served through a holistic approach combining scientific and alternative/ traditional medicine. A recognition that is not before time and includes a growing awareness of the significance of religious and spiritual issues.

Finally we have shown how religion plays a significant role in the life of every Muslim, physician, patient or carer, and how it guides their

Figure 16.1 Dimensions of health (adapted from Ewles & Simnett 1999).

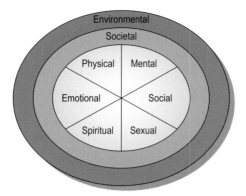

everyday activity in the same way that evidence-based clinical pathways and guidelines guide the contemporary physician through the intricacies of effective healthcare decision-making. However, it is self-evident that these healthcare decisions made by the Muslim patient and the provider are often made through an interpretation of divinely inspired and guided 'best evidence' which has been made available to them through the Hadith and the Qur'an.

REFLECTIVE QUESTIONS

1. There is a growing preference for patients to be better informed about the state of their illness or disease. How would you proceed with Muslim patients if 'fully informed' may mean providing them with negative information on their health status?
2. In which way does religion play a role, if at all, in your personal healthcare decision-making?
3. Do you find any agreement with the more extreme view of religion as the opium of the masses and that it has no place in modern medicine other than as a psychological crutch to sustain hope, specifically in end-of-life situations?

REFERENCES

Adib S M 2004 From the biomedical model to the Islamic alternative: a brief overview of medical practices in the contemporary Arab world. Social Science and Medicine 58(4):697–702

Ajlouni K M 2003 Values, qualifications, ethics and legal standards in Arabic (Islamic) medicine. Saudi Medical Journal 24(8):820–826

Al-Jauziyah Q 2003 Healing with the medicine of the Prophet. Darusallam, Riyadh

As-suyuti J 1994 As-suyuti's medicine of the Prophet. Ta-Ha Publishers, London

Aziz S 2000 Caring for Muslim patients. Radcliffe Medical Press, Oxford

Badri M B 1978 Islam and alcoholism. American Trust Publications. Washington

Browne E G 2001 Islamic medicine. Goodword Books, New Delhi

Davey Smith G 2003 Health inequality: lifecourse approaches. The Policy Press, Bristol

Davey Smith G, Morris N J, Shaw M 1998 The independent inquiry into inequalities in health. British Medical Journal 317:1465–1466

Durkheim E 1961 The elementary forms of the religious life. Collier Books, New York

El Kadi A 2003 What is Islamic medicine? Health an Islamic perspective. Online. Available: http://www.islamset.com

Ewles I, Simnett I 1999 Promoting health: a practical guide to health education. 4th edn. Harcourt, Edinburgh

Haralambos M, Holborn M 2000 Sociology: themes and perspectives. 5th edn. Harper Collins, London

Henley A, Schott J 2003 Culture, religion and patient care in a multi-ethnic society. Age Concern, London

Hofstede G 1991 Cultures and organizations: software of the mind. McGraw Hill, London

Jansen G 2000 Western medicine secularized and secularizing. Southern African Missiological Society. Online. Available: http://www.geocities.com. missionalia/articles.htm

Kemp C E, Rasbridge L A 2004 Refugee and immigrant health. Cambridge University Press, Cambridge

Khan M S 1986 Islamic medicine. Routledge & Kegan Paul, London

Koening H G, McCullough M E, Larson D B 2000 Handbook of religion and health. Oxford University Press, Oxford

Luna L J 1989 Transcultural nursing care of Arab Muslims. Journal of Transcultural Nursing 5(2):22–26

Macpherson W 1999 The Stephen Lawrence inquiry: report. Home Office, London

Mares P, Henley A, Baxter C 1985 Health care in multiracial Britain. Health Education Council and the National Extension College, Cambridge

Mogey J M 1956 Family and neighbourhood. Oxford University Press, Oxford

Moracco J 1983 Some correlates of the Arab character. Psychology 20:3–4

Mortimer E 1982 Faith and power: the politics of Islam. Vintage Books, New York

Naidoo J, Willis J 2003 Health promotion: foundations for practice. 2nd edn. Baillière Tindall, Edinburgh

Papadopolous I, Tilki M, Taylor G 1998 Transcultural care. A guide for healthcare professionals. Quay Books, Dinton

Pryce-Jones D 2002 The closed circle: an interpretation of the Arabs. Ivan R. Dee, Chicago

Rispler-Chaim V 1989 Islamic medical ethics in the 20th century. Journal of Medical Ethics 15(4):203–208

Sackett D L, Rosenberg W M C, Muir Gray J A et al 1996 Evidence-based medicine: what it is and what it isn't. BMJ 312:71–72

Scambler G 2003 Sociology as applied to medicine. 5th edn. Elsevier, Philadelphia

Shiloh A 1961 The system of medicine in Middle East culture. Middle East Journal 15(3):277–288

Shiner L 1967 The meanings of secularization, In: Matthes J (ed) International yearbook for the sociology of religion. Westdeutscher Verlag, Cologne, p 52–57

Tabbara K 1989 Cautery. Folk remedies and magic [editorial]. Annals of Saudi Medicine 9:433–434

Van Leeuwen A 1964 Christianity in world history. The meeting of the faiths East and West. Edinburgh House Press. London

References to Hadith

Abu Huraira. In: Sahih al-bukhari, *Volume 7, Book 71, Number 582. Online. Available:* http://www.usc.edu/ dept/MSA/ fundamentals/hadithsunnah/bukhari/

Aisha. In: Sahih al-bukhari, *Volume 7, Book 71, Number 634. Online. Available:* http://www.usc.edu/dept/MSA/ fundamentals/hadithsunnah/bukhari/

Islamic websites

Athar S. Information for healthcare providers when dealing with a Muslim patient. Available at http://www.islam-usa.com/e40.html

http://www.islamic-knowledge.com/Medicine

www.islamonline.net

Chapter **17**

Transcultural health care in Israel: past history and current issues

Vered Delbar

CHAPTER CONTENTS

LEARNING OBJECTIVES

After reading this chapter readers should be:
- aware of the unique causes and patterns for immigration of Jews to Israel
- knowledgeable about the cultural impact of the waves of immigration from different cultures on a small society and a new state
- aware of the professional and cultural issues related to healthcare workers who immigrate to Israel

- culturally sensitive to the healthcare needs of the various groups living in Israel
- able to make suggestions aiming at improving the cultural competence of Israeli healthcare providers and services
- able to comment on the applicability of the knowledge gained in this chapter to healthcare providers worldwide.

INTRODUCTION

Israel's citizens come from all over the world. Israel is also a meeting zone between Middle Eastern traditional healthcare practices and modern Western medicine. Patients and a substantial proportion of doctors, nurses and other healthcare professionals are from diverse ethnic backgrounds. Cultural effects can considerably complicate the assessment of how an individual is likely to react to various aspects of the hospital environment, medical condition, treatment, staff, fellow patients, and so on. Ideal care management includes the foresight to forestall problems that may arise and to create favourable conditions that help patients to respond positively to treatment.

The term Israeli citizen represents a broad and diverse group of people with different origins and backgrounds. In order to raise awareness about the diversity of the current Israeli society the chapter begins with the ethnohistory of the Israeli population. Some of the socio-economic and health-related issues of the various Jewish and non-Jewish groups living in Israel are discussed.

To illustrate the diverse cultural components in health care, four patient case studies are included in this chapter: (1) an Israeli-born Jew whose parents immigrated from Germany; (2) an Israeli-born Jew whose grandparents immigrated from Morocco; (3) an Israeli citizen who is an Arab Bedouin; (4) an Israeli Jewish child who immigrated with his parents from Ethiopia. The professional and cultural issues related to healthcare workers who immigrate to Israel are explored through the use of a final case study which discusses the case of a new immigrant nurse from the former Soviet Union. The chapter concludes with some suggestions aimed at improving the cultural competence of Israeli based healthcare providers and some comments on the applicability of the knowledge gained in this chapter to healthcare providers worldwide.

POPULATION, ETHNOHISTORY AND HEALTH SERVICES IN ISRAEL

When the state of Israel was declared on 14 May 1948, there were already some 650 000 Jews living in the 'Yishuv', the Jewish settlement in British governed Palestine. Motivated by a Jewish nationalist vision to reunite Jews from all corners of the earth in the Jewish state and to forge a new national identity ('Zionism'), successive waves of Jewish immigrants beginning in the 1880s had fled manifestations of European anti-Semitism and sought refuge and Jewish fulfilment in the 'Land of Israel'. New forms of settlement had been developed over the years, and certain regions had become a focus for the building of new communities. The Yishuv had developed its own political parties and quasi-government, labour union, school system, universities, Hebrew press, medical institutions, defence organizations as well as institutionalized bodies for dealing with finances, immigrant absorption and foreign affairs. Much of the ideological and social basis of Israeli society was laid during this pre-state period (Kaplan 2004).

Jews came to Israel in several different waves of immigration. Each wave had its own characteristics in terms of geographical origin, causes, dimensions, dominant ideas and achievements.

At the end of 2001, the population of Israel was officially reported to be 6 369 300. Of these, 77.8% (5 180 600) are Jews and 22.2% (1 188 600) are Arabs and others (Israel in Figures 2001). The population of Israel is now about 7 times larger than when the state was established in 1948. From 1955 to 1996, the Jewish population in Israel increased 2.9 times and the Arab population and others 5.6 times. During the period 1990 to 1995, 685 683 people immigrated to Israel (increasing the population by 14%): 87% of them came from Russia and 4.5% from Ethiopia (Statistical Abstract of Israel 1996). At the end of 2001 the Jewish population of 5 180 600 comprised: 61.9% born in Israel, 10.7% born in Asia and Africa, 27.4% born in Europe and America (Israel in Figures 2001). Between 1990 and 2004, 1 117 000 people immigrated to Israel (Statistical Abstract of Israel 2004).

Israel is unique in its official and long-standing encouragement of Jewish immigration. This openness to immigration has remained consistent even in times of economic stress and crises. As a result, Jews have continued to arrive from all over the world to settle in Israel. Naturally, the percentage of 'sabras' or native-born Israelis was relatively low when the state was established, reaching only 35.4% in late 1948. With time, the percentage of Israeli-born 'sabras' in society increased, and in recent years it has levelled off at just over 61%.

The new immigrants of the early years came from two main sources. Many were Holocaust survivors, most of whom were broken and passive, with few demands on the state. They wanted a shelter and were generally grateful for whatever they found. Most of the other immigrants were very different, however. They came from the Arab world – North Africa and the Middle East; while they made few demands on the new society they were migrating to, they certainly had expectations. These Jews were predominantly religious, holding conservative ideas regarding the character of a Jewish state; their family structure and way of life were traditional. The new wave of immigration during 1990–2000 from Russia and other parts of the former Soviet Union and from Ethiopia is unique (Delbar 1999) and will be discussed later in case studies 4 and 5.

The effect of a large number of immigrants ('olim') on a small society has been highly significant socially, economically and culturally. The need to absorb the newcomers placed a heavy burden on the young state, although once integrated, the immigrants contributed to a considerable economic growth of the country. Immigrants brought with them their values and traditions, and these in turn have influenced the emerging society in Israel.

In so far as these immigrant groups came from various geographical locations, spoke different languages, possessed diverse cultural values and maintained separate organizational frameworks, they resembled the phenomenon of ethnic groups. However, unlike the ethnic groups of modern immigrant societies, these 'edot' (communities) or ethnic subgroups also had much in common with the veteran Jewish residents. They were all Jewish. In addition, most had experienced manifestations of anti-Semitism such as discrimination, persecution and violent attacks (Kaplan 2004).

'EDOT' (COMMUNITIES OR ETHNIC SUBGROUPS)

Jewish communities were formed outside Israel for hundreds of years. In the Middle Ages, important Jewish centres were to be found in Babylonia, Spain and Franco-Germany. As members of a social and religious minority exposed to the cultural influences of the majority population, Jews took on certain elements of the local culture. They also created social patterns that suited the reality in which they lived. As a matter of course, Jews residing in different lands and living under different social, cultural and religious conditions developed different customs, manners and cultural expressions. These Jewish 'ethnic subgroups' are referred to in Israel as 'Edot'. They are characterized by a particular place of origin (e.g. Yemen) and a distinct culture which can include dress, cuisine, song, dance, crafts, religious traditions, language and even Hebrew pronunciation. Generally, 'Edot' are classified into one of the following categories.

ASHKENAZIM

These Jews are the descendants of the medieval Jewish communities in Franco-Germany. During the latter part of the Middle Ages, many Jews from this area moved eastward into Poland and other eastern European territories. Groups of orthodox Ashkenazi Jews came to Israel in the late eighteenth and early nineteenth centuries to form communities of Torah scholars in the holy cities of Jerusalem, Hebron, Safed and Tiberias. Large numbers of Russian Jews left for safer and more promising shores after the beginning of a period of pogroms (anti-Semitism manifested as persecution, and violent attacks) in the early 1880s. While most of these immigrated to the United States, Canada, Argentina and other countries, a small stream of ideologically motivated pioneers chose to live in Turkey, or, after 1917, in the British ruled Palestine. Here, they became the majority of the Jewish population, comprising some 80% of the Jewish settlement in 1948 (Kaplan 2004).

The epic immigration of Jews from the former Soviet Union during 1989–1992 brought 380 152 immigrants to Israel, swelling the country's population by nearly 10% (Statistical Abstract of Israel 1993). In 1999, a second epic immigration of Jews from the former Soviet Union brought 77 000 immigrants (Statistical Abstract of Israel 2004).

SEPHARDIM

These Jews trace their ancestry back to the Jewish population of medieval Spain. Following the persecution of Spanish Jews in the late fourteenth and fifteenth centuries, and their expulsion from the kingdom in 1492, these Jews settled in major ports and economic centres in Europe, the Middle East and even the New World. A centre of Sephardi Jews emerged in the Galilee town of Safed in the sixteenth century. Although Sephardi Jews, like their Ashkenazi brethren, came in limited numbers to live in the Holy Land throughout history, larger numbers of Sephardi Jews (e.g. from Bulgaria and Turkey) came to Israel only after its establishment in 1948).

ORIENTAL JEWS

Generally, Jews from Arab or Muslim countries (North Africa, the Middle East, Iran, Afghanistan and the Muslim republics of the former Soviet Union) are considered Oriental or Eastern Jews. A large wave of Jews from these areas came to Israel in the 1950s. As noted above, at the time of the establishment of the state of Israel, Ashkenazim made up about 80% of the Jewish population. Due to the large influx of Oriental Jews during the first decade of the state and their higher fertility rate, the percentage of Oriental Jews increased consistently until in 1965 they comprised the majority of Israeli Jewry. This trend was altered with the immigration of Jews from the former Soviet Union in the 1990s. Using the criterion of father's birthplace, as of December 1993, 39.9% of Israeli Jews were of European and American origin (Ashkenazim for the most part), 36.3% were of Asian or African origin (essentially Oriental Jews) and 23.8% were of Israeli origin. It would appear, at present, that there is a numerical balance between Ashkenazim and Oriental Jews (Kaplan 2004).

ETHIOPIAN JEWS

The population of Ethiopian residents in Israel is 80 000 (Almaya 2004). Most Ethiopian residents arrived in Israel as a group of 50 000 people during 1991 on Operation Solomon, which was organized due to the deteriorating political and economic situation in Ethiopia at the time. Those Jews had lived in rural northern Ethiopia for centuries. They were distinguished from their neighbours by their religious practices and codes of conduct, which allowed them to maintain their Jewish identity, even in difficult periods. The supportive extended family was the most meaningful social unit for Ethiopian Jews, extending its influence to all life spheres. The transition from a traditional Ethiopian society to an urban Israeli one has proven difficult for many Ethiopian immigrants. Although it has been twenty years since the beginning of immigration from Ethiopia, most of the community is still living in poverty. They continue to face difficulties in job training, and in finding suitable occupations (Levine-Rozalis 2004). This is also reflected by their various health problems in Israel and the transcultural coping strategies chosen to overcome them (Delbar 1999).

NON-JEWISH MINORITIES: ARAB CITIZENS

Israel's non-Jewish population is differentiated religiously, socially, culturally and nationally from the Jewish majority. Over 75% of Israeli non-Jews are Muslims, the rest being Christians, Druze and a few other smaller groups. The Muslims and the vast majority of the Christian Arabs are Palestinian Arabs who hold Israeli citizenship and have integrated considerably into the Israeli Western culture, but at the same time they also share feelings of solidarity with their Palestinian brethren outside Israel's borders. Among the Muslims, trends of Islamic fundamentalism have become more pronounced in recent years. It is very difficult for Arabs in Israel to accept the basic definition of Israel as a Jewish state and the reflection of this in the country's national symbols such as the national anthem, the flag, Remembrance Day for Fallen Soldiers, Independence Day and the Law of Return (Kaplan 2004).

THE NEGEV BEDOUIN – A SEMI-NOMADIC SOCIETY IN TRANSITION

The Negev, two-thirds of Israel's land area, contains 7% of the nation's population, 23% of whom are Bedouin Arabs. In 1996 the population of the Negev Bedouin Arabs was officially reported to be 88 300 (Statistical Abstract of Israel 1996). Before the state of Israel was established in 1948, it was estimated that there were between 50 000 and 70 000 Bedouin Arabs in the Negev. During the Independence war in 1948, many Bedouin left the area for Egypt and Jordan, becoming Palestinian refugees. Approximately 11 000 remained and became Israeli citizens (Marx 1981).

Bedouin Arabs have been in the Negev since the sixth century after Christ, having migrated from the Arabian Peninsula. Until recently, Negev Bedouin Arabs were a semi-nomadic population making their living herding sheep, goats and camels, and growing winter barley and wheat. Like numerous nomadic societies worldwide, the Israeli Negev Bedouin have been undergoing far-reaching transitions in recent decades. Some of these changes have been voluntary and spontaneous, others non-voluntary, having originated from the interrelationships between this minority group and the state government.

In the late 1940s some of the 11 000 Bedouin were relocated to a military-governed enclosure (known as the 'SEIG', occupying a region in the northern Negev desert). The rest of the Bedouin population remained on its lands. As a consequence of this relocation, some Bedouin tribes became landless (Ben-David 1986). Numerous tiny hamlets began to form within the SEIG during the 1950s and 1960s. These hamlets consisted of wooden barracks and tin shacks that replaced the traditional movable tent. Many of these were hastily erected on government-owned land, creating a conflict with the government over issues of ownership.

Consequently, the government began a programme of semi-urbanization consisting of seven planned towns designed to accommodate the entire Bedouin population (Meir & Ben-David 1989a).

THE SOCIO-ECONOMIC GAP

As noted earlier, immigrants from Asia and Africa during the 1950s began their life in Israel at a considerable social and economic disadvantage compared to the veteran Ashkenazi population. While a large proportion of the latter seized the opportunities offered by the mass migration to move from the working to the middle class, the new immigrants, lacking marketable skills, advanced education and connections with the authorities, had to accept lower paying jobs, often in marginal neighbourhoods and settlements which offered little economic promise. The effect of this was compounded by the fact that Oriental Jews tended to have large families. In many homes, parents were unable to provide the necessary educational support and assistance for their children, who lacked the space and resources needed for study. As a result, the first generation of Israeli-born Jews of Asian and African parents also grew up under disadvantaged circumstances.

Sadly, the socio-economic gap of the 1950s continued into the 1970s. This gap can be seen in the areas of income, occupational distribution, education and social influence.

NARROWING THE GAP

The continuing socio-economic gap led to violent outbreaks in the Moroccan populated Wadi Salib quarter of Haifa in July 1959 and to demonstrations by Oriental Jews who formed the Israeli Black Panthers in Jerusalem during the early 1970s. In the following years, head start programmes, integration in the schools alongside special classes for educationally disadvantaged students, leadership programmes, neighbourhood renewal (which built up the infrastructure of disadvantaged neighbourhoods through the cooperation of local residents), government housing assistance for young couples, research into the history and culture of Oriental Jewish communities as well as increased participation of Oriental Jews in politics led to a considerable narrowing of the socio-economic gap. No less important was the increasing social acceptance of Oriental Jews among young Israelis as evidenced by 'mixed' Oriental–Ashkenazi marriages. In 1968–1969, 17.4% of all first marriages in Israel were mixed, and this figure rose to 20.3% in 1980. By the 1990s, roughly a quarter of all new marriages were mixed (Kaplan 2004).

NARROWING THE GAP: THE NEGEV BEDOUIN

Currently, all seven Negev Bedouin towns are in various stages of development, the largest (Rahat) having a population of about 25 000. However, after three decades, only about 50% of the Bedouin have moved to towns, whereas another 40% still live in hamlets and the remainder are semi-nomadic (Meir & Ben-David 1989a, 1989b, Avicenne Initiative 1998,

Delbar 1999). In 1992 the Galilee Society (GS – the Arab National Society for Health Research and Services) commenced its activities in the Negev, following a measles outbreak which caused the death of nine Arab Bedouin infants in the unrecognized villages (Galilee Society 2004).

HEALTHCARE SERVICES IN ISRAEL

The healthcare system in Israel is now in the midst of a long process of reform, planning for which began in 1994, in both concepts and services. This process began only recently, after many years of political and professional debate, and comprises three main components:

- the National Health Insurance Law
- the withdrawal of the government from healthcare provision
- the reorganization of the Ministry of Health.

In June 1994, the Knesset passed a National Health Insurance Law. Under the new law, all residents of Israel must be insured by one of the authorized sickness funds that operate in the country. The funds must provide the basic package of services defined by the law. The National Insurance Institution (NII) handles the centralized collection of health insurance premiums and allocates resources to the various sickness funds according to a capitation formula. Every insured person has the right to choose his or her sickness fund. Each fund is obliged to accept any resident of Israel as an insured member, regardless of age or physical or mental condition (National Health Insurance Law 1994).

Since this process began only recently, the Ministry of Health still owns and operates 23% of the general hospitals, 50% of the mental hospitals and 4% of the geriatric hospitals. The remainder are non-profit or profit-making institutions. In the new system, the government hospitals have become self-financing non-profit institutions. In the future the Ministry of Health will continue to supervise and control hospitals, but not to run them. The Ministry will continue to be responsible for the following areas: developing policy, long-term planning, setting of standards, monitoring quality of services, and collecting and evaluating essential data.

OUTPATIENT HEALTH CARE

At the community level, primary health care is given in the following locations:

- sickness fund clinics
- hospital outpatient clinics and emergency rooms
- private clinics
- family health centres, which provide preventive health services.

In general, the sickness funds operate primary health care in Israel. Each fund organizes the ambulatory services through its clinics and physicians, or through purchased services. Each person is free to choose any physician, or specialist affiliated to the sickness fund. Usually an affiliated physician does not receive fees per visit from the patient, but a salary or reimbursement from the sickness fund.

Currently, some family health centres are still operated by the government, whilst the rest are operated by local authorities or sickness funds, according to an agreed geographical division. Israel has a network of these centres throughout the country. About 1000 are located in urban areas, and a public healthcare nurse visits small and peripheral localities at least once every two weeks. The services provided consist of physicians' examinations, developmental examinations, monitoring of breast-feeding, vaccination and the provision of guidance and advice to mothers. Local authorities are responsible for the provision of healthcare services for schoolchildren, which are funded by the parents (Rosen & Goldwag 2004).

The following sections examine some health issues in three cultural subgroups.

HEALTH PERSPECTIVES OF ETHIOPIAN IMMIGRANTS

Ethiopian immigrants visit traditional healers practising in Israel because they share the same cultural perceptions and beliefs regarding health and illness and therefore believe these healers can help them to solve their various health problems.

The treatments offered vary according to the type of healer and the patient's problem. Some of the healers have adapted their techniques to their new surroundings.

Often, different healing methods are combined. Herbal medicines are prepared to drink, to apply as an ointment mixed with butter, to inhale, or to put or sprinkle in a sick person's home. Scriptures prepared by a Dabtara (an unordained cleric) and amulets blessed by different healers are included in many treatments. Sick people may be instructed to move their place of residence to a more favourable one or to refrain from certain activities on specific unfavourable dates. Bathing in healing waters for a pre-established number of days, which was successful for many illnesses in Ethiopia, is also recommended in Israel (Delbar 1999). Because a large number of illnesses are believed to be caused by offending the Zar spirits, their cure will begin once the affected person and his family begin taking daily care of the Zar spirit. This includes performing the 'buna' (coffee) ceremony, burning incense, and taking other precautions. If the illness was caused by an important transgression, a special Zar ceremony is necessary. This is a big event with the participation of a balazar (Ba'al-Zar, meaning 'master of the strange'), which also includes the sacrifice of a sheep and the offering of gifts to the offended Zar spirit so that he will pardon the offender, thus enabling the cure of his illness. Ethiopian immigrants often use both medical systems simultaneously since illness can be due to a combination of natural and supernatural factors. Therefore, the Western doctor in the clinic can cure a wound and at the same time the traditional healer can deal with its supernatural cause (Delbar 1999).

Attitudes towards modern preventive treatments and Ethiopian parents' perception of their children's health have been studied by Ben-Natan (2000), who investigated the limited compliance of Ethiopian immigrants with modern preventive treatments. Twenty Ethiopian mothers of young children were interviewed. The findings indicated that the mothers can be divided into three different groups, regarding their knowledge of the language, learning a trade and finding a job, variables attesting to the extent to which an immigrant has become integrated in a new country. The findings of the study indicate that the subjects' integration in Israeli society affected their exposure to 'Western' thought processes in general and to 'Western' medicine in particular, and these affected their perceptions regarding disease prevention. The subjects who were more integrated in Israeli society adopted 'Western' preventive behaviours; in contrast, those who were poorly integrated in Israeli society adhered to the principles of traditional medicine.

HEALTH PERSPECTIVES OF FORMER SOVIET UNION IMMIGRANTS

Remennick (1999) examined the risk profile and preventive practice aimed at female reproductive cancer in a national sample of 620 women aged over 35 who immigrated to Israel from the former Soviet Union after 1989. The study setting typifies a more general problem of the encounter between eastern European immigrants and Western type health cultures and medical systems. It has shown that universal access to preventive care may not translate into its optimal utilization among marginalized population groups. Specifically, while being at moderate to high cancer risk, former Soviet Union immigrants avoid screening activities, gynaecological check-ups, breast examination and mammography. This is a reversal of the pre-emigration pattern: two-thirds of responders underwent cancer screening in their home country and only one-third in Israel. The risk groups for late detection of cancer are the women least integrated into the mainstream society: those over 60, unemployed or having unskilled jobs. Women without regular primary care providers showed the lowest cancer awareness and minimal screening activity. Even those who knew the key cancer facts and the benefits of early detection, in practice did little to avert the danger.

Three explanations for the discrepancy between cognition and practice are suggested: (a) the immigrants' low health motivation, reflecting their downward social mobility and preoccupation with resettlement problems; (b) low self-efficacy and external locus of control over health, typical of ex-Soviet citizens; and (c) communicative and other cultural barriers to healthcare services. This study adds to the evidence which links the difficulties immigrants face when trying to adapt and settle in the host country to negative effects on health (Papadopoulos et al 2004).

HEALTH PERSPECTIVES OF THE ISRAELI BEDOUIN ARABS

The Bedouin are religious Muslims who often combine the use of modern medicine with traditional preventive and curative medicine because they believe that each fulfils different needs. This approach results from the Bedouin perspective that illness can be due to a combination of natural and supernatural factors related to their religion and their culture. The healer (the 'darwish') is a religious learned man. Herbal medicines, music therapy, the reading of the Qur'an, and scriptures blessed by different healers are included in many treatments. Because a large number of illnesses are believed to be caused by offending religious rules, their cure will begin once the affected person and his family begin taking daily care of their religious duties. Combating the 'evil eye' is the duty of a grandmother, who will take three small pieces of alum (an aluminium compound) and will throw them into the fire; as the compound melts, she studies its shape and decides the origin of the evil eye. Once removed from the fire the shaped alum is placed in the tent for several minutes before it is crushed in the grandmother's hands; the ceremony is concluded when she circulates her hands several times around the affected person whilst praying to God to heal the sick person (Abu-Rabia 1983, Bailey & Danin 1981, Bailey 1982).

Access to health services for the Arab Bedouin has improved since the establishment of the Galilee Society (GS) in 1992. They began operating a mobile primary healthcare clinic in 1995. The clinic provides immunizations to Arab Bedouin infants and children in the 'unrecognized' villages, and mother and child care, as well as conducting core professional activities in the fields of education, and awareness in the fields of general health care (in conjunction with local professionals and community members). In 2001 the Ministry of Health established six permanent mother and child clinics in the 'unrecognized' villages and Ben-Gurion University Faculty of Health and the Galilee Society have been successful in reaching the Bedouin population (Delbar 1999, Galilee Society 2004).

Mortality rates have declined considerably among the Bedouin (Al-Krenawi et al 2001a, Meir & Ben-David 1989a, 1989b, Avicenne Initiative 1998, Weitzman et al 2000). However, the health services for the Bedouin still suffer from inadequate deployment of facilities and insufficient intercultural communication between medical staff and Bedouin patients (Al-Krenawi 2001, Al-Krenawi et al 2001b, Israel Cancer Association 2004, Meir & Ben-David 1989a, 1989b, Weitzman et al 2000)

This problem is further aggravated since marriages between first cousins are common in this traditional society, resulting in a high rate of fetal abnormalities (Weitzman et al 2000). The inferior status of Bedouin women, who are not allowed to approach the services independently, is also causing relatively high morbidity rates amongst children and women, low use of prenatal testing for fetal abnormalities and late breast cancer diagnosis. Bedouin women in Israel are not benefiting from the national early detection programme provided through breast cancer screening (Al-Krenawi 2001, Al-Krenawi et al 2001b, Israel Cancer Association 2004, Meir & Ben-David 1989a, 1989b, Weitzman et al 2000).

PATIENT CASE STUDIES

The term Israeli Jew or citizen represents a broad and diverse group of people with different origins and backgrounds. Therefore, it is important to be cautious in generalizing about health beliefs of Israeli citizens because numerous variables interact to influence their health practices.

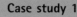

Case study 1

Mr DD was born in Israel 45 years ago to parents who emigrated from Germany after the Holocaust. He is an Ashkenazi, and works as a professor in a well-known university. He had a myocardial infarction 3 months ago. He joined a rehabilitation group, a relaxation therapy group, and a supportive group together with his wife. He searched for information on the internet, and then discussed it with his doctors. He is willing to change his lifestyle, since he is now convinced this was partly the cause of his health problem.

Mr DD believes in the biomedical model but also seeks alternative techniques and diets, which are very popular nowadays in Israel amongst the upper classes. 'He is a very compliant patient', reports the nurse in charge of the rehabilitation programme with satisfaction. 'He keeps a diary of his daily activity, attends his medical appointments, he stopped smoking, walks every day at least for an hour, has consulted our dietician and keeps a low cholesterol diet; one can see the results in his blood tests, it is really nice to have such a patient.' The nurse herself was born in Israel 30 years ago, to parents who emigrated from the USA 35 years ago; she is also an Ashkenazi in her ethnic origin. She has just finished her postgraduate studies and is aware that Mr DD's response to his illness is normative in a Western modern society. As long as Mr DD is cooperative with his rehabilitation programme, it is acceptable for him to use some alternative therapeutic options. The nurse knows that the larger and more complex the society in which the person is living, the more likely they are to exhibit medical pluralism (Papadopoulos et al 1998). Helman (1994) stated that within pluralist societies there are many groups or individuals, each offering the patient their own particular way of explaining, diagnosing and treating ill health.

Case study 2

Mrs CD was admitted to the oncology ward two weeks ago because of intolerable back pain; she was diagnosed with stage 4 invasive breast cancer. She was born in Israel in 1949. Her grandparents emigrated from Morocco in 1914. She is married, and has five children. One of them died from an acute illness (she could not name it) 25 years ago. Two of her daughters are married and have children. Mrs CD lives with her husband and two children aged 16 and 14 in a small flat in an ultraorthodox community in Jerusalem.

On hearing the bad news, Mrs CD immediately said: 'It's God's will' and after a while she said: 'It's the work of the evil eye'. The nurse was surprised because Mrs CD seemed to accept that her condition was both God's will or fate, and the result of the evil eye. She later asked Mrs CD to explain why she thought her illness was brought about by the evil eye. Mrs CD explained that 25 years ago she had had a big argument with her sister-in-law and had not spoken to her since. During that argument the sister-in-law had cursed her family. But now Mrs CD wanted her forgiveness because she believed in her magical powers; she needed her blessing to recover. The nurse who assessed the situation was sensitive to the cultural impact of the blessing for life and death and telephoned the sister-in-law, who arrived as soon as she could to give her blessing.

Since her diagnosis Mrs. CD has been surrounded by her family, who are praying constantly with her. For the ultraorthodox Jew, the family is the main source of support for both physical and emotional needs in the presence of illness. The traditional family is large. Decision-making about healthcare issues becomes a family matter as well as a religious matter; thus the involvement of a rabbi is very common (Al-Krenawi et al 2001a). Religion is very important to Mrs CD's community. This is expressed in the belief that God's will or fate controls life and health, and divine hope can overcome any eventuality. Religious Jews are more likely than non-religious Jews to believe strongly that illness is a matter of chance or fate and that the ability to recover faster or sooner from an illness is a matter of luck.

Even though Mrs CD's grandparents' emigration was more than 60 years ago, she seems to retain common Moroccan health beliefs that are deeply rooted in her original environment, emphasizing the power of the evil eye (Ben-Ami 1984, Kosansky 2001, Zaga et al 2003).

Very religious women in Israel, like Mrs CD, are not benefiting from the national early detection programme provided through breast cancer screening. Factors that prevent this in this population include the taboo of discussing certain female parts of the body with others, involving a male rabbi consultation in this matter, and the possible physical contact with male healthcare providers. Heler (2002) recommended that there is a need to prepare for encounters between medical caregivers and leading rabbis of ultraorthodox communities to promote screening and preventive medicine.

Case study 3

Mr MY is a 28-year-old Israeli Bedouin living 30 km from Beer-Sheva town with his tribe. He is married and has six children. He suffers from end-stage kidney disease and was advised to start CAPD (continuous ambulatory peritoneal dialysis) treatment. His family seems to be very close and supportive. He was admitted to the nephrology day-care unit to consider this treatment.

Mr MY inhabits a tent in the desert. He is an intelligent man with a formal education of 8 years; he works as a tractor driver on his farm. Mr MY understands the treatment and its side effects, but his doctor questions whether he can deal with the CAPD while living in a tent with no running water, adequate hygiene facilities, or privacy. The dilemma is whether to isolate this young man from his family and hospitalize him three times a week for haemodialysis or to try to improvise for CAPD in his tent. The social isolation far away from his village, which is located in the middle of the desert, with no regular transportation could also be very traumatic for him and for his family.

Mr MY's way of life and that of other chronically ill patients like him led to the establishment of a special healthcare unit for the Bedouin. This unit consists of a nurse and a social worker who are the link between the Bedouin, the Soroka Medical Centre and a pharmaceutical company which agreed to supply and deliver all the equipment regularly. These health workers drive into the desert three times a week with no exact addresses but descriptions of locations. Their job is to control the patients' symptoms and needs. The health team – nurses and social workers in this special unit – have to assess and decide when to teach the patient to be his own agent and when to teach his wife. For example, a sick man will never take care of his elimination needs by himself. He will never deal with continuous ambulatory peritoneal dialysis (CAPD) or a colostomy. It is not dignified. In this case the wife will be the care agent.

Mr MY is fortunate to be male. In the case of a young woman, her destiny will not be the same. Most likely her husband will take a second wife and she would return to her parents' family for support. If she were older she would have been cared for very warmly by her children. The strict tradition, and the status of Bedouin women, who are not allowed to approach the services independently, continues to cause relatively high morbidity rates among children and women (Al-Krenawi et al 2001b, 2001c, Delbar 1999, Heler 2002).

Case study 4

RT, aged 13, was diagnosed with diabetes three weeks ago. He has seven brothers and sisters and lives in the small immigrant town of Netivot. He was born in Ethiopia and immigrated to Israel in 1991. RT was admitted to the hospital with complaints of changes in bowel movements and eating habits, and weight loss. He started his treatment of insulin and appropriate diet in hospital and was discharged to his home after 5 days of hospitalization with a letter to his community clinic for further treatment. RT's illness reflects an increasing rate of diabetes incidence among Ethiopian children in Israel. One of the theories for this increase is the change in nutrition habits after immigration (Laron et al 1994, 'SATBA'-Diabetes incidence registry 2002, Shamis et al 1997, JDC 2004).

A week later RT was admitted again to the department with severe diarrhoea and hyperglycaemia. His mother had not implemented the recommended treatment. An Ethiopian translator assisted the medical team in understanding what had happened during the previous week. His mother had consulted a 'balazar', a traditional healer, who explained that his illness was provoked by a Ganal or Satan. His mother began a traditional treatment for him, which included herbal medicines and a visit to cold healing waters for a period of 7 days. The aim of it was to force the Ganal to abandon his body. Furthermore, the healer also explained that RT's ailments were due to a combination of two factors. In the first place they were living in a city, which according to 'The book' of his reference is not appropriate for his star Kokav. Second, in the small apartment where he and his family live, his mother had not set up a coffee tray to honour her Zar spirit.

This made Zar very angry, and he is punishing the family by making their son sick. The healer recommended that they move to another city and have a Zar ceremony to appease the angry Zar spirit. Under the circumstances, his mother could comply with only some of the healer's recommendations, which frustrated both her and her family, and she had to be taught sensitively to comply also with the treatment prescribed by the hospital (Delbar 1999, Ravid & Spitzer 1995).

TRAINING IMMIGRANT NURSES FROM THE FORMER SOVIET UNION

Case study 5

Mrs ND is a 50-year-old married woman who has worked for 32 years as an injections nurse (a common role for nurses who were trained especially for this function in the Soviet Union) in an oncology department in the former Soviet Union. Mrs ND has applied for a nursing job in an oncology day care department in Israel.

An unprecedented immigration wave of doctors and nurses to Israel, mainly from the former Soviet Union, between the years 1990 and 1995, and again in 1999, required a programme to induct these migrant health workers into the Israeli healthcare system and acceptable practice. The programme included an effort to provide every newcomer with an opportunity to thrive as much as possible in his or her profession. The National Licensing Examination (NLE) is required by Israeli law to be taken by all foreign graduates in order to assure quality within the healthcare system.

A 6-month programme, which was further expanded to 18 months, was launched in 1991 by the Recanati School of the Health Professions supported by the government of Israel. The programme was designed to provide effective responses to the specific problems of the immigrant population, who were lacking knowledge of the local language, whose professional specializations were often too narrow, who were in possession of nursing specialties (as injection nurse for example) that do not exist in Israel, who were insufficiently updated in medical and nursing sciences and technology, who were lacking awareness of the economic implications of health care and had difficulties in originating new nursing solutions to clinical problems.

This nursing programme was characterized by a protective environment, problem-oriented learning (both theoretical and clinical), small-group activities, and an emphasis on learning Hebrew and English. The clinical problems used in both the classroom and field are designed to emphasize the general nurse practitioner's role. The programme has achieved it goals, as judged by the success rate in the National Licensing Examination. From 1991 to 1999, approximately 250 registered nurses have participated in this programme in the Negev region alone (Delbar 1999, Nirel et al 1996, Romem & Benor 1993).

SUMMARY

Israeli society in the early twenty-first century is struggling toward a collective identity, caught in a web of internal tensions and contradictions. It is constantly moving, changing and developing. Therefore, it is important to be cautious in generalizing about health beliefs of Israeli citizens because numerous variables interact to influence their health practices.

In hospitals, clinics and other places where patients live, receive treatment, work or relax, there is a network of cultural factors that plays an important role in the well-being of patients. Several factors have been reported to affect immigrants' adjustments such as pre immigration problems, and the cultural gap between the country of origin and host country. Additional factors include a drop in professional status with its negative impact on self-esteem, loss of familial environment, language and people, and the emotional level of identification with the host culture and its values (Scott & Scott 1989, Shuval 1982). A recent study by Anson et al (1996) showed that the first 3 years after immigration to Israel were associated with inferior physical and psychosocial well-being as well as poor family functioning and social interaction but, with time, the differences between Israeli-born residents and immigrants tend to fade away.

Substantial proportions of doctors, nurses and other healthcare professionals are from different ethnic groups. The interaction between health providers and patients can prove frustrating for both sides and often this is blamed on cultural differences and difficulties in communication. The different cultural perspectives of patients and health providers often affect the nature and effectiveness of the health services.

These cultural effects can considerably complicate the assessment of how an individual will react to various aspects of the hospital environment, medical condition, treatment, staff, fellow patients, cure, rehabilitation and so on. Therefore cross-cultural sensitization is a necessary precondition to improving health services.

The whole sickness experience of patients should be considered. The health provider should relate not only to the disease organ, but also to the patient's own beliefs and feelings. The Israeli nursing code of ethics (Fogel 2004) states that preserving a person's dignity is a basic human right in life and in death. This code emphasizes the responsibility of nurses to protect the rights, values and beliefs of human beings and to give care according to their needs and the needs of their families without discrimination. However, the nursing core curriculum for licensing does not yet include transcultural competencies. Therefore the need to plan and support specific programmes that will train students in the skills necessary to give culturally competent nursing care is recommended. The evidence presented in this chapter makes the need to actively embrace transcultural nursing an imperative.

REFLECTIVE QUESTIONS

1. What are the unique causes and patterns of immigration to Israel?
2. Even though the causes and patterns of immigration to Israel are unique, can you find common health-related problems of immigrants, or ethnic subgroups worldwide?
3. This chapter illustrates some suggestions aimed at improving services to reach minority groups and ethnic subgroups' special needs; describe three of them.
4. The chapter deals with the professional and cultural issues related to healthcare workers who immigrate to a new country. Can you describe the reason for the special educational programme for healthcare practitioners who immigrated to Israel from the former Soviet Union?
5. Do you have any comments about the applicability of those educational programmes to healthcare practitioners who immigrated to your own country?

REFERENCES

Abu-Rabia A 1983 Traditional medicine versus modern medicine among Bedouin. Ben-Gurion University, The Desert Research Institution (in Hebrew)

Al-Krenawi A 2001 Women from polygamous and monogamous marriages in an out-patient psychiatric clinic. Transcultural Psychology 38(2):187–199

Al-Krenawi A, Graham J R, Ophir M, Kandah J 2001a Ethic and gender differences in mental health utilization: the case of Muslim Jordanian and Moroccan Jewish outpatient psychiatric patients. International Journal of Social Psychology 47(3):42–54

Al-Krenawi A, Graham J R, Izzeldin A 2001b The psychosocial impact of polygamous marriages on Palestinian women. Women and Health 34(1):1–16

Almaya 2004 Online. Available: http://www.almaya.org.il/beta.html 1 Nov 2004

Anson O, Pilpel D, Rolnik V 1996 Physical and psychological well-being among immigrant referrals to colonoscopy. Social Science and Medicine 43:1309–1316

Avicenne Initiative 1998 Evaluation and improvement of maternal and child preventive health resources and services to Bedouin Arabs in the Negev, Interim Report. Negev, Israel (in Hebrew)

Bailey C 1982 Bedouin religious practices in Sinai and the Negev. Anthropos 77:65–88

Bailey C, Danin A 1981 Bedouin plant utilization in Sinai and the Negev. Economic Botany 35:145–162

Ben-Ami I 1984 Saint veneration among the Jews in Morocco. The Magness Press, Jerusalem. (in Hebrew)

Ben-David Y 1986 The Negev Bedouin 1900–1960. Idan 6:81–99 (in Hebrew)

Ben-Natan M 2000 The limited compliance of Ethiopian immigrants with modern preventive treatments: The problem's foci, sources, extent and possible solutions. Tel-Aviv University, Faculty of Medicine, School of Health Professions, Department of Nursing (MN thesis in Hebrew)

Delbar V 1999 From the desert: transcultural aspects of cancer nursing care in Israel. Cancer Nursing 22:45–51

Fogel R 2004 Culture sensitivity of nursing students. Thesis submitted in partial fulfilment of the requirement for Master in Nursing, Ben-Gurion University of the Negev, The Faculty of Health Sciences, Leon, and Matilda Recanati School for Community Health Professions (in Hebrew)

Galilee Society 2004 Online. Available: http: www. gal-soc. org 12 Nov 2004

Heler H 2002 Early detection of breast cancer among the very religious community. Bamah-Journal of Health Professionals in the Field of Cancer 13:208–211

Helman C G 1994 Culture, health and illness. Butterworth Heinemann, London

Israel Cancer Association 2004 National breast cancer early detection program. Online. Available: http://www.cacer.org.il 12 Aug 2004

JDC-Brookdale Institute 2004 Health intervention program for Ethiopian immigrants in primary care clinic. Online. Available: http://www.jdc.org.il/brookheb/pages/briut-findings-rr-357–00-pa.htm 12 Sep 2004

Kaplan J 2004 The diversity of Israeli society. Online. Available: http://www.jafi.org.il/education/israel/culture.html 1 Nov 2004

Kosansky O 2001 Reading Jewish Fez: On the cultural identity of a Moroccan city. Journal of the International Institute. Online. Available: http: www.umich.edu/-iinet/journal/vol8no3/kosansky.htm 1 Jan 2001

Laron Z, Mansour T, Slepon R et al 1994 Incidence of diabetes mellitus in various population groups in 1989 and 1990. Israel Journal of Medical Science 30:770–774

Levine-Rozalis M 2004 Social representations: differences between the community of Ethiopian immigrants and the absorbing Israeli Society. Online. Available: http://www.almaya.org.il/beta.html 1 Nov 2004

Marx E 1981 Changes among the Bedouin. In: Berkovsky L, Faiman D, Gale J (eds) Setting the desert. Gordon & Breach, London, p 173–190

Meir A, Ben-David Y 1989a Changes in the status of Bedouin elders and their public implications. Submitted to the National Council for Research and Development, Ministry of Sciences and Technology. [research report in Hebrew]

Meir A, Ben-David Y 1989b Fertility behaviour among the Negev Bedouin. Israeli Academy of Sciences. [research report in Hebrew]

National Health Insurance Law 1994 Online Available: http://www.health.gov.il 1 Feb 2005

Nirel N, Rosen B, Gross R 1996 Immigration from the former Soviet Union: selected findings from a national employment survey. JDC-Brookdale Institute of Gerontology and Human Development, Jerusalem (in Hebrew)

Papadopoulos I, Lees S, Lay M, Gebrehiwot A 2004 Ethiopian refugees in the UK: migration, adaptation and settlement experiences and their relevance to health. Ethnicity and Health 9(1):55–73

Papadopoulos I, Tilki M, Taylor G 1998 Transcultural care. A guide for health care professionals. Quay Books, Dinton

Ravid C, Spitzer A 1995 Internal body perception of Ethiopians Jews who immigrated to Israel. Western Journal of Nursing Research 17(6):631–646

Remennick L I 1999 Preventive behavior among recent immigrants: Russian-speaking women and cancer screening in Israel. Social Science and Medicine 48(11):1669–1684

Romem Y, Benor D E 1993 Training immigrant doctors: issues and responses. Medical Education 27:74–82

Rosen B, Goldwag R 2004 Health care systems in transition, Israel 2003. Online. Available: http://www.who.dk./Countryinformation/Country?AreaCode=ISR 12 Nov 2004

Shamis I, Gordon O Albag Y et al 1997 Ethnic differences in the incidence of childhood IDDM in Israel (1965–1993) Diabetes Care 20:504–508

'SATBA'-Diabetes incidence registry, Israel 2002 Ethnic differences in the incidence of childhood IDDM in Israel. Israel Journal of Medical Science 141(9):789–791(in Hebrew)

Scott W, Scott R 1989 Adaptation of immigrants: individual differences and determinants. Pergamon, Oxford

Shuval J T 1982 Migration and stress. In: Goldberger L Breznitz S (eds) Handbook of stress: theoretical and clinical aspects. Free Press, New York, p 677–691

Statistical Abstract of Israel 1993 Central Bureau of Statistics, 44: 85–89, Jerusalem

Statistical Abstract of Israel 1996 Jerusalem National Statistic Office

Statistical Abstract of Israel 2004 Jerusalem National Statistic Office. Online. Available: http://www.cbs.gov.il 12 Aug 2004

Weitzman D, Shoham-Vardi I, Elbedour K et al 2000 Factors affecting the use of prenatal testing for fetal anomalities in a traditional society. Community Genetics 3:61–70

Zaga C, Delbar V, Farkash M, Cohen M 2003 Meningiomas and the evil: health and illness beliefs. Abstract, 7th Quadrennial Congress, European Association of Neuroscience Nurses, Copenhagen Denmark

Chapter **18**

Transcultural nursing: the way to prepare culturally competent practitioners in Australia

Akram Omeri

LEARNING OBJECTIVES

After reading this chapter you should be able to:
- discuss the nature of Australia's diversity including social, economic and cultural variations
- discuss the challenges faced by nurses, midwives and other health practitioners in provision of health and social care
- analyse cultural diversity and issues that influence health access and outcomes for people of culturally and linguistically diverse backgrounds (CLDB)

- identify the implications of multicultural policies for health and social care
- examine the major health and welfare issues as reported by the Australian Institute of Health and Welfare (AIHW 2004) and ways to promote culturally competent practice in health and social care
- understand the importance of utilizing knowledge and strategies to enhance delivery of culturally competent healthcare practice
- understand and address inequalities in the provision of health care in Australia and in contemporary nursing practice.

INTRODUCTION

Multiculturalism is a worldwide phenomenon. As multiculturalism grows so does the realization that traditional ideologies are no longer applicable or functional in dealing with health and social care in a changing world. In every part of the world, populations with new demographics and cultural milieus need to be redefined. Worldwide migration and cultural trends have given rise to a new world culture. This new culture phenomenon reflects diversity of values, beliefs and practices relating to health and social care, in every part of the world.

Contemporary philosophers and proponents of multiculturalism such as Jacques Derrida (1987, 1997a, 1997b, 2000), Deutcher (1998), Paul de Mon (cited in Ruffin 1991) and Michel Foucault (1976, 1980) challenge Eurocentric traditions. In spite of differences in interpretation of the term multiculturalism, the philosophical stance of Foucault, Derrida and de Mon highlights the significance of cultural knowledge as the basis for understanding and accepting the new and emerging cultures of the world (Omeri 1996).

The new world culture is characterized and underpinned by globalization, wars, poverty and fear of terrorism. Furthermore, diverse cultural groups are searching for cultural identity as well as demanding their rights to equal opportunity in humanistic and fair ways. One emerging characteristic of the new world culture is the obvious disparity in health and social care.

Nursing in multicultural Australia reflects the overall and deeply rooted monocultural ideology of the dominant culture, namely white Anglo-Saxon or, as it is more commonly called, Anglo-Australian. Reflected in day-to-day practices in health and social care, the influence of this ideology is evident in nurse education, research and administration. In essence the ideology reflects the biomedical and monocultural nature of contemporary Australian society (Bates & Linder-Pelz 1990, Martin 1978, Omeri 1996, Omeri & Ahern 1999, Omeri & Atkins 2002, Pittman & Rogers 1990). The nature of Australian society's cultural diversity creates an urgent need for healthcare professionals to examine their knowledge and attitudes relating to cultural diversity and its importance in education and practice. There is also a need for reconsideration of health and social policies in order to reduce disparities in health care and promote equal opportunity in health care, or, to use an Australian phrase, to enable a 'fair go for all'.

With the aim of examining issues and trends that impact upon the health and social well-being of people of culturally and linguistically diverse backgrounds, this chapter will identify barriers to transcultural nursing education, research, administration and practice in nursing, health and social care in Australia. In an attempt to encourage the discovery of pathways to advance culturally competent health and nursing practice, it raises questions that need to be answered by healthcare providers.

CULTURAL DIVERSITY AND POPULATION TRENDS IN AUSTRALIA

The diversity of Australia's population is evident in the most recent population Census statistics (Australian Bureau of Statistics (ABS) 2001). With a total population of 18 972 350 in 2001, nearly 22% were born overseas and 2.2% were identified as Indigenous, being of Aboriginal or Torres Strait Islanders origin. Changes in immigration patterns were also observed in this Census. The traditional source of immigrants, England, remained dominant; however, in 1996–1997, 31% of immigrants were born in Asia. The change in population mix is reflected in the languages spoken in the home other than English. The three most prominent after English were listed at that time as Chinese languages (2.1%), Italian (1.9%) and Greek (1.4%).

In Australia it has been the practice to distinguish immigrants according to whether their backgrounds are English speaking (ESB) or non-English speaking (NESB). In the face of increasing diversity and complexity in the immigrant population, it has been suggested that this classification may be too broad to be useful (Iredale & Nivison-Smith 1995), as it does not reflect the diverse linguistic backgrounds of an increasing proportion of immigrants.

A closer look at the complexities in Australian society is provided when immigrant populations are compared with the non-immigrant populations on social, demographic and economic indicators (ABS 2001, Castle et al 1998). Compiled from 2001 Census data, the proportion of immigrant males to females is estimated as equal, with 101 males to 100 females. Immigrants tend to concentrate in urban areas and have higher levels of home ownership than non-immigrants. NESB immigrants are more likely to be married to someone from the same cultural background and less likely to divorce. NESB immigrants tend to have higher fertility rates than either ESB immigrants or the non-immigrant population and are more likely to have dependent children. Mortality rates are lower for both ESB and NESB immigrants than for non-immigrants; NESB immigrants are less likely to experience illness, take medication or attend hospital in the immediate post-migration phase, which has been identified as being approximately the first 5 years (Castle et al 1998, Martin 1978, Reid & Trompf 1990).

A higher proportion of young immigrants than non-immigrants attend educational institutions. In 1992, 60% of NESB persons aged 15–24 years attended educational institutions compared with 50% of both ESB immigrants and non-immigrants. However, NESB persons tend to experience a disproportionate level of unemployment.

Immigration raises issues of social cohesion and social justice and fundamental concerns relating to the ultimate size and mix of Australia's population. The current policy of multiculturalism is intended to enhance and foster social integration and fairness, yet respect difference (Castle et al 1998). Its reach has not extended to the health system where monoculturalism remains dominant and disparities and inequalities in service provision remain.

MULTICULTURALISM AND RELATED POLICIES

ETHNIC HEALTH POLICY: ROOTS AND DIRECTIONS IN AUSTRALIA

A shift in community views and policy directions on ethnic relations has been in train since World War II (WWII). The shift has been away from Anglo-conformity (assimilation) to integration of the immigrant and related experiences arising during and following migration and settlement as a 'distinct set of experiences to be solved by government' (Martin 1978). More recent phenomena underpinning policy development are the concepts of multiculturalism and equity.

In recent decades three themes have come into prevalence in ethnic relations ideology and are reflected in ethnic health policy and the health and welfare service planning and allocation. The themes are social cohesion, cultural identity and social equality. In more recent times, the notion of 'productive diversity' predominates (Lewins 1984, cited in Reid & Trompf 1990, National Multicultural Advisory Council (NMAC) 1999). Productive diversity (PD) is a public policy that promotes and supports utilizing Australia's language and cultural diversity for the economic and social benefit of all Australians (Department of Immigration, Multicultural & Indigenous Affairs (DIMIA) 2003a) 'Benefits for all' is one of the four principal objectives of the Australian Government's multicultural policy (DIMIA 2003b).

Of the several waves of immigration since WWII the two most significant for ethnic health policy occurred just after WWII and after the Vietnam War. Health screening was the initial health policy response, designed to protect the Australian population from 'imported' diseases and to ensure a healthy immigrant population able to work and procreate. Covert and overt racial discrimination against refugees was rife at this time. By the 1980s health service programmes reflected more closely community needs and more recent arrivals were offered a broader range of health and welfare services. As ethnic affairs policy developed, debate on ethnic health policy changed (Garrett & Lin 1990).

The social reforms of the Whitlam government (Labour) in the 1970s were directed towards structural change to provide for greater equality and participation in community life of marginalized and disadvantaged groups including ethnic groups. A major change was the introduction of universal health insurance, which by removing financial barriers aimed to provide equal access to health services for all members of the community, including immigrants.

However, the Commission of Inquiry into Poverty (1973–75), known as the Henderson Report (Henderson 1975), found that immigrants were unable to use the health system effectively due to cultural differences being ignored and a lack of information. The report also brought into focus other aspects of social inequality experienced by NESB immigrants. These included: 12% with incomes below the poverty line; disadvantage in employment due to language barriers resulting in lower employment status and a disproportionate number in unskilled jobs where they tended to remain. Some of the recommendations made in the report included: grants for hostel care of those with a psychiatric illness; group homes; employment of ethnic staff in community health; and more bilingual educators in early childhood centres (Garrett & Lin 1990: 346).

Over the past 30 years in Australia, a range of multicultural policies have been developed and enacted which provide a guiding framework for dealing with cultural diversity. Two policy principles have become dominant in the national agendas: (1) access and equity; and (2) inclusiveness (Office of Multicultural Affairs (OMA) 1989, National Multicultural Advisory Council (NMAC) 1999). In practical terms, in the health and welfare sector the first principle translates into equality of access to services for all, and the second into the provision of culturally appropriate services to meet the needs of people from culturally and linguistically diverse backgrounds. In spite of these initiatives an integrated approach to meeting the health and nursing care needs of diverse groups has not evolved (NMAC 1999). There is a substantial gap between policy and practice, specifically nursing education and practice.

CRITIQUE OF MULTICULTURAL POLICIES

The failure of government policy to keep up with the cultural diversification of Australian society as a result of the post-war immigration programme was demonstrated by Martin (1978). She concludes that multiculturalism was never 'the cause' of policy change but a necessary response to cultural diversity. Castle et al (1998) write of change in the form of citizenship to accommodate the transnational backgrounds of many settlers in Australia and elsewhere. These authors recommended four fundamental objectives, one of which is to foster: 'multicultural citizenship and transnational belonging as a means of including permanent residents into the rights and obligations of citizenship' as a means of developing a fairer and more democratic society. Castle (1999) has argued that the policy of basing citizenship upon residence in Australia, and not on ethnicity or culture, is a major step in realizing this objective. He argues that a right to full participation, in all areas of society, is a crucial part of multicultural citizenship (Castle 1999: 39). For many immigrants, citizenship based upon actual societal membership irrespective of origins is still a long way off.

The problem with the policy of inclusiveness in Australia was that it reflected the early post-war notion of integrating ethnic groups into

Australian society to homogenize the population (Castle et al 1998). Integration policy was designed to avoid cultural change (Castle et al 1998) rather than accommodate it as the later multicultural polices were designed to do; the policy of integration was open to misinterpretation and, in the provision of health and welfare services, this could lead to cultural blindness, stereotyping and discrimination (Leininger & McFarland 2002).

The pitfall with policies of 'inclusiveness', in the Australian context, is that they tend to make all the same and reduce the significance of difference. As a consequence the aim to provide culture-specific nursing care congruent with the culture care needs of people is undermined together with the value of transcultural nursing practice.

HEALTH STATUS OF AUSTRALIANS

Overall, Australians enjoy one of the highest life expectancies in the world (WHO 2003). However, the health and social care of Indigenous people and immigrants, particularly those of culturally and linguistically diverse backgrounds and refugees, leaves much to be desired.

INDIGENOUS PEOPLE IN AUSTRALIA

In 2001 the population of Aborigines and Torres Strait Islanders, the Indigenous peoples of Australia, comprised 2.4% (458 520) of the total Australian population (Australian Institute of Health & Welfare 2004), with approximately 10% of Indigenous people of Torres Strait Islander origin. More than half of all Indigenous people live in Queensland and New South Wales. Most of the Indigenous population live in major cities and inner and outer regional areas, but 27% live in remote or very remote areas, compared with 2% of the non-Indigenous population.

The health status of the Indigenous population for all ages is much worse than that of non-Indigenous Australians. They are affected by Western lifestyle diseases (e.g. heart and respiratory diseases, diabetes and hypertension) in addition to those diseases common to developing countries, such as trachoma, malnutrition, anaemia, and chronic ear infections that result in hearing loss (AIHW 1990, National Aboriginal Health Strategy 1989, Omeri & Ahern 1999). Kidney disease is significantly more prevalent among Indigenous people than among non-Indigenous people.

The estimated life expectancy at birth for Aboriginal and Torres Strait Islander people is approximately 15–20 years less for men and women than the national average. For the period 1999–2001, the life expectancy at birth was estimated to be 56 years for Indigenous males, and 63 years for Indigenous females. In contrast, the life expectancy at birth for all Australians in 1999–2001 was 77 years for males and 82 years for females. Indigenous people suffer a much greater burden of ill health (AIHW 2004) together with obesity, smoking, drug and alcohol abuse, lower incomes than other Australians, poorer education and lower rates of home ownership (ABS 2003).

HEALTH OF IMMIGRANTS FROM CULTURALLY AND LINGUISTICALLY DIVERSE BACKGROUNDS (CLDB)

Health requirements for immigration ensure that migrants generally enjoy good health status known as the 'healthy migrant effect' (Young 1992). Immigrants often have lower death and hospitalization rates, as well as lower rates of disability and prevalence of certain lifestyle-related risk factors compared with the non-immigrant population (AIHW 2004). However, as the length of residence in Australia increases, the relative advantage that migrants have over Australian-born people tends to decrease (Young 1992).

The health status of refugees is a concern as they are the most disadvantaged compared with the rest of the community except for Indigenous Australians. Multiple factors contribute to their state of ill health. Some may have experienced torture and trauma prior to their entry to Australia, which can have a severe impact upon health and well-being.

Under Australia's Humanitarian Program some 12 000 places a year (a figure that has remained stable for some years) are available for people from refugee-like situations. The Humanitarian Program 2003–2004 has three categories. Broadly these are: refugees, those outside their own countries seeking to escape persecution; the special humanitarian category, for those seeking protection from violation of human rights; and the special assistance category for those with family connections in Australia who are in a vulnerable position in their own country. Australia also has a population of people who have attempted unauthorized entry to the country who are known as asylum seekers and for whom the government has made special provision outside the mainland of Australia. Some refugees and asylum seekers may be afforded temporary protection (TPV) (DIMIA 2002).

Diverse factors impact upon the health of refugees. Family tensions, marital difficulties, the uncertainty of living under TPV constraints, exacerbated by language, employment and other issues of daily living were linked to the process of migration by participants in a recent study of Afghan refugees (DIMIA 2002, Omeri et al 2004a, 2004b, 2005a, 2005b).

In this study, Omeri et al (2004a) identified barriers to accessing healthcare and support services by Afghan people. The main barriers were culturally based, including a lack of cultural knowledge relating to health and illness on the part of healthcare providers. This led to discriminatory and culturally incongruent healthcare services; lack of services and treatment modalities congruent with Islamic religious beliefs; and the need for health and other information in the Dari language and the dearth of Dari speaking interpreters.

ADVANCED NURSING PRACTICE IN AUSTRALIA: REFLECTIONS AND INTERPRETATIONS

In Australia, the term 'advanced nursing practice' has only recently begun to be defined and recognized (Jamieson & Williams 2002, Pearson & Peels 2002). Changes in the profession and the healthcare system have interfered with the development of the concept of advanced practice.

In the UK and the USA, advanced practitioners are required to be competent in clinical practice, research, teaching, consultancy and leadership. The minimum qualification is a Master's degree plus competence in an area of specialist practice (Pearson & Peels 2002).

The cost-effectiveness of the advanced practice role in care delivery is one of the issues raised by a number of authors (Byers & Burrell 1998, Schroeder et al 2000a, 2000b). The main issues, however, relate to measuring nurse competencies and standards of care, and the notion of nurse practitioners as doctor substitutes (Schroeder et al 2000b).

In Australia, Sutton & Smith (1995) differentiate between advanced nurse practitioners and expert and specialist nurses on the grounds that advanced nursing practice is based upon an holistic approach to care. They argue that the roles of expert and specialist nurses, on the other hand, are driven by technological developments and are dominated by the medical model of care.

National nursing organizations in Australia have developed 'position statements' on advanced nursing practice, with no apparent universally agreed definitions or guidelines. The Australian Nursing Council (ANC 2002a, 2002b), which has developed National Competency Standards for the registered and enrolled nurse, is yet to develop competencies for advanced nursing practice.

The Royal College of Nursing Australia (2002a: 2) position statement on 'Advanced practice nursing' states that: 'advanced practice nurses fulfil an essential function within the Australian health care system' and defines an advanced practice as: 'a level of nursing practice that utilizes extended and expanded skills, experience and knowledge in assessment, planning, implementation, diagnosis and evaluation of the care as required' (RCNA 2002a: 2). Experience, knowledge, skill and postgraduate educational preparation are recognized by the College as the essential basis for advanced practice, together with the capacity to demonstrate a list of qualities in practice recognized by the College as integral to the advanced nursing practice role (RCNA 2002a). The College also supports the principle of health as a right for all Australians. Integral to realizing this right the College expands cultural diversity beyond ethnicity, and advocates equality of access and appropriate health services (RCNA 2002c).

The International Council of Nurses (ICN) Health Policy Network have developed a definition and guidelines for standards of practice for advanced practice roles. These were formulated into a position statement designed to facilitate a common understanding of the role and to guide further development.

The ICN Position on Advanced Nursing Roles, published in October 2002, defines an advanced nurse practitioner/advanced practice nurse as: 'a registered nurse who has acquired the expert knowledge base, complex decision-making skills and clinical competencies for expanded practice, the characteristics of which are shaped by the context and/or country in which s/he is credentialed to practice. A Master's degree is recommended for entry level' (ICN 2002).

The National Review of Nurse Education (2002) and the guidelines issued by the ANC, RCNA, ANF and Nurses Registration Board of New

South Wales highlight a number of issues and challenges relating to advanced practice nursing and transcultural nursing care.

PREPARING NURSES FOR ADVANCED TRANSCULTURAL PRACTICE ROLES

The National Review of Nurse Education (2002) explored the ways in which multicultural health is currently addressed in nursing education in Australia at both the undergraduate and postgraduate levels. Strategies were recommended aimed at enhancing cultural competence in nursing including the need for a multicultural framework for nursing education. It also raised a number of related issues in respect of culturally competent nursing education such as: the potential impact of multicultural nursing education on nursing practice in a diverse nation; the need for a definition of culture in nursing education; and the diversity of interpretation of theoretical frameworks used in teaching and practice nationally and internationally.

Looking forward the review noted that the nurse of the future would be flexible and one who respects and understands different value systems and adapts to changing needs. Nurses of the future will engage: 'with cultural diversity as a core practice rather than an optional extra' (National Review of Nurse Education, Department of Education, Science and Training (DEST), Section 8 Conclusion 2002: 1).

The review identified the following questions that need to be answered in respect of advanced transcultural nursing care practice:

- Who are advanced transcultural nurses?
- What educational preparation is required for advanced transcultural nursing practice, beyond diversity and ethnospecific services?
- What commitments do faculties of nursing have to prepare advanced transcultural practice nurses?
- What are the implications of the diversities in definition, theory, and models of transcultural nursing for advanced transcultural nursing practice in Australia?
- What transcultural nursing care competencies are needed to meet the challenges of the 'productive diversity' as specified in the New Agenda for a multicultural Australia?
- What is the role of national nursing organizations in promoting advanced practice in transcultural nursing?

(The National Review of Nurse Education in Australia: Multicultural Nursing Education: Section 5.1 (2002) describes the Abrums & Leppa 2001 model for multicultural education.)

CULTURALLY COMPETENT PRACTICE: THE WAY FOR THE FUTURE

Leininger & McFarland (2002) argue that transcultural nursing underpins the discipline of nursing whilst culture-specific care knowledge is essential knowledge for the provision of culturally congruent and competent nursing care.

In emphasizing the importance of transcultural nurse specialists, Leininger wrote that, for this role, graduates need preparation in transcultural nursing in order to develop new knowledge or reconfirm existing knowledge; to communicate and disseminate knowledge in the discipline and apply knowledge in the care of people; to practise and consult other nurses in the care of people; and to give noteworthy leadership to advance transcultural nursing practices in order to improve care to people of different cultures (Leininger 1989a, 1989b).

Transcultural nurse specialists require in-depth knowledge of culture with a comparative focus on human care, health and the environmental context, and new, innovative and specific skills, to be able to provide such a level of care (Leininger 1989a, 1989b). Cultural care nursing assessment would be considered essential in the provision of culture-specific care for people of diverse cultural backgrounds.

Transcultural nursing has been defined as 'a formal area of study and practice focused on comparative human-care (caring) differences and similarities of the beliefs, values, and patterned lifeways of cultures to provide culturally congruent, meaningful, and beneficial health care to people' (Leininger & McFarland 2002: 5–6). Leininger & McFarland (2002) postulate that the theory of 'culture care diversity and universality' provides the substantive knowledge to know, explain, interpret, predict and legitimize nursing as a discipline and profession. Leininger also holds that: 'culture care knowledge could provide the truest knowledge base for culturally congruent care, so that people would benefit from and be satisfied with nursing care practices held to be healthy ways of serving them' (Leininger 1991: 36) and that: 'Care is the essence of nursing and the central, dominant, and unifying focus of nursing' (Leininger 1991: 36).

TRANSCULTURAL NURSING COMPETENCIES: GUIDE TO CULTURAL SENSITIVITY AND AWARENESS

The issues of defining what cultural competence is and how it may be achieved and maintained are in need of urgent attention by the nursing profession. The two concepts culture and competence are brought together in the term cultural competence. Culture encompasses the values, beliefs, traditions customs actions, belief systems of a racial, ethnic, religious or social group. Competence implies a capacity to function effectively within a context. The term cultural competence therefore implies the capacity to work effectively within an integrated pattern of behaviour as described by a designated group, community or an institution. There are a number of definitions of cultural competence and some are given below.

Papadopoulos (2003: 5) defines cultural competence as: 'the capacity to provide effective healthcare taking into consideration people's cultural beliefs, behaviours and needs. . . . cultural competence is the synthesis of a lot of knowledge and skills which we acquire during our personal and professional lives and to which we are constantly adding'.

Papadopoulos et al (1998: 178) describe the four stages of the transcultural skills development model as: cultural awareness, cultural knowledge, cultural sensitivity and cultural competence. The model places equal emphasis on the importance of culture and the effects of societal structures. In order to reduce health inequalities, healthcare practitioners must understand the significance that culture has on health as well as the impact that social structures and professional power have on the healthcare users. Based on their assertions, the authors state that the achievement of cultural competence can only be effective within an anti-discriminatory and anti-oppressive practice framework. Therefore, empowerment (an essential component of anti-oppressive praxis), of both clients and healthcare practitioners, is an important element in transcultural care.

Cultural competence has also been defined as 'a set of congruent behaviors, practices, attitudes, and policies related to embracing cultural differences that are integrated into a system or agency or among professionals. It is a state of being able to function effectively in this area' (Mays et al 2002: 139).

Others have viewed cultural competence as respect for difference with a desire to learn and accept diversities. Yet others speak of cultural competence as cultural openness in professional care contexts, achieved through cultural self-awareness and continuing development of transcultural skills (Campinha-Bacote 1999, Wenger 1999).

Maintaining competency (otherwise known as continuing competence) in nursing is measured by nurses demonstrating that they possess the requisite skills and knowledge and have the right attitude to function in ways which guarantee the safety of the client/s in a context of care. Currently continuing competence in culture care is assumed and there is no provision in Australia for continuing education for faculty members or nurse administrators, for example to study transcultural nursing, nor any means for nurses to demonstrate continuing competence in this area.

A GLIMPSE AT MODELS OF CULTURALLY COMPETENT NURSING CARE

There appears the same degree of variability in defining cultural competence in nursing in Australia and overseas as there is in defining the field of transcultural nursing. There are many models for cultural competence by which cultural care competence may be taught and demonstrated by practitioners – some are noted here.

Campinha-Bacote (2002: 181) states that cultural competence is a 'process' incorporating five integrated constructs: cultural awareness, cultural knowledge, cultural skills, cultural encounters and cultural desire. Her model assumes that: 'there is a direct relationship between the level of competence of health care provider and their ability to provide culturally responsive health care service' (Campinha-Bacote 2002: 181).

Andrews & Boyle (2003) describe a model that focuses on a combination of cultural assessment skills and critical thinking skills of nurses to provide the necessary knowledge on which to base culturally competent care.

To guide student nurses in developing competence in culture care, nursing faculty need to have the opportunity and the choice to undertake core studies in transcultural nursing to inform their teaching and research. Transcultural knowledge is essential to guide students towards safe, responsive, meaningful and culturally competent care, congruent with the culturally diverse population in Australia and elsewhere.

In the USA Boyle (2000) has developed guidelines to shift the focus of undergraduate curricula from the more usual individuals and groups to economic and political systems. Her guidelines foster the development of transcultural knowledge in undergraduates and she asserts that nurses thus prepared have the potential to bring about real change in healthcare policy, thereby transforming the health system of the USA.

To facilitate culturally competent health and nursing care Leuning et al (2002) proposed standards for transcultural nursing based on the American Nurses Association (ANA) Standards for Nursing Practice (ANA 1986, revised edition 1996). Seven sets of standards were developed relating to: theory, cultural information gathering process, caring and healing system, cultural health patterns and caring practices, healthcare planning, evaluation, research and professional development (Leuning et al 2002).

'Sensitivity' to cultures was one aspect of cultural competence identified by the American Academy of Nursing (AAN) Expert Panel on Culturally Competent Nursing Care. This panel identified a range of issues and barriers relating to the acquisition of cultural knowledge for the provision of culturally competent health care. Included in these issues were:

- limited access to principles to guide the selection of culturally appropriate research designs and cultural context
- limited access to guidelines for developing and using research definitions congruent with cultural diversity
- lack of readily available articulated principles for selecting culturally sensitive research questions congruent with the needs of populations and the priorities of the discipline (AAN 1992).

A number of culture care models are recommended for practice including culture brokering and culturally sensitive models for health promotion and wellness.

Recognizing the considerable impact of culture and language on access to healthcare services, the US Department of Health and Human Resources, Office of Minority Health in 2001 released a set of national standards to promote cultural competence in health care. The document included recommendations for national standards and an outcomes focused research agenda.

Efforts are in place to promote the development of competency standards relevant to the discipline of transcultural nursing and suited to the Australian context. However, as yet, there are none in place.

CONCLUSION

There appears to be some degree of variability in defining cultural competence in nursing in Australia and overseas, just as there is in defining the field of transcultural nursing. Australian nursing is in the midst of a dilemma as to how best to incorporate *cultural care* into its practice domains and how best to prepare nurses with transcultural knowledge and skills. In the absence of a consensus about the knowledge and skills required to improve the care of people in culturally meaningful ways, the Australian health policy guidelines are limited to improving cultural sensitivity and awareness. Some initiatives that would improve this situation include the following:

- the establishment of a national body to develop, revise and evaluate national transcultural nursing competency standards
- transcultural nursing units of study should become core units of study in the undergraduate as well as graduate nursing programmes
- faculties of nursing should demonstrate ongoing commitment to the development and revision of units of study in transcultural nursing;
- faculty members should be prepared in advanced graduate studies in transcultural nursing, and certification of transcultural nursing practitioners by accrediting bodies should be established to ensure safe, accountable and culturally congruent and competent nursing care.

A strategy to meet the diverse health needs of the nation's population in culturally congruent and meaningful ways is to develop transcultural knowledge and skills among advanced transcultural nurse practitioners (Omeri 2002, 2003, Omeri et al 2003, Omeri et al 2004a, 2005a, 2005b). As such, the notion of a 'fair go for all Australians' may become reality.

REFLECTIVE QUESTIONS

Let us give some thought to the following questions to find ways to promote culturally competent nursing care:

1. What are the sociocultural dimensions of Australia?
2. Who are diverse populations in Australia? What are the differences/similarities with populations in other parts of the world?
3. How does research-based transcultural nursing knowledge contribute to the re-education of health disparities?
4. How do Indigenous people and their health vary from the rest of Australia's diverse populations. Compare and contrast similarities and differences.
5. Identify reasons for health disparities in Australia and examine possible stratagems to improve health outcomes.

ADDITIONAL READING

INDIGENOUS HEALTH

A number of publications dealing with Indigenous health and social issues are listed for reference and research knowledge (Eckermann et al

1995, Goold 2001, Gray & Pratt 1995a, 1995b, Omeri & Cameron-Traub 1996, Reid & Trompf 1990).

IMMIGRANT HEALTH

In addition to information available on the website and internet, a few additional references are given for in-depth reading and research on the evolution of multicultural policies and immigrant health in Australia. These are Gray & Pratt 1995a, 1995b, Omeri 2002, 2003, Omeri & Cameron-Traub 1996, Reid & Trompf 1991.

Acknowledgement

I acknowledge and am grateful for the editorial assistance of Helen Hamilton, Consulting Editor and co-editor of the following publication: Clare J, Hamilton H (eds) (2002) *Writing Research. Transforming Data into Text*. Churchill Livingstone, Edinburgh.

REFERENCES

Abrums M E, Leppa C 2001 Beyond cultural competence: teaching about race, gender, class, and sexual orientation. Journal of Nursing Education 40(6):270–276

American Academy of Nursing (AAN) 1992 Expert Panel Report: Culturally competent health care 1992 The AAN Expert Panel on Culturally Competent Nursing Care. Nursing Outlook 40(6):277–283

American Nurses Association (ANA) 1986 Standards of community health nursing practice. In: Leuning C J, Swiggum P D, Balmore Wegert H M, McCullough-Zander K 2002 Proposed standards for transcultural nursing. Journal of Transcultural Nursing 13(1):40–46

Andrews M M, Boyle J S 2003 Transcultural concepts in nursing care. 4th edn. Lippincott, Philadelphia

Australian Bureau of Statistics (ABS) 2001 Census basic community profile. Online. Available: http://www.abs. gov.au/ausstats/abs%40census 27 July 2004

Australian Bureau of Statistics (ABS) 2003 Population characteristics: Aboriginal and Torres Strait Islander Australians 2001 ABS Cat. No. 4713.0. Canberra NSW, Australia

Australian Institute of Health (AIHW) 1990 Australia's health 1990, AGPS, Canberra NSW, Australia

Australian Institute of Health and Welfare (AIHW) 2004 Australia's health, population health: Indigenous population. Online. Available: http://www.aihw.gov.au/ publication/index.efm 31 July 2004

Australian Nursing Council ANC Media Release 2002a ANC principles of assessment guide nursing profession, Online. Available: http://www.anc.org.au/ Media%20Release%20Nov ember.htm 28 Nov 2002

Australian Nursing Council ANC 2002b Position statement continuing competence in nursing. Online. Available: http://www.anc.org.au/Media%20Release%20Novembe r.htm 28 Nov 2002

Australian Nursing Federation ANF 1997 Competency standards for the advanced nurse, ANF Publications, Melbourne

Bates E, Linder-Pelz 1990 Health care issues. 2nd edn. Allen & Unwin, Sydney, Australia

Boyle J S 2000 Transcultural nursing: where do we go from here? Journal of Transcultural Nursing 11(1):10–11

Byers J F, Burrell M L 1998 Demonstrating the value of the advanced practice nurse: an evaluation model. Advanced Practice in Acute and Critical Care 9:296–300

Campinha-Bacote J 2002 The process of cultural competence in the delivery of health care services: A model of care. Journal of Transcultural Nursing 13(3):181–184

Castle S 1999 Globalization, multicultural citizenship and transnational democracy. In: Hage G, Couch R (eds) The future of Australian multiculturalism: Reflections on the 20th anniversary of Jean Martin's The Migrant Presence Star Printary. NSW Research Institute for Humanities RIHSS, The University of Sydney, NSW

Castle S, Foster W, Iredale R, Withers G 1998 Immigration and Australia: myths and realities. Allen & Unwin, Sydney

Department of Immigration, Multicultural & Indigenous Affairs DIMIA 2002 Refugees and humanitarian issues: Australia's response. Online. Available: http://www. immi.gov.au/refugee/publications/refuhumiss.htm 30 Oct 2003

Department of Immigration, Multicultural & Indigenous Affairs 2003a Productive diversity: Australian's competitive advantage. Fact Sheet 7. Online. Available: http://www.immi.gov.au/facts/pdf/07productive.pdf 25 Aug 2004

Department of Immigration, Multicultural & Indigenous Affairs 2003b Multicultural Australia: united in diversity, updating the 1999 New Agenda for Multicultural Australia: Strategic directions for 2003–2006. Online. Available: http://www.dimia.gov.au/multicultural_inc/ pdf-doc/united_diversity 25 Aug 2005

Derrida J 1987 Deconstruction and philosophy: the texts of Jacques Derrida. University of Chicago Press, Chicago.

Derrida J 1997a Cosmopolities detous les pays, encore un effort. Galilee, Paris.

Derrida J 1997b Questions d'étranger: Venue de l'étranger; Pas d'hospitalité. In: Derrida J, Dufourmantelle A (eds) De l'hospitalité. Calman-Levy, Paris.

Derrida J 2000 Of hospitality: Anne Dufourmantelle invites J Derrida to respond. (Translated by Rachel Bowl.) Stanford University Press, Stanford, CA

Deutcher P 1998 Already mourning the other's absence: Deconstruction, immigration, colonialism. Paper presented at the 'Future of Australian multiculturalism', Research Institute for Humanities & Social Sciences RIHSS, The University of Sydney, December 1998.

Eckermann A, Dowd T, Martin M et al 1995 Binaj Goonj: Bridging cultures in Aboriginal health, University of New England Press, Armidale

Foucault M 1976 The will to know. Gallimard, Paris

Foucault M 1980 Power/Knowledge: Selected interviews and other writings 1972–1977. Harvester Press, Brighton

Garrett P, Lin V 1990 Ethnic health policy and service development. In: Reid J, Trompf P (eds) The health of immigrant Australia: A social perspective. Harcourt Brace Jovanovich, Sydney, Australia, p 339–342

Goold S 2001 Transcultural nursing: can we meet the challenge of caring for the Australian Indigenous person? Journal of Transcultural Nursing 12(2):94–99

Gray G, Pratt R (eds) 1995a Issues in Australian nursing 4: The nurse as clinician. Churchill Livingstone, Melbourne

Gray G, Pratt R (eds) 1995b Issues in Australian nursing 5: The nurse as clinician. Churchill Livingstone, Melbourne

Hage G, Couch R 1999 The future of Australian multiculturalism: Reflections on the 20th Anniversary of Jean Martin's The Migrant Presence Star Printary. NSW Research Institute for Humanities RIHSS, The University of Sydney

Henderson R F 1975 Poverty in Australia: First main report of the commission of inquiry into poverty. Australian Government Printing Service AGPS, Canberra

International Council of Nurses (ICN) 2002 International Council of Nurses announces position on advanced nursing practice, Press Release, October 2002. Online. Available: http://www.icn.ch/PR/02 18 Dec 2002

Iredale R, Nivison-Smith I 1995 Immigrants' experience of qualifications recognition and employment: Results from the prototype longitudinal survey of immigrants to Australia. AGPS, Canberra. In: Jamieson S, Williams L 2002 Confusion prevails in defining 'Advanced' nursing practice. Collegian 9(4):29–33

Jamieson L, Williams L 2002 Confusion prevails in defining 'Advanced' nursing practice Collegian 9(4):29–33

Leininger M M 1989a Transcultural nurse specialist: imperative in today's world. Nursing and Health Care 10(5):25–27

Leininger M M 1989b Transcultural nurse specialist and generalists: new practitioners in nursing. Journal of Transcultural Nursing 1(1):4–16

Leininger M M 1991 Culture care diversity and universality: a theory of nursing. National League for Nursing, New York

Leininger M M, McFarland M 2002 Transcultural nursing concepts, theories, research and practices. 3rd edn. McGraw Hill, New York

Leuning C J, Swiggum P D, Wegert H M, McCullough-Zander K 2002 Proposed standards for transcultural nursing. Journal of Transcultural Nursing 13(1):40–46

Lewins F 1984 Putting politics into ethnic relations. In: Jupp J (ed) Ethnic politics in Australia. Allen & Unwin, Sydney

Martin J I 1978 The migrant presence: Australian responses 1947–1977, research report for the National Population Inquiry. Allen & Unwin, Sydney

Mays R M, De Leon Siantz M L, Viehweg S A 2002 Assessing cultural competence of policy organizations. Journal of Transcultural Nursing 13(2):139–144

National Aboriginal Health Strategy 1989 Australian Government Printing Office AGPS, Canberra, Australia

National Multicultural Advisory Council 1999 Australian Multiculturalism for a New Century: Towards Inclusiveness. Commonwealth of Australia. Online. Available: http://www.immigration.gov.au 25 Nov 2004

National Review of Nurse Education 2002 Multicultural nursing education, October 2002; Section 5.1. Commonwealth Department of Education, Science and Training, DEST Online. Available: http://www.dest.gov.au/highered/nursing/pubs/multicultural/2htm 28 Nov 2002

Nurses Registration Board of New South Wales 2002 NRB Board Works: Newsletter of the nurses registration board of NSW, November 2002 10: 2–4

Office of Multicultural Affairs (OMA) 1989 National agenda for a multicultural Australia . . .Sharing our future. AGPS, Canberra

Omeri A 1996 Transcultural nursing care values, beliefs and practices of Iranian immigrants in NSW Australia. Unpublished doctoral thesis, Faculty of Nursing, The University of Sydney, NSW, Australia

Omeri A 2002 Reflections on Australia and transcultural nursing in the new millennium. In: Leininger M, McFarland M (eds) Transcultural nursing concepts, theories, research and practice. 3rd edn. McGraw Hill, New York, p 517–523

Omeri A 2003 Meeting diversity challenges: Pathway of 'advanced' transcultural nursing practice in Australia. In: Daly J, Jackson D (eds) Advances in contemporary transcultural nursing. Contemporary Nurse: Special issue: 15(3):175–187

Omeri A, Ahern M 1999 Utilising culturally congruent strategies to enhance recruitment and retention of Australian Indigenous nursing students. Journal of Transcultural Nursing 10(2):150–155

Omeri A, Atkins K 2002 Lived experience of immigrant nurses in NSW Australia: Searching for meaning. International Journal of Nursing Studies 39:495–505

Omeri A, Cameron-Traub E (eds) 1996 Transcultural nursing in multicultural Australia. Royal College of Nursing Australia, Canberra ACT

Omeri A, Malcolm P, Ahern M, Wellington B 2003 Meeting the challenges of cultural diversity in the academic setting. Nurse Education in Practice 3:5–22

Omeri A, Lennings C, Raymond L 2004a Access to and appropriateness of health services for Afghan refugees in NSW Australia: implications for policy and practice. The University of Sydney, Australia

Omeri A, Lennings C, Raymond L 2004b Hardiness and transformational coping in asylum seekers: the Afghan experience. Journal of Diversity in Health and Social Care in Community 1(1):21–30

Omeri A, Lennings C, Raymond L 2005a Beyond asylum: the Afghan experience. Research report, Transcultural Mental Health TMHC, Sydney

Omeri A, Lennings C, Raymond L 2005b Beyond asylum: implications for nursing and health care delivery for Afghan refugees in Australia. Journal of Transcultural Nursing (in press)

Papadopoulos I 2003 The Papadopoulos, Tilki and Taylor model for the development of cultural competence in nursing. Journal of Health, Social and Environmental Issues 4(1):5–7

Papadopoulos I, Tilki M, Taylor G 1998 Transcultural care. A guide for health care professionals. Quay Books, Dinton

Pearson A, Peels S 2002 Advanced practice in nursing: international perspective. International Journal of Nursing Practice 8(2):51

Pittman L, Rogers T 1990 Nursing: a culturally diverse profession in a monocultural health system. Australian Journal of Advanced Nursing 8(1):30–38

Reid J, Trompf P (eds) 1990 The health of immigrant Australia: a social perspective. Harcourt Brace Jovanovich, Sydney

Reid J, Trompf P (eds) 1991 The health of Aboriginal Australia. Harcourt Brace Jovanovich, Sydney

Royal College of Nursing Australia RCNA 2002a Position statement: Advanced practice nursing. Online. Available: http://www.rcnarg.au 28 Nov 2002

Royal College of Nursing Australia RCNA 2002b Position statement: Nursing research. Online. Available: http://www.rcna.org.au 28 Nov 2002

Royal College of Nursing Australia RCNA 2002c Position statement: Nursing practice in a culturally diverse Australian society. Online. Available: http://www.rcna.org.au 28 Nov 2002

Ruffin R 1991 Multiculturalism: what it means to SVSU. The Interior 10–14

Schroeder C, Trehearne B, Ward D 2000a Expanded role of nursing in ambulatory managed care. Part 1: Literature, role development and education. Nurse Economics 18(1):14–19

Schroeder C, Trehearne B, Ward D 2000b Expanded role of nursing in ambulatory managed care. Part II: Impact on outcomes of costs, quality, provider and patient satisfaction. Nursing Economics 18(2):71–78

Sutton F, Smith C 1995 Advanced nursing practice: new idea and new perspectives. Journal of Advanced Nursing 21(6):1037–1043

US Department of Health and Human Resources, The Office of Minority Health, Public Health Services 2001 Assuring cultural competence in health care: recommendations for national standards and an outcome-focused research agenda. Online. Available: http://www.OMHRC.gov/clas/cultural1a.htm 18 July 2005

Wenger A F Z 1999 Cultural openness: intrinsic to human care. Journal of Transcultural Nursing 10(1):10

WHO 2003 The world health report 2003. WHO, Geneva

Young C 1992 Mortality, the ultimate indicator of survival: the differential experience between birthplace groups. In: Donovan J et al (eds) Immigrants in Australia: a health profile. AGPS, Canberra, NSW

Chapter **19**

Culture and health: discourses and practices in the Canadian context

M. Judith Lynam

LEARNING OBJECTIVES

On completion of this chapter the reader will be able to:
- describe how patterns of migration have contributed to the cultural diversity of Canada
- appreciate how the social and health policy context has shaped the discourse on culture and health in Canada
- identify the ways priorities in health for immigrants and refugees in Canada are delineated
- understand the ways selected social processes mediate the health of immigrant groups.

INTRODUCTION

My orientation to, and interest in, culture and health arises out of clinical practice and a programme of research with new immigrants to Canada. As I have explored different theoretical perspectives on culture and engaged with healthcare providers in examining what it is that we need to know to practise effectively with patients from different cultural backgrounds to our own, I have moved towards the realization that while there are 'cultural' influences, these are largely influenced by the social context in which we are living. This became more evident when I completed my PhD in Britain. My research involved first-generation immigrants to Britain and to Canada.

As the goal of this book is to enable healthcare professionals to consider culture and diversity in their work with individuals and in policy and programme development, I have written this chapter with a view to sharing a 'Canadian' perspective. To introduce culture and diversity in the Canadian context I begin by providing a brief overview of the ways history has shaped Canada's story of migration and in turn how policy decisions have set the context for the ways the discourse on culture and health has been taken up. I then draw upon my programme of research and practice to trace the ways the discourses on culture and health have developed, to introduce the nature of health issues faced by immigrants and refugees and the ways these have been responded to.

Cultures and cultural practices are shaped by geography, resources and social conventions. Canada is the second largest country in the world in terms of its geography, and has a total population of approximately 31 million people (Canada 2001b). It is geographically, environmentally and ecologically diverse. These conditions have also had important influences on how Canadians organize their lives and the resources they draw upon.

CANADA – IMMIGRATION POLICIES

Canada's policies on immigration have had an important influence on the patterns of settlement. Policies set the rules for 'who' may take up residence and apply for citizenship. Currently, there are several ways people may qualify to immigrate.

Immigrants: Persons applying to immigrate are assigned 'points' on the basis of their skills or competencies such as knowledge of English or French, or being educated or trained in particular trades, disciplines or professions. Persons may also immigrate under the 'family class' or family reunification aspect of the policy. Such persons are considered on the basis of their relationship (such as spouse, parent or child) to others already in Canada.

Once an immigrant is granted 'landed immigrant status', he or she is eligible to work and to benefit from a range of social programmes including universal systems of health care and education. Landed immigrants who meet specific criteria, including a period of residency, are eligible to apply for Canadian citizenship.

Refugees: Canada is signatory to the United Nations Convention on the Status of Refugees and accepts both Convention refugees (such as refugees from Vietnam, most of whom arrived in the 1970s) and refugee claimants. The latter are individuals or families who present themselves to Canada and make a case for protection as refugees so they may legally take up residence in Canada.

The most recent statistics suggest that 25% of Canadian residents report speaking only English or French at home, with the remaining number speaking one or more of over 100 different languages. Of these the most prevalent are Chinese, Punjabi, Italian and Arabic (Canada 2004a). This profile does not, however, provide the full picture. To understand what contributes to the diversity of Canada and what shapes the current experiences of immigrants and health care, we must step back.

CANADA – COLONY AND COLONIZER

In recent years a number of scholars have drawn upon postcolonial theory to illustrate the ways in which historical relations influence current policy and practice. What is particularly important is the way this history contributes to what are largely taken-for-granted assumptions about groups within society and how such assumptions are taken up, or acted upon, in day-to-day encounters. Those who have drawn upon this perspective in health have illustrated the frequently negative impact this can have on the ways healthcare interactions are structured and also how programmes and policies are framed and enacted (see, for example, Anderson 2000, 2002, Reimer Kirkham & Anderson 2002).

Thinking of Canada in the context of its history as both a colony and colonizer helps to illustrate the ways this history has contributed to both our successes and challenges in addressing diversity. These two aspects of Canada's history have an ongoing influence on Canada's systems of governance, the definitions of individuals' rights and freedoms and the ways issues of culture and diversity are conceptualized or framed.

CANADA THE COLONY

As suggested above, the Canadian ethnocultural profile is characterized by diversity. The profiles of settlement and source countries of immigrants have changed over the years and have been influenced by our own, and other governments', economic and social policies, world events such as war or famine and more recently by what we generally refer to as the global economy.

For example, in the early Canada, settlers—primarily from Britain and France—were fishermen, hunters and explorers. Later the majority moved to Canada as an alternative to living in 'poor houses' or as tenant farmers on land they could not own. For example, during the mid 1800s thousands of Irish and other poor of the British islands immigrated to escape the 'potato famine' and to take advantage of opportunities to work and own land.

In the early years of settlement Canada had two forms of colonial government. 'Lower Canada', the region that is generally the province of Quebec, was a colony of France. France sent representatives to establish systems of colonial government, establish French as the language of education and commerce and to formalize trade agreements. Similarly, 'upper Canada', the region that is generally the province of Ontario, was a colony of Britain. As such, the King also sent representatives to establish systems of governance, establish English as the language of education and commerce and to formalize trade agreements. Migration was not, however, restricted to these two arenas and, despite laying formal claim to territories, immigrants from both countries settled in all regions. After the war of 1812, when Britain defeated France, Britain laid claim to the French region. However, despite formal rule by Britain, French continued to be the language of choice for the majority of the population and the social systems in place in that region continued to reflect the French heritage of the region.

At the time of confederation – 1867 – when Canada was officially 'created' by combining provinces under a federal government, the legislative Act passed in Britain recognized French and English as the two official languages and made provisions for the continuance of Quebec's National Assembly and other provinces' Legislative Assemblies that model Britain's parliamentary system of governance and legal system of common law.

A number of events in history have influenced the source countries for immigrants to Canada. For example, in the years surrounding Confederation (1867) Canada was engaged in building a national railway. Major contributors to this undertaking were Chinese labourers. This group is unique in that, unlike those immigrating from other, mainly northern European countries, Chinese were required for many years to pay a 'head tax' to gain entry to Canada. This tax was eventually removed but it is an early example of systemic exclusion of particular groups. Many Chinese Canadians can trace their family history to this era.

Similarly, although not often recognized as having a long history in Canada, many blacks immigrated to Canada from what we know as the United States to escape slavery. Following the First and Second World Wars considerable numbers of eastern Europeans migrated to take up offers of hectares of virtually free farm land in the prairie region. Of note in this era are the families of Jewish background who chose to immigrate from countries that had denied them the opportunity to own land.

These groups, although all of different ethnocultural backgrounds and with different histories, combined with a host of others and with their descendants to develop Canada's current systems of government, education and health care, to establish and build cities and to develop its economy largely from its resources such as fishing, logging, mining and farming and more recently from oil and gas explorations.

In the past thirty years events of history have shifted the source countries for migration from Europe to the East and the south. In these years the top source countries for migration have been countries in Asia (such as Hong Kong, China and Vietnam) and south Asia (such as India, Sri Lanka and Pakistan). There has also been a considerable migration from countries in the south (particularly Commonwealth countries in the Caribbean and Africa) and from Central and South America (such as Guatemala and Colombia).

The profiles of migration to Quebec are somewhat different because French continues to be that province's first language. Quebec has therefore received more migrants from French speaking countries such as those in North Africa (e.g. Morocco, Algeria) than other parts of Canada.

As with many other countries, new immigrants have tended to migrate to larger city centres. Currently, Montreal, Toronto and Vancouver are host cities for the largest proportion of immigrants and refugees. For those interested in examining the settlement profiles and ethnocultural make up of Canada and its neighbourhoods, such information is available at the following web link: http://www.statcan.ca. But as with other statistical data, numbers only tell part of the story.

There are several important consequences of the recent shift in source countries and the distribution within the population. One is that more immigrants speak languages other than English and French and more of them are visibly different to the broader population. Additionally, however, in the major centres the notions of 'minority–majority' are challenged as proportions of newcomers to Canadian-born in many neighbourhoods approximate 1 : 2. These changes in the composition of communities have created challenges for healthcare delivery, and have prompted healthcare professionals to consider alternative ways of conceptualizing health, illness and treatment, and have drawn attention to the ways 'culture' and history shape the ways healthcare relationships are structured and enacted.

CANADA THE COLONIZER

While Canada is represented in literature and history as a new frontier, and uncharted territory open to settlement, Canada has an indigenous population. It was first settled by a number of what we now refer to as First Nations (FN) or Aboriginal groups. These groups have, over the course of history, been referred to as 'Indians', Natives, or by such tribal names as Cree, Sioux, Iroquois, Haida, Innu or Mohawk to name a few. The relationships between Aboriginals, explorers, settlers, colonial governments and more recently the provincial and federal governments are complex and multifaceted. While I cannot possibly do justice to it in this space, the history of these relationships has had, and continues to have, important implications for the health of First Nations people and must be mentioned. For those who may be interested in examining in greater depth the ways this history has influenced this population in general and their health in particular I refer you to the Royal Commission on

Aboriginal Peoples (RCAP). This inquiry, completed in 1994, and reports and publications related to it, can be accessed at the following internet link: http://www.ubcic.bc.ca/RCAP.htm.

At the outset First Nations peoples were used as resources by newcomers. They shared their technology and knowledge of the land with explorers, traders and trappers. However, as more settlers arrived to claim territory, different views of 'ownership', approaches to settlement and use of the land created conflicts that were resolved in a number of ways that ranged from violence to the establishment of treaties that delineated rights and responsibilities while also defining territorial boundaries. As these treaties can be viewed as treaties between nations, the federal government rather than provincial governments have assumed primary responsibility for relationships with First Nations.

Under the terms of this relationship as set out in what is referred to as the 'Indian Act' (Canada 1985), the government was committed to ensuring such services as health care and education were provided. There was a considerable period of history, however, where the strategies for implementing this commitment have been labelled assimilationist. For example, policies that required First Nations children to attend residential schools away from their families had the effect of erasing children's knowledge of their traditional languages and First Nations cultures. Residential schools for Aboriginal children were the norm in much of the country between 1950 and 1969.

Although there has been some shifting in the nature of the relationship it is still one that draws attention to the power imbalances that characterize colonial relationships. At the forefront of First Nations and Canadian government relations is achieving some form of resolution of, and restitution for, the negative impact of residential schools on First Nations communities and cultures and the completion of treaty negotiations including land claims and agreement on issues of governance.

One manifestation of the negative impact of colonial relationships and the marginalization and exclusion associated with them is evident in the health status of First Nations. Although there is considerable diversity within the First Nations communities, and lives and lifestyles vary considerably, as a population this group has the poorest health profile of all Canadians. For all indicators of mortality and morbidity this population fares worse than the broader population (British Columbia 2000, Canadian Institute of Health Information 2004).

The reasons for this are complex but it is being increasingly argued that the poor health profile accrues from the broader social conditions under which many First Nations people live (Dion-Stout et al 2001). This is a population that has, through policy and associated practices, been politically, socially and economically marginalized.

This brief overview is meant to introduce you to Canada as a country that has been ethnoculturally diverse from its outset and although I will argue it has taken steps towards ensuring equality rights, language protection and valuing diversity, it is a country living through change and this is evident in the ways the discourse on culture and health has developed.

CANADIAN HEALTH POLICY CONTEXT

In the last thirty years a number of important decisions that have shaped the Canadian discourse on culture and health have been made. These include the institution of a national healthcare plan that is universally available, adopting an official policy of 'multiculturalism', establishing a Canadian Charter of Rights and Freedoms and maintaining a policy that encourages immigration to promote growth and development.

The legislative process in Canada must comply with the Charter of Rights and Freedoms that defines the rights of citizenship and explicates the domains of responsibility allocated to different levels of government. In particular it delineates *equality rights*.

It has been argued that the ideology of community (versus individualism) informed many policy decisions at the inception of Canada's system of medicare – the term used in the general population to refer to Canada's system of universal health care (Badgeley & Wolfe 1967). The roots of the national healthcare system are traced to programmes initiated in the prairie provinces by the Co-operative Commonwealth Federation (CCF), who were in power in Saskatchewan's provincial government years earlier. In this region, where people lived in small and isolated farming communities, faced severe winters and relied upon one another to help at peak periods of harvest, collective action was a familiar concept. 'The settlers of the "last best west" – became used to helping each other through collective and co-operative action' (Badgeley & Wolfe 1967: 3). This commitment to communities sharing the costs of ill health was reiterated in the Royal Commission on Health Services Report (Canada 1964), which served as a precursor to the Canada Health Act (Canada 1984). In this report the concepts of *universality* and *accessibility* were identified as key components of a national system of health care.

Even in the early years, the link between poverty and health and access to health care was being made by analysts, much as the relationship between health and poverty had been documented in the UK (Badgeley & Wolfe 1967, Canada 1997a). From its outset Canada's national health system was based upon the premise that a healthy society is a necessity for a healthy economy and was designed to ensure that the burden of ill health was shared, thereby diminishing the impact of the cumulative burden associated with ill health on individuals (Badgeley & Wolfe 1967). As well as seeking to provide illness care, the Canadian system also includes health promotion (originally public health) programmes as a component of its mandate.

The 1960s, then, ushered in the era of a universal system of healthcare provision. Policy initiatives undertaken in subsequent decades influenced the ways in which services were delivered.

As the 1980s continued to be a time of substantial immigration to Canada and as the source countries for migration changed, so did the demographic profile. As a number of health issues became evident, for newcomers and health practitioners, the federal government established a Task Force on Mental Health of Immigrants and Refugees. Their report published in 1988 drew attention to the unique health challenges faced by new immigrants and refugees. This report (Canada 1988a) and the mental health policy (Canada 1988b) developed in the same year made recommendations regarding ways of upholding principles of accessibility and universality of health care for immigrant and refugee populations.

ERA OF REFORM

The 1990s marked a transition in government priorities. Canada, like other countries, entered a period of economic retrenchment. The shift in emphasis from spending to reducing debt prompted a review of government financial commitments. Expenses related to health care at both the provincial and federal levels are major components of the government budget. In this era the continued commitment to collective versus individual responsibility for health was called into question. However, it has been since reiterated as a central premise of the Canadian health system. The importance of this has been underscored by the most recent health-care accord, an agreement reached between the provinces and the federal government in September 2004 (Canada 2004b).

FOCUS ON UNDERREPRESENTED GROUPS: A RECOMMITMENT TO EQUITY

In the same decade the federal government commissioned its 'National Forum on Health' in an effort to identify (from the viewpoint of professionals, healthcare organizations and citizen groups) the central elements of the system that were most valued and areas where costs could be trimmed. An additional mandate for this commission was to assess the currency of the founding principles of medicare. Their report affirmed that medicare is deemed essential by Canadians (Canada 1997a, 1997b). Indeed, it concluded that Canada's system of medicare is a defining feature of Canada.

This report, like many of the provincial studies being undertaken, documented that certain groups, including most particularly FN people, but also new immigrants, women, children, youth and the elderly, were not receiving the same consideration in services as other sectors of the population. As a consequence these groups had inequitable access to health services and many had poorer health profiles.

The report reaffirmed a commitment to a view of health that was broader than illness care and one that recognized the social determinants of health.

We believe that the social and economic determinants of health merit particular attention. This is not to diminish in any way the important contribution made by . . . (the system of illness care). Rather, our goal is to raise awareness of the far reaching implications of the social and economic factors and to propose concrete actions to improve the health prospects of Canadians. (Canada 1997a: 1)

Thus, the National Forum reaffirmed that the remit of Canada's health system extended beyond illness care. It identified groups requiring particular attention in research and programme development and proposed strategies to foster broader-based participation in the design and delivery of healthcare services while upholding equality rights and maintaining a commitment to universality and accessibility.

KEY ISSUES OF THE HEALTH POLICY CLIMATE

The concern about cost in this era has meant that when groups are identified as requiring different approaches to care, any initiatives must be justified on a basis of cost (and evidence). Also, in the insurance risk assessment model, some population groups are portrayed as commanding 'more than their share' of resources. This era, then, has seen a shift towards discourses emphasizing efficiency and a re-emergence of health discourse that characterizes health as a reward for pursuing a healthy (morally good) lifestyle. Along with this there was pressure from a number of groups to consider the implementation of a 'two tier' system of public and private health care with and without (private or public) insurance, as is in place in a number of other countries. Those arguing against this model cite the considerable body of research which has documented that such systems tend to provide different levels of care to different population groups and be associated with markedly different health outcomes (Abel-Smith 1994, Evans 1992, Feinstein 1993, Hsiao 1992, Frank & Mustard 1994, Reinhardt 1992, Stroik & Jensen 1999).

There are, however, a number of conceptual issues and associated assumptions that underlie the ways in which issues faced by different population groups have been taken up in policy. While *universality* aims to ensure cost is not a barrier to access health services there is considerable evidence, much of it produced in the UK (Cooper et al 1999, Gordon et al 1999, MacIntyre 1997, Whitehead 1992) but also in Canada and elsewhere (Evans et al 1994, Haan et al 1987), that material circumstances, social position and the capacity to mobilize such societal resources have important influences on health status.

Further, as has been noted, some groups, notably women and particularly women heading families and new immigrants, have access to fewer such resources. As such, the health policy discourse includes an exploration of tensions between policies driven by efficiency and policies driven by equity.

Several authors (Arber & Cooper 2000, Graham 2000) have also illustrated the ways in which assumptions about women, and men are taken up and acted upon in policy. So, too, the ways in which issues of culture, race and ethnicity have been conceptualized, or overlooked, have had an impact upon how policy has been framed (Anderson 2000, Anderson et al 2003, Browne & Smye 2002, Lynam 2005, Ramsden 1993, Williams 1989). In the next section, therefore, I examine the ways in which the discourse on culture has developed and how, in turn, this influences both our understanding of culture and health in the Canadian context and strategies for addressing issues of culture and health.

THE CANADIAN POLICY DISCOURSE ON CULTURE AND HEALTH

In Canada, the approaches to inequalities in health have been introduced by drawing upon core principles of health policy such as universality and accessibility and the equality rights provision of the Canadian Charter of Rights and Freedoms. For example, in the last two decades, initiatives in health for immigrant populations have been influenced by legislative and policy initiatives in three major arenas. These include the Canada Health Act (Canada 1984) and associated national health policy initiatives including 'Achieving Health for All' (Canada 1986), the Canadian Multiculturalism Act of 1988 and associated policies, and the Canadian Constitution Act of 1982. These legislative and policy initiatives have shaped the ways in which the discourse on culture and health has been framed and have, in turn, influenced how identified issues are responded to in policy and programme development.

Changing patterns of migration to Canada have drawn attention to different perspectives on health held by professionals and cultural communities and raised awareness of the ways in which immigration influences individuals' capacities to access healthcare resources and to mobilize personal resources to manage health and illness. In Canada, therefore, particularly in provinces with high rates of immigration, such as British Columbia (BC), introducing a provincial multiculturalism policy (British Columbia 1996a) provides evidence that it has been argued, with some degree of success, that attention must be paid to the examination of the ways migration and culture can be addressed in all government departments including health. In the same time period Quebec mandated health and social services to develop 'accessibility plans' as a strategy for ensuring barriers to accessing services were addressed at all levels.

Additionally, many initiatives to address health needs of immigrant groups and cultural communities have for several decades been framed in relation to the Canadian Charter of Rights and Freedoms (Canada 1982), which states under Section 15 (Equality Rights):

> *Every individual is equal before and under the law and has the right to equal protection and equal benefit of the law without discrimination and, in particular, without discrimination based on race, national or ethnic origin, colour, religion, sex, age or mental or physical disability. (Canada 2001a)*

As such, since its inception, the Charter has been drawn upon by those arguing for changes in all sectors of society, including the ways in which health services are organized, and to ensure that the delivery of care fosters *equity*.

In the past two decades Canadian health policy has shown evidence of having broadened the view of health – beyond the traditional biomedical view – and according explicit recognition of the social determinants of health including gender, age, migration status and income. The theoretical and empirical work drawn upon to inform these national policy initiatives is described by Evans and colleagues (Evans et al 1994). The current policy, developed from what is commonly referred to as the Epp Report completed in 1986, recognized the links between income and poor health that required attention (Canada 1986):

> Within the low-income bracket, certain groups have a higher chance of experiencing poor health than others. Older people, the unemployed, welfare recipients, single women supporting children and minorities such as natives and immigrants all fall into this category . . . So far, we have not done enough to deal with these disparities. As we search for health policies which can take this country confidently into the future, it is obvious that the reduction of health inequalities between high- and low-income groups is one of our leading challenges. (Canada 1986: 4)

During the 1980s much of the Canadian literature related to culture and health, or the health of immigrants, was informed by the portrayal of Canada as a multicultural society with an attendant focus on understanding and celebrating diversity. A parallel literature focused attention on difficulties practitioners faced in attempting to deliver care to persons who did not speak English or who were unfamiliar with the system of healthcare delivery and hence faced barriers to access (Masi et al 1993). The publication of the report of the Canadian Task Force on Mental Health Issues of Immigrants and Refugees in 1988 (Canada 1988a) drew widespread attention to the impact of migration on mental health. This report took early steps towards refining our understanding of some of the social determinants of health and contributed to a reconceptualization of the root causes of many of the problems health professionals identified as mental health issues. Those identified include the impact of the *lack of community*, *social isolation* and *discrimination* faced by immigrants and refugees. Thus new perspectives were introduced into the discourse on culture and health and attention was drawn to the ways social context can potentially foster or impede health.

In addition to making visible the extent of change faced by new immigrants, this report identified subgroups within the immigrant populations whose needs for support and care had been greatly overlooked. The subgroups identified include youth, women and the elderly (Canada 1988a). The issues raised in this report resonate with experiences of marginalization described by participants in my own research (Lynam 1985, 2004) and point to mental health consequences of marginalization.

The health policy of this era focused on *community building* initiatives and accorded recognition to the need for healthcare services to be *inclusive* and to recognize ways social conditions influence health. This perspective influenced how health policy was implemented and programmes were developed. At the federal level it led to the identification of priorities in programmes and resulted in a number of projects being funded that fostered community building and enhanced the awareness of health professionals regarding these issues.

The national mental health policy that was subsequently developed identified *partnership* and *mutual aid* as key concepts. This policy led to a number of initiatives to address isolation and the marginalization of persons within communities. These policy frameworks challenged professionals to move beyond biomedical views of health, illness and treatment and articulated a role for the informal sector as a resource for health.

It is at the programme development stage that the *equity* principle has shown its value. For, at the implementation stage, there can be a requirement to demonstrate that resources have been allocated equitably, according to need, and to demonstrate the impact upon the population, or benefit in terms of desired health outcomes. As such, a number of initiatives, in health, in education, in social service programme development and in industry, explicitly recognized multiculturalism, and the diversity associated with it, as a feature of society and sought to take these up in an effort to redress inequities.

APPROACHES TO CONCEPTUALIZING CULTURAL INFLUENCES ON HEALTH

With the recognition that there are cultural influences on health and health practices the conceptualization of culture and cultural traditions has been central to the work of a number of theorists. Nurse researchers have drawn upon a number of theoretical traditions in anthropology, sociology, philosophy and feminist theory in framing their studies. Work grounded in each perspective has contributed in different ways to the discourse on culture and health. Each perspective calls for different research approaches and each is built upon different, sometimes competing, assumptions. Work derived from these viewpoints has, therefore, contributed to an ongoing debate about the nature of culture and its impact upon health.

A number of theorists outside of nursing have sought to make visible the ways in which cultural viewpoints shape and influence how health is defined (Helman 2000, Eisenberg & Kleinman 1980, Good & Good 1980). Culture and associated systems of meaning also suggest the nature of roles different people in families or communities play in assuming responsibility for ensuring the health of family members or managing illness events (Helman 2000).

Additionally, while in some contexts nurses have found it helpful to use an approach that identifies culture-specific beliefs or practices in order to provide care, in the Canadian context this has not proved to be particularly effective in addressing practice issues for a number of reasons.

First, as is evident from the description of the Canadian context, there is considerable diversity across the population. Even within ethnocultural groups there is considerable diversity because of their migration histories, and their experiences in the communities to which they migrate. For example, while there are many first-generation Chinese Canadians there are also many fourth-generation Chinese Canadian families. As such, their experiences, needs and knowledge of resources are likely to be entirely different.

A number of theorists have identified that oppression is central to the experience of cultural groups, particularly those shaped by colonial relations. Work in this area has been strongly influenced by feminist theory, which has sought to make visible the ideologies and structures that have historically privileged men on the basis of gender (Anderson 2000, Smith 1987). A central premise of feminist analysis is that the processes of assigning and exerting power are based on gender and that the social context in which we live is structured to privilege groups on the basis of gender. It is argued, therefore, that women are more vulnerable to oppression and in response, in recent years, there have been revisions to social policies to correct such imbalances (British Columbia 1996b).

Some theorists have identified parallels between the experiences of women and immigrant groups. A number of analysts (Anderson 2000, Browne & Smye 2002, Lynam 2005) have drawn upon feminist theory and the work of such theorists as Foucault and Bourdieu to illustrate the ways policies and practices of societies create and sustain power imbalances between groups, thereby contributing to social inequities.

In recent years a number of researchers have drawn upon perspectives that focus attention on the ways power relations are manifest in how healthcare interactions are structured, priorities in programme and service delivery determined, and resources drawn upon. This work has identified areas where initiatives in hospital and community have successfully fostered access and overcome barriers while also illustrating contexts where inequities persist (Anderson 1998, 2002, Browne & Smye 2002, Lynam 2005, Lynam et al 2003, Reimer Kirkham & Anderson 2002).

In providing this historical overview and illustrating the Canadian policy commitment to make healthcare services universally and equitably accessible for the multicultural population I have argued that the discourse on culture and health has been framed to emphasize inclusion rather than difference. The policy context has recognized social conditions, such as social and material resources, that have an impact upon health profiles and has framed issues related to culture and health in terms of equity and access.

FRAMING HEALTH ISSUES

What, then, are the health issues of concern in this culturally and linguistically diverse society? First, it must be noted that Canada does have one of the healthiest populations in the world. Having said this, there are disparities in health within the population. As has been suggested earlier in this chapter, immigrants and refugees along with the Aboriginal population are among those who seem to face higher risks for health disparities, or to use the British term, health inequalities. Despite being healthier than their Canadian-born counterparts at the time of immigration, as elsewhere, there are studies that show that the health of immigrants declines to match that of broader Canadian society (Chen et al 1996).

In the Canadian context health issues are framed as issues of access, issues of equity (i.e. striving to ensure different sectors of the population receive needed services) and also the identification and dismantling of barriers to access and the equitable delivery of services. Barriers include such factors as language barriers, lack of knowledge of available services or programmes, or lack of awareness on the part of healthcare providers about the lives and challenges faced by immigrants or refugees as they cope with resettlement, seek to establish new networks of support in communities and work to balance demands of work, home and family. Given that the health profile of new Canadians shifts over time towards poorer health, we must ask what it is about being Canadian, or being an immigrant to Canada, that adversely impacts on health, and how health issues are being responded to in the Canadian context. What is it that contributes to this poorer health profile? As evidence has shown in a number of contexts, disparities in health are associated with socio-economic standing but the impact of few material resources can be mediated by social conditions. Marmot and colleagues (1997), for example, compared results of studies undertaken in the UK and the USA that examined material resources and indicators of mental and physical health. They concluded:

> There is worse health among those at the bottom of the socioeconomic distribution than those at the top. Perhaps more important, all three studies show a social gradient that runs right across the whole population: the lower the social status the greater the physical and mental ill health and the worse the psychological well-being. (Marmot et al 1997: 905)

What must be considered with this observation is 'who' is more likely to be living in poverty. While the disparities are not as great as they are in other countries (Wilkinson 1996) it has been shown that immigrants to Canada experience downward mobility in the workforce and as a consequence many have lower incomes than their Canadian-born counterparts (British Columbia 1998); as such, they are more likely to be among those who are living in poorer material circumstances.

MITIGATING INFLUENCES: WHY INCLUSION IS HEALTHIER THAN EXCLUSION

There are, however, a number of studies that suggest the impact of poor material circumstances can be mediated by other conditions in the social environment. For example, in addition to corroborating findings of research in the UK related to poverty and health, the Alameda County study undertaken in the USA was one of the first studies to draw attention to the links between social environment, particularly social networks, and health status. Haan and colleagues undertook a 10-year follow-up of the original study participants and concluded:

> Overall these research results, supported by similar findings elsewhere . . . suggest that . . . the persistent and pervasive link between socio-

economic position and disease should include assessment of the social and physical environmental demands to which persons of lower socioeconomic position are exposed. (Haan et al 1987: 995).

Other studies have since shown the importance of integrated networks of support to health status (Berkman & Kawachi 2000, Cooper et al 1999) and provided evidence that some communities are better at creating a sense of belonging or inclusion while others foster marginalization or exclusion (Kawachi & Kennedy 1997, Lynam 2004) or limit access to diverse groups for support (Berkman & Clark 2003).

Wilkinson (1996) offers a refinement of the material deprivation explanation for health inequalities and focuses attention on the relative rates of poverty within a population as influencing the extent of health inequalities. Based on comparative analyses of a number of countries worldwide, he advances the view that income inequality is an indicator of a 'fragmented society' and proposes that such societies are characterized by an erosion of social capital or unsustainable development.

DOES THE BROADER POLICY CONTEXT IMPACT ON INDIVIDUALS AND THEIR HEALTH?

I have spent considerable space delineating the Canadian social and health policy context and the principles that underpin it. But, I imagine you are asking; does the broader health and social policy context and the principles that inform it make a difference to people?

In what follows I draw upon examples from my own research that offer insight into the ways these policy positions are taken up at the 'local' level and in doing so illustrate health issues of importance. This study was undertaken in Britain and Canada with first-generation immigrant teens and their mothers (Lynam 2004, 2005). All participants were 'visible minorities' in the sense that they were visibly different to the broader society because of language and physical features such as colour. They were also all living in households of modest means. The focus of the research was on the nature of relationships established within the formal and informal sectors of the healthcare system and the ways these relationships were drawn upon to foster health. This study, then, focused attention on issues of equity and access to services within the formal sector and on moderating conditions that have been shown to have a protective function such as connection and support, the converse of which is to be 'on the margins' or excluded. As noted earlier, these latter conditions have been shown to be associated with poorer health profiles over the life course.

Marginalization was central to the experiences of the 'working class' immigrant women and their adolescent daughters who participated in my research in Britain and Canada (Lynam 2004). In recounting their experiences, however, it became evident that there were characteristics of their social environments, and the opportunities within them, that augmented or diminished this experience and its largely negative consequences. I argued that the broader social policy context contributed to the creation of contexts for inclusion or exclusion (Lynam 2004, 2005).

In what follows I draw briefly upon some data examples that illustrate ways the participants themselves see broader social conditions as influencing their day-to-day experiences. A Canadian immigrant teen described the ways she interprets Canada's policy of multiculturalism as one that 'invites her in' and how her school offered avenues for participation in activities that extended to involvement in, and connections with, the broader community. What is of particular interest is that although teens were aware of their different histories, in the Canadian context, they were more likely to have some aspects of these differences, such as language abilities, viewed as assets, or capital for which they received recognition. So, for many teens, constructing 'difference' in this way was affirming. This teen's comments were echoed by most other teen participants in Canada. As such, in this case it can be argued that a context for inclusion has been created, one that would take steps towards fostering connection and building networks of support within the broader community.

The parents' accounts were somewhat different in that although they too viewed the Canadian multicultural context as 'inviting them in', many of them faced difficulties accessing work roles that took into account their education or experience in their countries of origin. As such, they spoke about being 'on the margins'. Nonetheless, many of them indicated life was still better than the life they had in their countries of origin and that the future for their children was brighter.

However, some families struggled and as the following account indicates, it is sometimes difficult to separate the issues out. In the case that follows the teen speaking lives with several siblings in a single-parent household headed by her mother. His comments illustrate some of the ways the family's social circumstances placed limits on opportunities to participate in activities, but also how their circumstances shape their relationships, in both positive and negative ways, with the broader community.

Teen: . . . *so being a big family* (single parent) *is, just difficult, – period – and whatever, right? . . . I guess people try to pay more attention, I don't know, towards us because we're a big family like they always try to, they'll give us like programmes* (i.e. free enrolment in community summer camps, or classes) *where we can put our little brothers in and . . . Sometimes it's very difficult, some people are really ignorant and rude and they don't understand our situation, they always say like why can't, they criticize and you know, like make judgements and stuff, and that's kind of hard because some friends will want to do this and we can't* (afford it). *Also money situations, like there's a lot of programmes in* (area) *that help with money like they're low cost and everything but there's other programmes that you want to put people* (from the family) *into and it's just*

Researcher: *you can't?*

Teen: *and you can't* (afford it). (Canada, interview 2.)

While the family situation was one that challenged a number of conventions, the daughter (who was 16) demonstrated she was able to navigate a number of social domains very effectively. She was popular at school with both teachers and other students. For example, as well as doing well academically, she had been invited to participate in a number of school-sponsored activities, like sports or band tours. Unlike many of the other participants she did therefore have a number of adults who were in a position to be resources for her. Additionally, for this teen, knowing Spanish had become an asset as she was able to capitalize on it, particularly in school. It also helped her to define her 'place' in Canada as well as to maintain connections with her heritage.

Teen: *I was just going to say bilingual, like being bilingual it's um, I think it's really*
Researcher: *an asset?*
Teen: *It's a good advantage especially in this country because it's so many cultures – multiculturalism – so it's really good to know.* (Canada, interview 2.)

A number of other participants successfully transformed their first language skills into assets for the workplace and also saw this as a skill for their children to develop.

Woman: *But, for me it's pretty important, you know, to have the credentials, you know, to know more experience, you know and speak two or three language, even for my job, it's very good . . . you can have more opportunity.*
Researcher: *So you see learning different languages as a skill for work?*
Woman: *Oh yes, yeah, I can see them going to apply for a, you know, for a job, they ask how many language do you speak,*
Researcher: *when you apply for a*
Woman: *for a job.* (Canada interview 2.)

One Canadian family is involved in a church where the priest and much of the congregation are Spanish speaking. The teen describes the importance of this for her mother.

Teen: *I think it is* (important) *because it would be very strange if you don't, if my mom didn't have any friends because her family doesn't live here, they all live in El Salvador and different places in the US, but I think she needs someone to talk to as well, right?*
Researcher: *Yes.*
Teen: *Because I've made my friends in schools. She makes her friends in wherever she gathers . . . she also went to school . . . and she made a lot of like non-English speaking friends and, well, which is pretty cool because like that she gets adapted to having a multicultural relationship with people, you know, because they speak a different language but they could be in the same situation except with a different country.* (Canada, interview 1.)

So, in these examples we hear teens and parents speaking of ways they establish connections in the community and the impact that valuing diversity – multiculturalism – has on their views of self and their abilities to establish connections. These views are, however, intertwined with other challenges such as being poor, managing multiple responsibilities with few resources and coping with others' misconceptions.

By contrast, the following quote illustrates one woman's view of the ways tensions between gender and British society's taken-for-granted constructions of 'race' set her apart. She comments that despite citizenship she and her children are visibly different and can be singled out at any time. She found she was continually challenging others' assumptions about her abilities and discusses how she sought to respond by challenging assumptions and gaining skills for 'repositioning'. This woman, like others in the British context, spoke in terms of their differences, which in turn influenced the valuing of their abilities. As this woman speaks we hear how gender and 'race' intersect to create the social conditions with which she must contend. She describes how she furthered her own education and sought to prepare her daughters by gaining the credentials she viewed as necessary in the new cultural context.

Mother: *For two reasons I'm doing it or I've been trying to achieve . . . as a woman, um, in any society women are always, you know, kind of like second citizen, um, but the other one was because you, – woman from ethnicity minority – have it worse, I think people don't give you credit . . . and it's a shame, it is a shame really, because that's the way people perceive other people. But if, you, you know, are white and well dressed right away they think, you know, she's educated.* (Britain, interview 1.)

This account draws attention to the ways unchallenged assumptions about women and people of colour lead her to observe that 'people don't give you credit'. But also, she takes up the discourse on 'ethnic minority' which emphasizes difference. Such assumptions, she observes, can disadvantage some while creating conditions of privilege for others.

These very brief examples are intended to prompt reflection on the ways the broader social context shapes how we view and take up issues of culture and health in our day-to-day practice. I have used examples from research undertaken in a community context that focused on relationships as resources for health.

SUMMARY

Canada's history as a colony and as a colonizer draws attention to how the Canadian systems of government, health care and education have been shaped by its relationships with Britain and France. It also draws attention to the ways power relations between groups are formalized in these institutional structures and the policies developed to enact them.

In recent years a number of scholars have drawn upon what is broadly referred to as postcolonial scholarship as a way of drawing attention to the ways current practices and relationships are rooted in history and the ways current assumptions about others are shaped by what are often unchallenged assumptions about individuals or groups.

In the Canadian context, disparities in health have been noted for immigrants, refugees and most particularly First Nations populations. So, too, there is evidence that many people within these groups have fewer social and material resources to draw upon, in part because of social processes, rooted in historical relations, that make it more difficult to become part of or establish a range of connections within the broader community and because the social processes involved in assigning value are rooted in taken-for-granted assumptions about people and the nature of their abilities.

Since the 1980s the overriding discourse on culture has been shaped by Canada's commitment to multiculturalism. An assumption inherent in this view is that everyone has culture and 'our' Canadian culture is multifaceted. There are some who credit this policy with creating a context for inclusion while others argue it masks disparities within the population. Within the Canadian health policy framework with its commitment to universality and equality, equity has become the premise guiding initiatives. While equality makes the provision for all to have the same services, equity recognizes all may not have the same ability to mobilize resources or may face barriers to achieving a similar outcome. In the 1990s the focus of many initiatives related to culture and health was to identify and dismantle barriers to health. While the examples included in the chapter illustrate that Canada has taken steps towards fostering inclusion and addressing issues of access, there is still work to do.

REFLECTIVE QUESTIONS

1. In this chapter I have argued that there is a need for critical reflection on the ways we view 'others'. We all make assumptions, but it is important from time to time to think through these assumptions; what are our assumptions based upon and how do they shape our actions?
2. Given the intersections between health and broader social conditions I would encourage those practising in hospitals or other health settings to ask how are assumptions about patients, the resources available to them and the goals of care manifest in your practice setting?
3. Are these assumptions well founded? For example, do you systematically ask about the nature of resources available to a person upon discharge? Or have you, as many do – albeit often incorrectly – assumed that all 'immigrants' have extended families?
4. What similarities and differences are there between Canadian policies on culture and health and those of your own country? As countries in the European Union redefine their relationships to one another, what issues related to culture and diversity are likely to emerge and how are they being taken up in policy?

REFERENCES

Abel-Smith B 1994 An introduction to health policy, planning and financing. Longman, London

Anderson J M 1998 Speaking of illness: issues of first generation Canadian women – implications for patient education and counseling. Patient Education and Counseling 33:197–207

Anderson J M 2000 Gender, 'race', poverty, health and discourses of health reform in the context of globalization: a postcolonial feminist perspective in policy research. Nursing Inquiry 7:220–229

Anderson J M 2002 Toward a post-colonial feminist methodology in nursing research: exploring the convergence of post-colonial and Black feminist scholarship. Nurse Researcher 9(3):7–25

Anderson J M, Perry J, Blue C et al 2003 Rewriting cultural safety within the postcolonial and post national feminist project: toward new epistemologies of healing. Advances in Nursing Science 26(3):196–214

Arber S, Cooper H 2000 Gender and inequalities across the life course. In. Annandale E, Hunt K (eds) Gender and inequalities in health. Open University Press, Buckingham, p 123–149

Badgeley R F, Wolfe S 1967 Doctors' strike: Medical care and conflict in Saskatchewan. Macmillan, Toronto

Berkman L F, Breslow L 1983 Health and ways of living: The Alameda County study. Oxford University Press, New York

Berkman L F, Clark C 2003 Neighbourhoods and networks: The construction of safe places and bridges. In Kawachi I, Berkman L (eds) Neighbourhoods and health. Oxford University Press, New York, p 288–302

Berkman L F, Kawachi I (eds) 2000 Social epidemiology. Oxford University Press. New York

British Columbia 1996a Multiculturalism Act. RSBC, Ch. 321. Victoria. Online. Available: http://www.mcaws.gov. bc.ca/amip/prgs/policy.htm 20 Jan 2005

British Columbia 1996b Report on the health of British Columbians. Provincial Health Officers' annual report, 1995. Feature report, women's health. BC Ministry of health and Ministry responsible for seniors, Victoria

British Columbia 1998 Unfulfilled expectations: Missed opportunities. Poverty among immigrants and refugees in British Columbia. A report of the working group on poverty by Marin Spigelman Research Associates. BC Ministry responsible for multiculturalism and immigration, immigration policy and research division. Victoria

British Columbia 2000 Report on the health of British Columbians. Provincial Health Officer's annual report, 1999. BC Ministry of health, Victoria

Browne A J, Smye V 2002 A postcolonial analysis of health care discourses addressing Aboriginal women. Nurse Researcher: The International Journal of Research Methodology in Nursing and Health Care 9(3):28–41

Canada 1964 Royal Commission on Health Services report, vol 1 (Hall report). Queen's Printer, Ottawa

Canada 1982 Charter of Rights and Freedoms. Queen's Printer, Ottawa

Canada 1984 Canada Health Act, consolidated statutes & regulations. Chapter C-6. S. 1. Online. Available: http:// laws.justice.gc.ca.en/C-6/17077/.html 31 Aug 2004

Canada 1985 Department of Justice, Revised Statute (RS) Indian Act. Online. Available: http://laws.justice.gc/ca/ en/I-5 28 Sep 2004

Canada 1986 Achieving health for all: A framework for health promotion. Department of Health and Welfare, Ottawa

Canada 1988a After the door has opened. Mental health issues affecting immigrants and refugees in Canada. A report of the Task Force on mental health issues affecting immigrants and refugees. Minister of Supply and Services. Cat. No. Ci96–38/1988E. Ottawa

Canada 1988b Mental health of Canadians: Striking a balance. Ministry of National Health and Welfare. Ministry of Supplies and Services Canada. Cat. H39–128/1998E

Canada 1994 Royal Commission on Aboriginal Peoples (RCAP). Online. Available: http://www.ubc.ic.bc.ca/ RCAP.htm

Canada 1997a Canada health action: Building on the legacy. Report of the National Forum on Health Volume 1. The final report. Online. Available: http://wwwnfh.hc-sc.gc. ca/publicat/finvol1 28 Sep 2004

Canada 1997b Canada health action: Building on the legacy. Report of the National Forum on Health. Volume 2. Synthesis reports and issues papers. Online. Available: http://wwwnfh.hc-sc.gc.ca/publicat/finvol2 30 Sept 2004

Canada 2001a The health of Canadians – the Federal role. Interim report. Vol 1 – The story so far. The Standing Senate Committee on Social Affairs, Science and Technology. Ottawa. March. Online. Available: http:// www.parl.gc.ca/3711/parlbbus/commbus/senate/con. e/soc1-E/vep-e/reprintmar01-e-htm 30 Sept 2004

Canada 2001b Canadian statistics, population and demography. Online. Available: http://www.statcan.ca/ english 30 Sept 2004

Canada 2004a Statistics Canada. Census tables. Online. Available: http://www.statcan.ca/ 30 Sept 2004

Canada 2004b Health care renewal. First Ministers meeting on the future of health care. Online. Available: http://www.hc-sc.gc.ca/english/hca 2003/ 20 Jan 2005

Canada 2005 Canadian statistics, population and demography – 2001 data. Online. Available: http:// www.statcan.ca/english 30 Sept 2004

Canadian Institute of Health Information (CIHI) 2004 Improving the health of Canadians. Ottawa, Ontario

Chen J, Ng E, Wilkins R 1996 The health of Canada's immigrants 1994–95. Health Reports 7(4):33–45. Statistics Canada, Ottawa Cat. No. 82–003

Cooper H, Arber S, Fee L, Ginn J 1999 The influence of social support and social capital on health: A review and analysis of British data. Health Education Authority, London

Dion- Stout M, Kipling G D, Stout R 2001 Aboriginal women's health research: Synthesis project final report. Ottawa, Ontario, Canada: Centres of excellence for women's health

Eisenberg L, Kleinman A 1980 Clinical social science. In: Eisenberg L, Kleinman A (eds) The relevance of social science for medicine. Reidel Publishing, Boston, p 1–23

Evans R 1992 Canada: The real issues. In: Hsiao W, Morone J (eds) Comparative health policy. Journal of Health Politics, Health Policy and Law 17(4):739–762

Evans R G, Barer M L, Marmor T R (eds) 1994 Why are some people healthy and others not? The determinants of health of populations. Aldine de Gruyter, New York

Feinstein J S 1993 The relationship between socioeconomic status and health: a review of the literature. Milbank Quarterly 71(2):279–322

Frank J W, Mustard J F 1994 The determinants of health from a historical perspective. Daedalus 123(4):1–20

Good B, Good M J 1980 The meaning of symptoms: a cultural hermeneutic model for clinical practice. In Eisenberg L, Kleinman A (eds) The relevance of social science for medicine. Reidel Publishing, Boston, p 165–196

Gordon D, Shaw M, Dorling D, Davey Smith G (eds) 1999 Inequalities in health: the evidence. The Policy Press, Bristol, p 138–147

Graham H 2000 Socioeconomic change and inequalities in men and women's health in the UK. In: Annandale E, Hunt K (eds) Gender inequalities in health. Open University Press, Buckingham, p 90–122

Haan M, Kaplain G, Camacho T 1987 Poverty and health: prospective evidence from the Alameda County study. American Journal of Epidemiology 125(6):989–998

Helman C 2000 Culture, health and illness: An introduction for health professionals. 4th edn. Butterworth Heinemann, Oxford

Hsiao W C 1992 Comparing health care systems: what nations can learn from one another. Journal of Health Politics, Policy and Law 17(4):612–636

Kawachi I, Kennedy B 1997 Health and social cohesion: why care about income inequality? British Medical Journal 314:1037–1040

Lynam M J 1985 Support networks of immigrant women. Social Science and Medicine 21(3):327–333

Lynam M J 2004 Marginalization of first generation immigrant women: an experience with implications for health. PhD thesis, Kings College University of London

Lynam M J 2005 Health as a socially mediated process: theoretical and practice imperatives emerging from research on health inequalities. Advances in Nursing Science 28(1):25–37

Lynam M J, Henderson A, Browne A et al 2003 Health care restructuring with a view to equity and efficiency: reflections on unintended consequences. Canadian Journal of Nursing Leadership 16(1):112–140

MacIntyre S 1997 The Black report and beyond: What are the issues? Social Science and Medicine 44(6):723–745

Marmot M, Ryff C D, Bumpass L L et al 1997 Social inequalities in health: next questions and converging evidence. Social Science and Medicine 44(6):901–910

Masi R, Mensah L, McLeod K (eds) 1993 Health and cultures exploring the relationships, vol 2. Mosaic Press, Oakville

Ramsden I 1993 Kawa Whakaruruhau; Cultural safety in nursing education in Aotearearoa (New Zealand). Nursing Praxis, New Zealand 8(3):4–10

Reimer Kirkham S, Anderson J M 2002 Post colonial nursing scholarship from epistemology to method. Advances in Nursing Science 25(11):1–17

Reinhardt U 1992 The United States: breakthroughs and waste. In: Hsiao W, Morone J (eds) Comparative health policy. Journal of Health Politics, Health Policy and Law 17(4);637–666

Smith D 1987 The everyday world as problematic: a feminist sociology. University of Toronto Press, Toronto

Stroik S, Jensen J 1999 What is the best policy mix for Canada's young children? CPRN, Study no. F109, Renouf Publishers, Ottawa

Whitehead M 1992 The health divide. In: Inequalities in health. 2nd edn. Penguin Books, London

Wilkinson R G 1996 Unhealthy societies: the afflictions of inequality. Routledge, London

Williams F 1989 Social policy: a critical introduction. Policy Press, Cambridge

Chapter 20

Reflections and conclusions

Irena Papadopoulos

We must be the change we wish to see. (Mahatma Gandhi)

On an aeroplane travelling to Berlin, where I was invited to speak at a conference about transcultural care, I sat next to Dominic. He was a bright, lively 4-year-old who, speaking in Somali, constantly asked his Somali mother question after question. He was also very happy to hold a conversation with me in English. He told me that he was going to meet his daddy at the airport and was very excited about it. According to his mother, Dominic's German father was temporarily living in Germany due to work commitments. Their permanent home was in the USA. She also told me that Dominic spoke fluent German, something I was very jealous of as I was about to deliver my speech in English to a German audience with the help of an interpreter.

The conference was successful, and the audience seemed to appreciate my contribution. Since I had no formal script but only a number of Powerpoint slides to which I spoke, I had to trust that the interpreter was as accurate as possible during his double act with me. During lunch a number of the participants spoke to me in English, and I quickly felt comfortable in their company and was able to joke about my inability to speak German.

On my return to London I sat next to an elderly woman. When I tried to talk to her I realized she could not speak English. The flight was not smooth and turbulence soon made us all feel as though we were in a blender! The elderly woman appeared very frightened and uncomfortable and tried to gain the attention of the flight attendants. As far as I could tell she was not speaking in German either but, as it turned out, she was speaking in Bosnian. This presented a challenge to the crew who disappeared for a few minutes to return with a passenger who acted as their interpreter. I could not help hearing that this was the first time she was travelling by air and thought that the aeroplane was going to crash. She was duly reassured by the flight attendant through the interpreter.

I am telling this short story for a number of reasons which relate to the aims of this book. I hope that the preceding chapters raised your awareness around many of the issues which health and social care professionals will continue to face during the twenty-first century. Without wishing to stereotype the actors in my story and for the sake of using them to help me reflect on the themes of this book, I will argue that they represent the different people whom health and welfare practitioners will continue to come in contact with in their daily work. In many ways Dominic represents an increasing number of people, of mixed heritage, who are exposed from a young age to a number of cultures and languages and are able to function effectively within multicultural environments. I, on the other hand, represent those people who migrated from a specific culture and who, through the passage of time, adapted successfully to the host culture. The process of acculturation has given me enough skills to be able to function adequately in a variety of cultural environments. The elderly Bosnian woman represents those people who find themselves for the first time in a strange environment or a foreign land, unable to communicate and faced with the unknown.

You may conclude that the differences in the three actors in my story are due to personal circumstances and characteristics rather than culture. In many ways you will be correct. People like Dominic are multilingual because they are growing up in an environment which provides the opportunities for them to be so. As they grow within three cultures (their parents' and that of the society they are born into), they will come in contact with people from even more cultures, will eat food that has its origin from many different countries, will have at least 10 years of education, will surf the internet, will travel by air and so on. In contrast, people like the elderly Bosnian woman may have had far fewer opportunities with regard to education, technology, travel, living in multicultural communities. Their different structural elements influence their life chances and shape their lives. But irrespective of how strong and influential the structural forces are, we cannot deny that the family and the societies they each live in have their own customs, values, ways of understanding and explaining their world, in other words, their own culture. The way they care for themselves will depend both on their cultural values and beliefs as well as on their ability to access and process information about health and illness, to access health promotion including preventive and screening health services, and to access illness services they can afford and when they need them. By 'ability' I do not just refer to their personal characteristics and responsibility but I also refer to the availability of these services which, as we all know, depends on policy-makers and service providers. However, it is quite likely that despite their 'ability' differences, they will both (as I have) experience discrimination, culturally insensitive and incompetent care. Why? Because as the preceding chapters have demonstrated, many of the existing services have some way to go before they fully integrate the principles of cultural competence within their everyday decision-making systems. Further, many of the front line service providers have not been provided with adequate training and resources to enable them to be culturally competent.

It is for this reason that this book has been written. A considerable amount of positive change has occurred during the last thirty to forty years in many of the developed countries, mainly through legislation and government policy. The World Health Organization and other international bodies like the United Nations High Commission for Refugees have highlighted over the years the negative impact of poverty, ethnic conflict and cultural misunderstandings on people's health. Despite national and international policy and legislation, culturally incompetent care continues to be experienced by health and social care service users as evidenced in the chapters of this book. This is an area that needs our continuous attention and our efforts in order to improve the experience and health outcomes of our service users. If we want to change things we must start by changing ourselves and must lead by example. I hope that the principles of the cultural competence model which run through the chapters of this book as well as the knowledge and skills you have gained from it will empower you to make a small contribution towards this change.

Index